Macular Disorders
An Illustrated Diagnostic Guide

Macular Disorders
An Illustrated Diagnostic Guide

Edited by

Anthony A. Cavallerano, O.D.
Dean of Clinical Affairs and Professor of Optometry, New England College of Optometry, Boston; Consulting Staff Optometrist, Medical Department, Massachusetts Institute of Technology, Cambridge

Rodney K. Gutner, O.D.
Chief, Optometry Section, Ambulatory Care Service, Department of Veterans Affairs, Edith Nourse Rogers Memorial Veterans Hospital, Bedford, Massachusetts; Associate Professor of Optometry, New England College of Optometry, Boston

Leonard J. Oshinskie, O.D.
Chief, Optometry Section, Surgical Service, VA Connecticut Health Care System, Newington, Connecticut; Adjunct Clinical Professor of Optometry, New England College of Optometry, Boston

With illustrations by Laurel Cook Lhowe
Medical Graphics, Cambridge, Massachusetts

Butterworth–Heinemann
Boston • Oxford • Johannesburg • Melbourne • New Delhi • Singapore

Every effort has been made to ensure that the drug dosage schedules within this text are accurate and conform to standards accepted at time of publication. However, as treatment recommendations vary in the light of continuing research and clinical experience, the reader is advised to verify drug dosage schedules herein with information found on product information sheets. This is especially true in cases of new or infrequently used drugs.

Recognizing the importance of preserving what has been written, Butterworth-Heinemann prints its books on acid-free paper whenever possible.

Library of Congress Cataloging-in-Publication Data

Cavallerano, Anthony A.
Macular disorders : an illustrated diagnostic guide / Anthony A. Cavallerano, Rodney K. Gutner, Leonard J. Oshinskie ; with illustrations by Laurel Cook Lhowe.
p. cm.
Includes bibliographical references and index.
ISBN 0-7506-9224-3
1. Macula lutea--Diseases--Atlases. I. Gutner, Rodney K. II. Oshinskie, Leonard J. III. Title.
[DNLM: 1. Macula Lutea--pathology--atlases. 2. Retinal Diseases--diagnosis--atlases. WW 17 C377m 1997]
RE661.M3C38 1997
617.7'35--dc21
DNLM/DLC
for Library of Congress 96-39906
CIP

British Library Cataloguing-in-Publication Data
A catalogue record for this book is available from the British Library.

The publisher offers discounts on bulk orders of this book.
For information, please write:

Manager of Special Sales
Butterworth-Heinemann
313 Washington Street
Newton, MA 02158-1626
Tel: 617-928-2500
Fax: 617-928-2620

For information on all B-H medical publications available, contact our World Wide Web home page at http://www.bh.com/med

10 9 8 7 6 5 4 3 2 1

Printed in the United States of America

To Susan

Jenny

Lisa

Nicole

—AAC

To Jamie

Tristan

Cassidy

Gloria and Leonard

In memoriam, Martha and Phil

—RKG

To Dore

Emy

Ali

Nancy and Len

—LJO

Contents

Contributing Authors

Leland W. Carr, O.D.
Associate Dean for Clinical Programs, The Pacific University College of Optometry, Forest Grove, Oregon

Anthony A. Cavallerano, O.D.
Dean of Clinical Affairs and Professor of Optometry, New England College of Optometry, Boston; Consulting Staff Optometrist, Medical Department, Massachusetts Institute of Technology, Cambridge

Jerry D. Cavallerano, O.D., Ph.D.
Associate Professor of Optometry, New England College of Optometry, Boston; Staff Optometrist, Beetham Eye Institute, Joslin Diabetes Center, Boston

Gerald R. Friedman, O.D.
Retina Associates, Boston

Rodney K. Gutner, O.D.
Chief, Optometry Section, Ambulatory Care Service, Department of Veterans Affairs, Edith Nourse Rogers Memorial Veterans Hospital, Bedford, Massachusetts; Associate Professor of Optometry, New England College of Optometry, Boston

Timothy Harkins, O.D.
Clinical Optometrist, Veterans Affairs Medical Center, Kansas City, Missouri

John L. Henahan, O.D., P.O.C.
Instructor in Ophthalmology and Director of Low Vision Services, Department of Ophthalmology, Louisiana State University School of Medicine in New Orleans

Leonard J. Oshinskie, O.D.
Chief, Optometry Section, Surgical Service, VA Connecticut Health Care System, Newington, Connecticut; Adjunct Clinical Professor of Optometry, New England College of Optometry, Boston

Michael T. Porter, O.D.
Private Practice, Advanced Eyecare, P.C., Vermont, New York, and Massachusetts

Susan A. Primo, O.D., F.A.A.O.
Clinical Instructor in Ophthalmology, Emory University School of Medicine, Atlanta

Stuart P. Richer, O.D., M.S., Ph.D.
Adjunct Associate Professor of Optometry, Department of Clinical Education, Illinois College of Optometry, Chicago; Staff Optometrist, Surgical Service, Veterans Affairs Medical Center, North Chicago

Preface

Macular disease is a common cause of severe vision loss. Increasing longevity and the likelihood of a greater risk for developing acquired macular disease has increased the responsibility of the primary eye care clinician for making timely and accurate diagnoses if visual function is to be preserved.

This book is designed to enhance the clinical decision-making skills of the primary eye care clinician in the area of macular disease. The intent is to provide the necessary information for the clinician to make appropriate and timely clinical judgments regarding the management of patients with or suspected of having macular disease. Clinical decision-making skills are derived from an assortment of factors:

- Good observational and listening skills
- An understanding of tissue response
- Identification and assessment of risk factors
- An appreciation of problem-solving techniques
- And finally, experience

Most experienced clinicians employ a problem-solving approach to dealing with clinical situations, a process that is necessary for developing and refining decision-making skills. By promoting a problem-specific method of examining the patient, refining cognitive skills, and furthering decision-making skills, the clinician is better prepared to engage in the accurate, timely diagnosis and effective management of more challenging and complicated clinical cases.

An understanding of tissue reaction is important in predicting the response and outcome of a disease state, so that a prognosis can be established for each patient and condition. This enables the clinician to determine and develop a management and treatment strategy and helps to determine how aggressive the treatment should be, especially if surgical treatment is an option.

Observational skills are important in the detection of abnormal findings. A clinician must have the proper tools available to make these observations, and the best equipment providing the highest resolution is imperative when examining the posterior segment.

The retina, and in particular the macula, is a complex structure capable of responding to insult in a variety of ways. Early detection of potentially sight-threatening lesions and prompt treatment may prevent significant vision loss. This can only be accomplished by painstaking stereoscopic examination of the macula and by careful attention to a patient's symptoms. The highly sensitive nature of the macula and its important role in providing good central vision will often lead the patient to advise the practitioner of functional changes in vision. Therefore, patient education and counseling are an important responsibility of the clinical practitioner when managing patients with macular disease.

This text is designed as a practical guide to detecting, evaluating, diagnosing, and managing congenital and acquired macular disorders. Special consideration is given to developing decision-making skills and establishing treatment plans and strategies based on predictive measures. Whether one has extensive knowledge of or limited experience with macular disease, this text provides a foundation and serves as a reference for understanding the etiopathogenesis of a disease entity and predicting outcomes based on observed macular incompetence. Unlike many books that presume the reader knows the diagnosis, this book is designed to chart the diagnostic course for the clinician. Part I provides the reader with anatomic, physiologic, and diagnostic information relating to the retina in general and specifically, the macula. This section is designed to provide a foundation for understanding how the macula responds to insult and how to approach macular disease from the standpoint of examination and testing procedures. In Part II information is provided in such a way that the clinician can make decisions and apply differential diagnostic principles based on the appearance of the observed clinical finding. Additional information is provided in the latter parts of the book to expand the knowledge base in specific clinical entities.

It is our hope that this work will not only provide the reader with the necessary information to comfortably manage patients with macular disorders but will also stimulate the clinician to pursue additional avenues of knowledge in the area of retinal disease. Creating interest in this important area of ophthalmic care will greatly enhance the ability of the clinician to make critical decisions in the management of posterior segment disorders.

Anthony A. Cavallerano
Rodney K. Gutner
Leonard J. Oshinskie

Acknowledgments

This text is the culmination of an exceptional effort that would not have been possible without the encouragement and support of many people. We would like to thank those who have helped to make this project a reality.

First and foremost we would like to thank our families for their continued patience, unfailing love, and generous support. We would also like to acknowledge Drs. Florence Milch and Steve Sinclair for their insight and encouragement, for their promotion of intellectual curiosity, and for their willingness to share their knowledge and information with us. A special thanks to Dr. Tom Freddo for his expertise in reviewing the first section of this atlas. Additionally, thanks to Dr. Franklin Watters of the Department of Veterans Affairs. Finally, thanks to our patients, who have allowed us to use their cases to educate others.

Our gratitude is extended to Andrew Bell for his outstanding clinical photographs and for his intense desire to share his wisdom by teaching others. Additional thanks to those whose photographs have added greatly to the richly visual nature of this text.

Finally, to others, who both know us and to whom we are unknown, for their direct and indirect furtherance of this project: to R.A. Zimmerman for his inspiration, to Neil, Leonard, Lou, and many others for their accompaniment, to the GD for keeping us tuned, and to J. Rice for starting the whole thing.

Macular Disorders
An Illustrated Diagnostic Guide

PART

I

Anatomy, Physiology, and Examination of the Macula

CHAPTER

1

Anatomy, Histology, and Morphology

Anthony A. Cavallerano

The macula is the histologically and clinically distinct area of the retina sometimes referred to as the *posterior pole* or *area centralis*. It is characterized by a unique arrangement of cells and tissue that separate it in form and function from the adjacent retina. Clinicians and anatomists sometimes differ in their description and interpretation of the macula; this text discusses anatomy from the clinician's viewpoint.

For the purposes of this text, the normal macula measures 5.5–6.0 mm in diameter (approximately 4 disc diameters). The center of the macula lies approximately 4 mm temporal and 0.8 mm inferior to the center of the optic disc. There is a change in the surface of the retina where a slope or hill of clivus is formed, corresponding to the *fovea centralis*. This 1.5-mm wide pit creates a change in the appearance of the macula, often producing an annular reflex that may be observed with the light of an ophthalmoscope. The floor of this pit is referred to as the *foveola,* which measures 0.33–0.35 mm; its deepest point is called the *umbo*. This area acts like a concave mirror, producing a foveal light reflex observed with the ophthalmoscope or condensing lens in fundus biomicroscopy. The foveola is part of the *foveal avascular zone* (FAZ), sometimes referred to as the capillary-free zone, which measures approximately 0.35–0.50 mm or 350–500 μ in diameter.

The retina is approximately 0.55 mm thick at the foveal margin, equaling the maximal retinal thickness, and is of minimal thickness, 0.13 mm, at the umbo (Figures 1.1 and 1.2).

The macula is unique compared with the remainder of the retina for a number of reasons.

1. The macula contains five main layers:
   The internal limiting membrane
   The outer plexiform layer (OPL)
   The outer nuclear layer
   The external limiting membrane
   The photoreceptors

   The OPL of the macula is fibrous rather than reticular, thicker in the macula (although almost absent in the fovea), and referred to as *Henle's fiber layer*. There are no horizontal cell processes in the foveal area. The nerve fibers run parallel to the surface of the macula, becoming obliquely oriented rather than perpendicular to the surface, as found in the adjacent area and throughout the retina. Exudates settle and accumulate in this layer (Figure 1.3).

   The photoreceptors are primarily cones in the fovea, and each cone is connected to only one ganglion cell. Elsewhere in the retina there can be up to 100 rods connected to each ganglion cell.

2. Müller cells span the entire thickness of the retina from the internal limiting membrane to the level of the photoreceptor outer segments. These cells lend support to the retinal structure, and their appearance varies in different retinal layers. There is an abundance of Müller cells in the foveal floor.

3. The ganglion cell layer is multicellular in thickness (versus a single row outside of the macula), and cells are more numerous in the macular area.

4. Nerve fibers are oriented obliquely rather than horizontally in the macular area.

5. The internal limiting membrane is thicker in the macular area and is attached to the hyaloid membrane of the vitreous. The hyaloid membrane of the vitreous is thinnest at the macular area.

6. Retinal pigment epithelial (RPE) cells are more tightly packed in the macular region, are regular, taller, and more columnar, and contain more melanin granules. RPE cells serve as the outer blood-retinal barrier. The RPE cells interdigitate with the outer segments of the

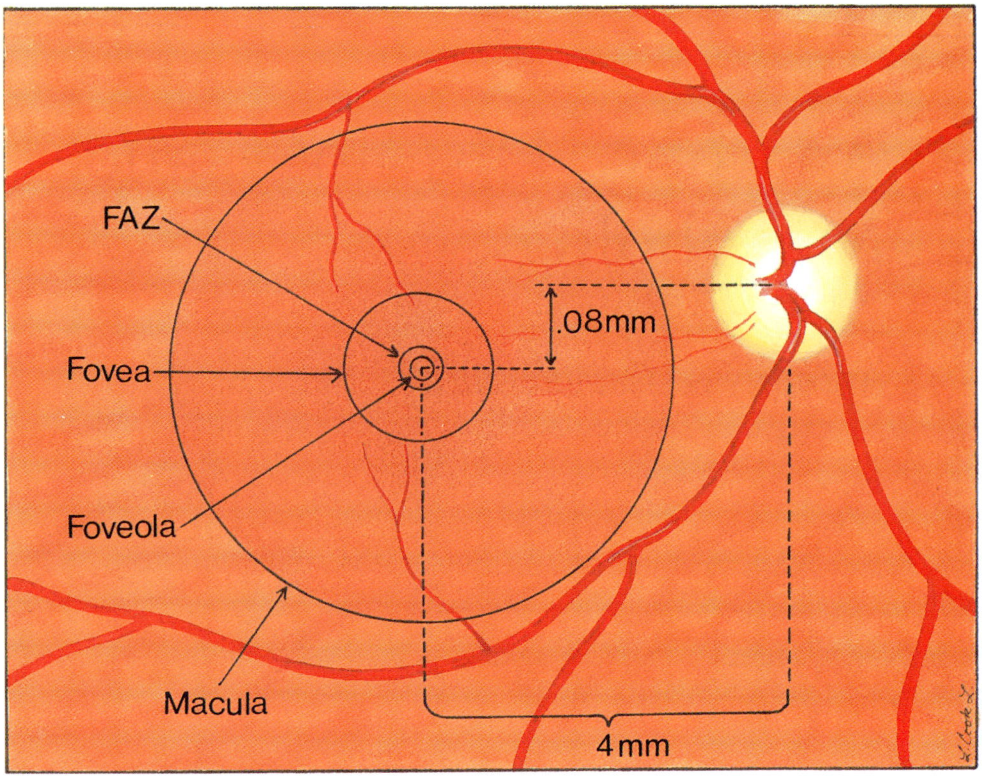

FIGURE 1.1. Anatomic location and geographic extent of the normal macula. (FAZ = foveal avascular zone.)

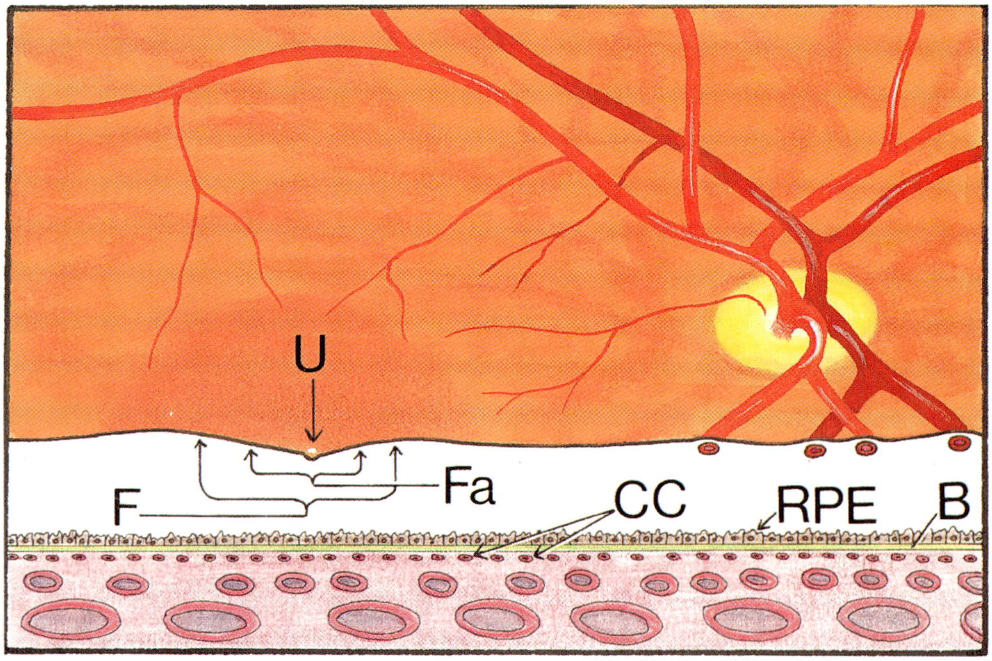

FIGURE 1.2. Anatomic section of the normal macula and underlying choroidal complex. (U = umbo; Fa = pit of the foveola; F = anatomic fovea.) The foveal avascular zone comprises 350–500 μ of this area. Also represented are the retinal pigment epithelium (RPE), Bruch's membrane (B), and the choriocapillaris (CC).

photoreceptors via a potential space. The RPE cells are interconnected by the continuous zonulae occludentes, which prevent passage of macromolecules between RPE cells into the neurosensory retina. These cells block the diffusion of small molecules (including fluorescein) from the extravascular space of the choroid to the retina.

The RPE is one of the most active cellular layers in the body and plays a vital role in maintaining integrity to the photoreceptors. It is responsible for engulfing photoreceptor discs on a daily basis with a resultant buildup of metabolic waste within the cell. The RPE cells are nondividing, and an accumulation of lipofuscin and other

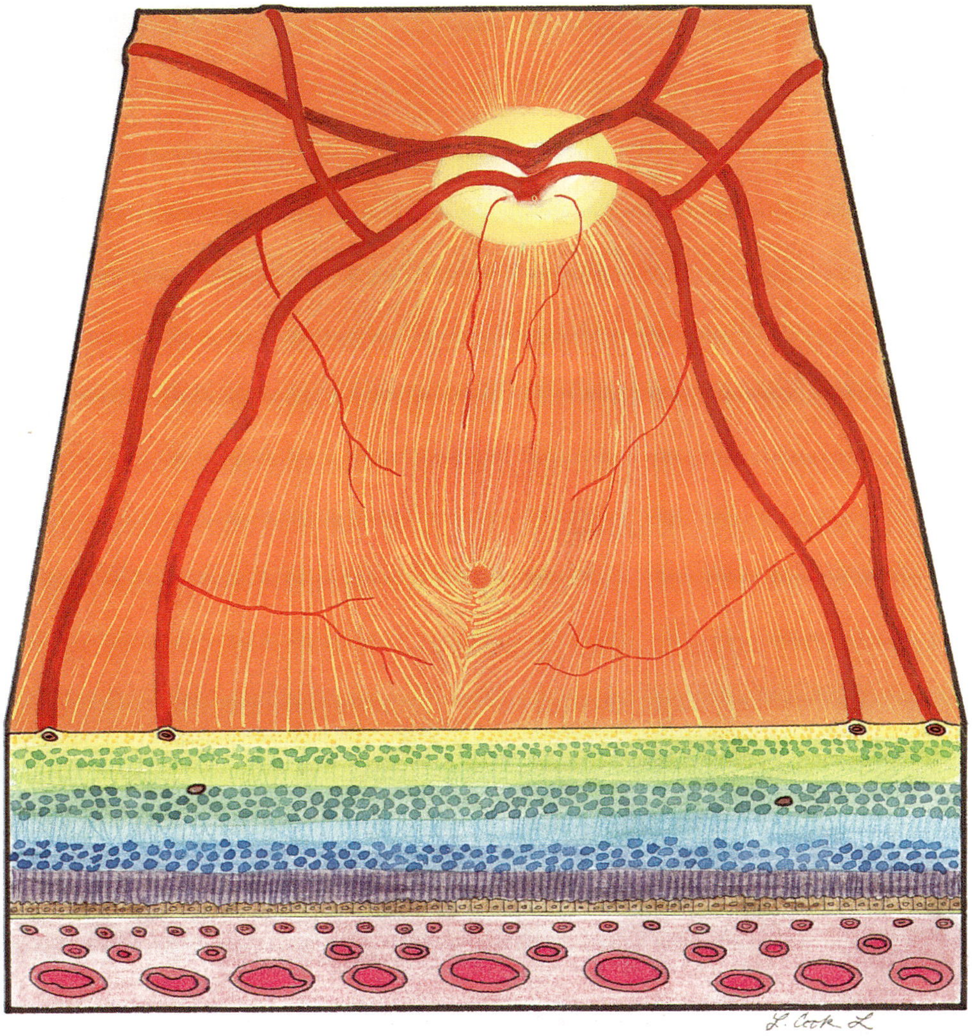

FIGURE 1.3. Cross section of the macula demonstrating the distribution of the nerve fibers, which run obliquely and then perpendicularly to the retinal surface in the macular area.

breakdown products leads to changes associated with aging that may lead to age-related macular degeneration (AMD) and other macular anomalies. Table 1.1 summarizes the function of the RPE cells.

7. Lipofuscin is an orange pigment seen in abundance in the macular area with age. It is an indigestible by-product of the breakdown of free radicals that form peroxide and unsaturated fatty acids. Accumulation of lipofuscin leads to metabolic compromise and eventual breakdown of the RPE.

8. Xanthophyll, a soluble protein, gives the macula its yellow color (macula lutea). It is abundant in the inner nuclear and ganglion cell layers, acts as a barrier to transmitted fluorescence, and is a chromophore which absorbs laser energy. Xanthophyll also serves as a protective barrier to the macula, absorbing potentially damaging ultraviolet wavelengths.

9. The FAZ depends on the choriocapillaris and the perifoveal retinal vessels for nourishment.

RETINAL VASCULATURE AND CIRCULATION

The retinal vasculature is a closed system with end-artery circulation that is confined to the inner half of the retina, serving the nutritional needs of the inner five retinal layers. Larger vessels are present in the nerve fiber and ganglion cell layer. The deep capillary plexus is found at the inner nuclear–outer plexiform layer junction, and the superficial capillary plexus lies in the nerve fiber and ganglion cell layers (Figure 1.4).

The inner layers of the retina are served by branches of the central retinal artery (CRA), whereas the outer layers are served by the choroidal circulation. The main circulation arises from the CRA. Arborizing branches emanate from the temporal arcade and vault over and under the macula in the same fashion as the nerve fiber layer. Small branches of these twigs serve the macula and run radially, forming a ring around the macula, delin-

TABLE 1.1. Function of Retinal Pigment Epithelium

Physical

- Serves as the outer blood-retinal barrier protecting the neurosensory retina from the passage of unwanted molecules from the choroid
- Active transport of fluids serves as the prime force in adhering the neurosensory retina to the retinal pigment epithelium
- Synthesizes acid mucopolysaccharides, which accumulate in subretinal space. Minor role in adhesion
- Microvilli of retinal pigment epithelial cells have intimate structural relationship with outer segments of photoreceptors. May play a minor role in adherence

Optical

- Melanin granules absorb light energy
  - Reduces light scatter
  - Concentrates light and improves resolution
- Pigment barrier prevents excess light from coming through the sclera
- Serves as a chromophore for laser photocoagulation

Metabolic

- Phagocytizes outer segments of photoreceptors
- Metabolizes vitamin A
- Synthesizes acid mucopolysaccharides
- Lysozomes degrade outer segment membranes
- Contains tyrosinase for synthesis and replacement of melanin

Source: Revised from American Academy of Ophthalmology. Basic and Clinical Science Course. Section 11: Retina and Vitreous. San Francisco: American Academy of Ophthalmology, 1991.

eating the FAZ (Figure 1.5). There are three layers of capillaries in the perifoveal zone.

The endothelial cells of the retinal blood vessels are joined by continuous zonulae occludentes (tight junctions), which prevent them from leaking. This comprises the inner blood-retinal barrier.

CHOROID

The choroid is the highly vascularized coat of the eye that provides nourishment to the outer retina. It is highly pigmented and consists of layers. Bruch's membrane, the complex acellular basement membrane, is elaborated in part by the RPE. Waste products accumulate on the inner aspect of this membrane, decreasing permeability and interfering with nutritional support and metabolic elimination of the RPE and photoreceptors. The basal laminar deposits increase with age (see Figure 1.2).

The outer retina is served by the choriocapillaris, which is an open vascular system. The choriocapillaris is comprised of discrete lobules with limited interconnections that arise from the short posterior ciliary arterial system. Drainage occurs via postcapillary venules that empty into the vortex system. The choriocapillaris is composed of fenestrated vessels, thus allowing for leakage into the extravascular space of the choroid. The larger vessels of the choroid are not fenestrated.

Components of the Retinal and Choroidal Structure

Preretinal area. The preretinal glial membrane exerts an influence on retinal circulation. Hemorrhage may accumulate in this area.

Sensory retina. Deep and superficial vascular layer.

Avascular sensory retina. Site of intraretinal edema and exudate accumulation, especially OPL.

RPE. One of the most metabolically active tissues in the body. Typical response of the RPE is proliferation, migration, depigmentation, and detachment, both with and without neurosensory detachment. The RPE may tear following hemorrhagic or exudative detachment.

Choroidal circulation. Larger choroidal vessels and choriocapillaris.

Bruch's membrane/photoreceptor/choriocapillaris complex functions as a unit; any disruption or defect in one layer will lead to potential abnormalities in the others. This intimate relationship is important in the understanding of the pathogenesis of macular disease, especially choroidal neovascular membrane formation and AMD.

VITREOUS

The vitreous plays an important role in the pathogenesis of many retinal anomalies, including macular disease. The vitreous occupies a volume of 4 ml, weighs 4 g, and makes up four-fifths of the total volume of the globe. In healthy, young patients, the vitreous body is a homogeneous, transparent gel composed of 99% water. The vitreous provides a clear media for the passage of light and is supported by collagen fibers and hyaluronic acid.

The vitreous has a unique relationship with the posterior pole by engaging in close approximation and sometimes attachment in a 4-mm annular ring encircling the macular area. The attachment of the vitreous to the macular area is responsible for producing the annular reflex sometimes observed with direct and indirect ophthalmoscopy, especially in younger patients. The tenaci-

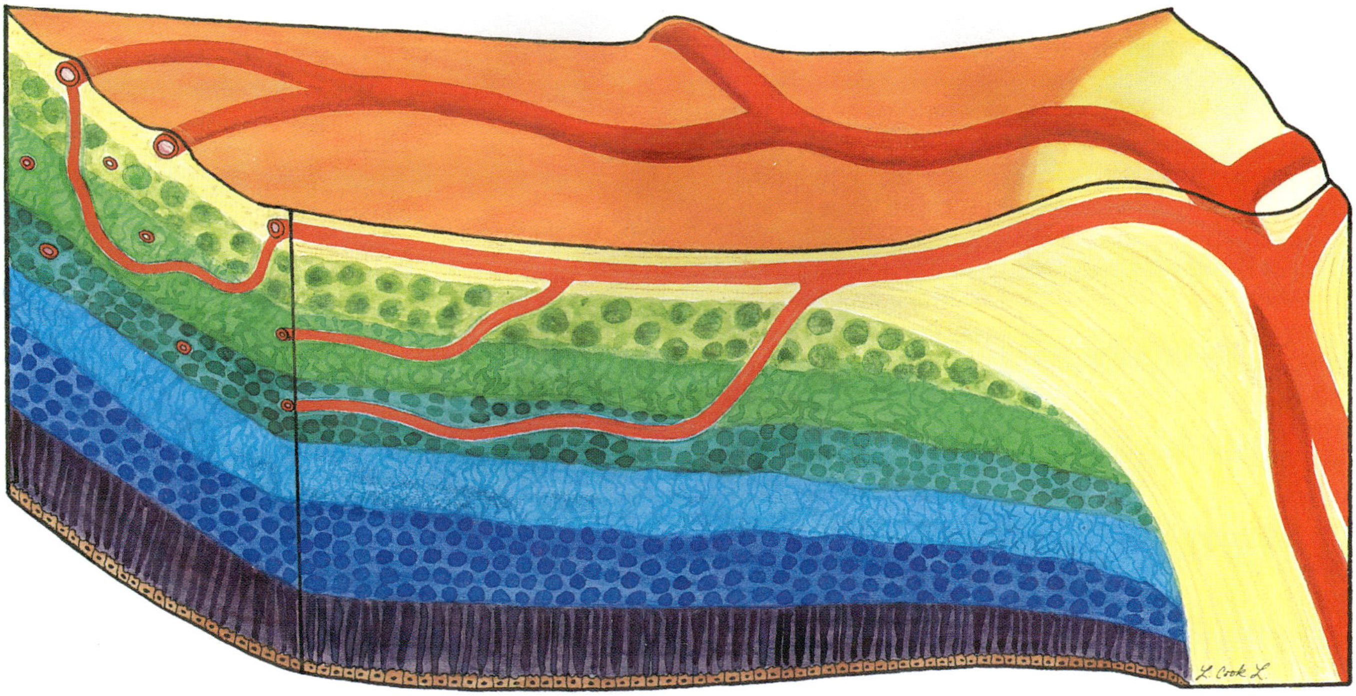

FIGURE 1.4. Retinal vessels arise from the central retinal artery, with larger vessels running in the nerve fiber layer. The deep capillary plexus is distributed throughout the inner nuclear and outer plexiform layer.

FIGURE 1.5. Cross section of the macula with arborizing branches from the temporal arcades. The small branches run radially and form a ring around the macula, delineating the foveal avascular zone.

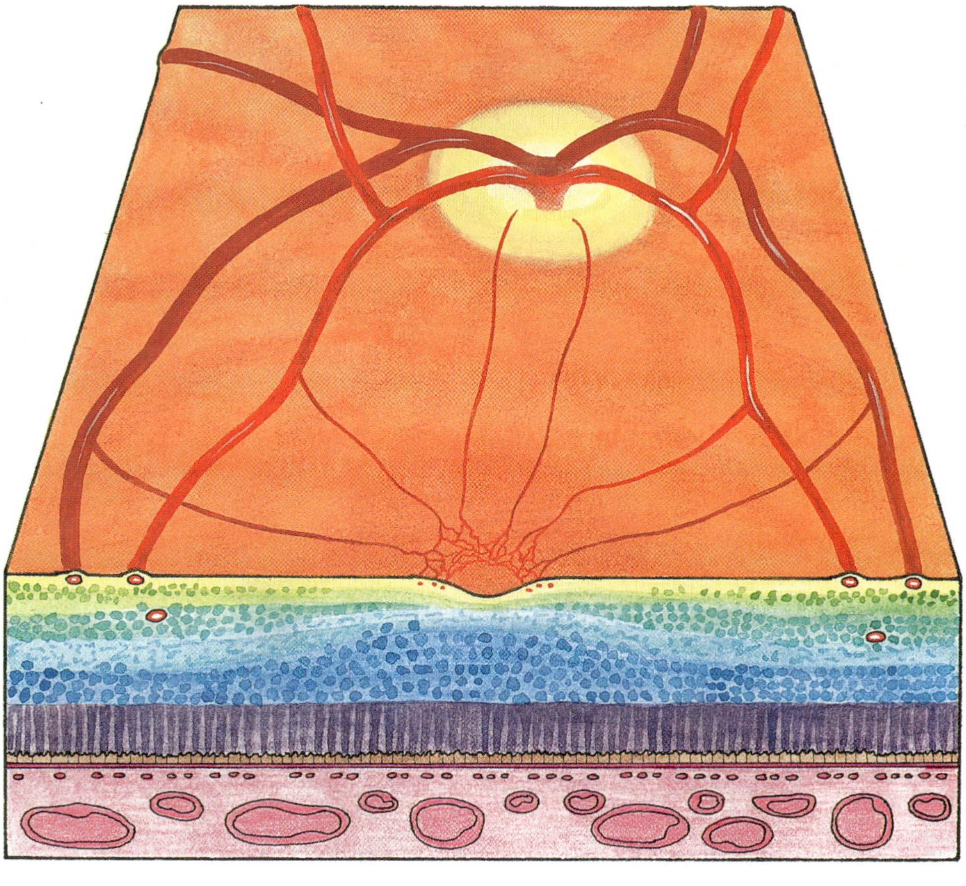

ty of the attachment varies, and it is known that the vitreous can attach to the fovea as well, a phenomenon demonstrated by a tiny operculum sometimes observed in front of the macula in macular holes. The posterior hyaloid membrane of the vitreous tends to be thinner at the macular area and, therefore, liquefied vitreous can communicate with the retina in this area if the membrane ruptures. In certain disorders, the posterior hyaloid membrane of the vitreous may become thickened and opacified and may attach more firmly to the macula.

In addition to its attachment around the macula, the vitreous is adherent to the margins of the optic disc, a likely site of separation of the vitreous with age. The firmest attachment occurs at the ora serrata, the vitreous base, and there are tenuous attachments of the vitreous to the equatorial retina, especially around retinal vessels. The vitreous is also adherent to the crystalline lens via Wieger's ligament, but this attachment weakens with age.

SUGGESTED READING

American Academy of Ophthalmology. Basic and Clinical Science Course. Section 11: Retina and Vitreous. San Francisco: American Academy of Ophthalmology, 1991.

Apple DJ, Rabb MF. Clinicopathologic Correlation of Ocular Disease: A Text and Stereoscopic Atlas. St. Louis: Mosby, 1990.

Hogan MF, Zimmerman LE. Ophthalmic Pathology, An Atlas and Textbook (2nd ed). Philadelphia: Saunders, 1962.

Yanoff M, Fine BS. Ocular Pathology: A Text and Atlas (3rd ed). Philadelphia: Lippincott, 1989.

CHAPTER 2

Clinical Examination of the Macula

Anthony A. Cavallerano and Rodney K. Gutner

A detailed examination of the posterior pole is critical in detecting macular abnormalities. A number of methods are available for direct examination of the macula, and each has its advantages. Since each method relies on a bright light source, psychophysical testing such as visual acuity and Amsler grid testing should be conducted prior to introducing a bright light source to the retina.

Stereoscopic examination using a bright light source and the slit beam of the biomicroscope is the most definitive means for examining the macula. Brightness is an important requirement in obtaining high resolution when examining the fundus. A stereoscopic view may be obtained by a number of different systems, including binocular indirect ophthalmoscopy or fundus biomicroscopy with either hand-held condensing lenses or fundus contact lenses. Stereopsis is crucial in determining the elevation and depth of lesions, the presence of edema, cystic changes, vascular anomalies, and retinal pigment epithelial (RPE) changes. Localization of changes within the layers of the retina is better observed with the biomicroscope using a slit beam with variable magnification to meet the observational needs of the examiner. Table 2.1 summarizes the differences between the examination systems.

WHAT TO LOOK FOR

The overall appearance of the macula should be evaluated for elevation, depression, and pigment changes. The appearance of drusen, RPE variations, hemorrhage, or exudate should be noted, as well as the presence of a foveal reflex. Absence of a foveal reflex may represent a normal anatomic variation relating to the concavity of the umbo; however, absence of a reflex where one was once present may indicate early macular disease.

Direct Ophthalmoscopy

Direct ophthalmoscopy provides the easiest, most utilitarian view of the macula. An acceptable view is usually obtained through the undilated pupil, and the examiner is able to make preliminary determinations with this method. Magnification is fixed and image quality is limited by the amount of illumination obtainable with this system. However, the magnification (14.5× in an emmetropic eye) obtained by this system is useful in identifying subtle macular changes such as fine drusen and variations in the appearance of the RPE. Since stereopsis is not possible, the examiner must rely on monocular clues to locate the depth of macular lesions. With direct ophthalmoscopy, the image is erect with a field of view of 10–15 degrees in an emmetropic eye (Figure 2.1).

The view of the macula is enhanced through a dilated pupil using direct ophthalmoscopy. However, the examiner must contend with peripheral aberrations and distortions encountered through the enlarged pupil. For this reason it is helpful for the examiner to obtain a view through the undilated pupil with the direct ophthalmoscope prior to dilation. It is sometimes difficult to observe macular and retinal detail through media opacities, even through the dilated pupil. Delicate changes that sometimes take place at the vitreoretinal interface in the macular area, with the exception of epiretinal membrane formation, may be difficult to observe with the direct ophthalmoscope. Therefore, the direct ophthalmoscope should be reserved for a quick screen of the macula prior to dilation.

Binocular Indirect Ophthalmoscopy

Binocular indirect ophthalmoscopy (BIO), although not ideal for macular evaluation, will provide a stereoscopic overview of the posterior pole, including the vascular

TABLE 2.1. Direct Examination of the Macula

Technique	*Advantages*	*Disadvantages*	*What to look for*
Direct ophthalmoscopy	Magnification Detection of discrete changes Subtle changes in the level of the RPE Ease of use Applicable through an undilated pupil	Small field of view Limited illumination Diffuse light source does not allow for easy detection of macula edema No stereopsis Poor view through media opacities	Fine drusen RPE changes in the macular area Microaneurysms and fine vascular changes
Binocular indirect ophthalmoscopy	Wide field of view Stereopsis Bright light source Enhanced resolution Better view through media opacities	Interpretation of reversed, inverted image Pupil dilation mostly required Insufficient magnification for subtle maculopathies	Diffuse macula edema Neurosensory detachment RPE detachment Overview of the vessel arcades Equatorial and peripheral lesions resulting in macular anomalies
Fundus biomicroscopy			
Hruby precorneal lens	Ease of use Slit beam with variable magnification Stereopsis	Poor view through hazy media Requires constant focusing and adjustment Surface reflections	All of the above plus: Macular edema Elevation of the neurosensory retina RPE detachment
Hand-held condensing lenses: 60 D, 78 D, 90 D	Ease of use Excellent stereopsis Bright light source Slit beam with variable magnification Increased field of view over Hruby lens Uniform illumination Excellent for slit lamp photodocumentation	Interpretation of reversed, inverted image 60 D and 78 D require maximum dilation for optimal view (90 D provides acceptable view through smaller pupil) Limited field of view	All of the above plus: Fine drusen and subtle RPE changes
Universal fundus lenses including 3-mirror lens (Goldmann type)	Same as hand-held condensing lenses, plus: Erect image Excellent stereopsis	Topical anesthetic and intervening fluid required	All of the above

RPE = retinal pigment epithelium.

arcades. The relatively low degree of magnification, 2.5–3.0× magnification with a 20 D condensing lens in an emmetropic eye, makes it difficult to observe subtle changes in the macular and foveal regions. However, the broad view afforded with BIO sometimes reveals entities such as an edematous or elevated macula and vascular occlusive disease and will show caliber and distribution changes of the retinal vessels. The field of view is estimated at 35–40 degrees in an emmetropic eye using a 20 D condensing lens. A 14 D condensing lens is available, which provides more magnification and is designed specifically for examining the posterior pole. The resultant aerial image obtained with BIO is reversed and inverted, and both the field of view and magnification are directly influenced by the power of the condensing lens and, to a lesser extent, the patient's refractive error.

The instrument should be used to evaluate the equatorial and peripheral retina when macular disease is detected. Certain macular entities may be associated with disorders elsewhere in the retina, such as rhegmatogenous and nonrhegmatogenous retinal detachment, retinoschisis, and intermediate or posterior uveitis. Scleral indentation, a useful adjunct in peripheral retinal examination, may be performed in conjunction with BIO.

BIO also permits examination of the fundus through a hazy media. Larger opacities in the central vitreous cavity are readily seen. The bright light source and

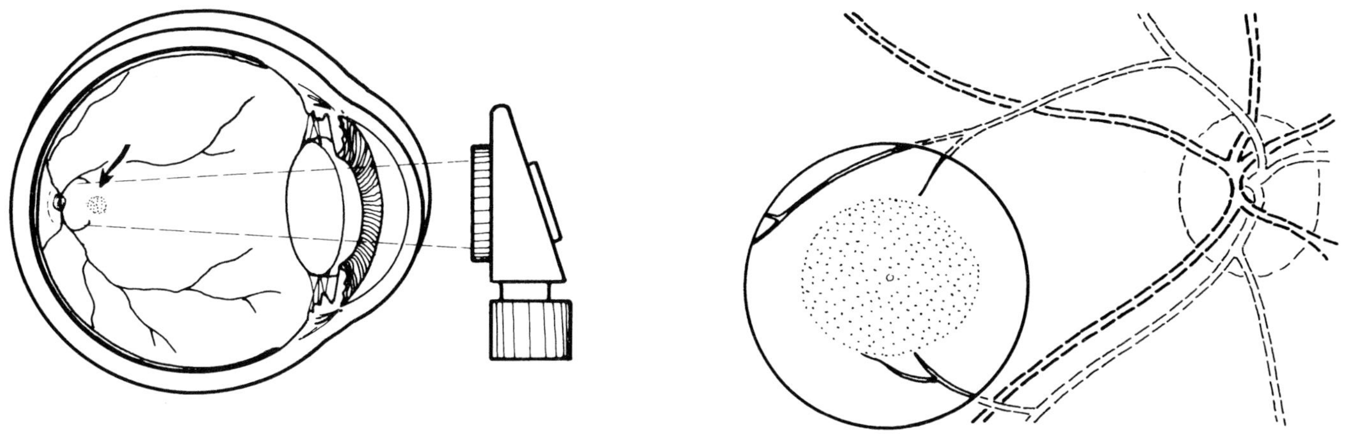

FIGURE 2.1. Average field of view obtained with the direct ophthalmoscope in an emmetropic eye. The entire foveal avascular zone is visible, and approximately one-half of the anatomic macula is observed in one field.

TABLE 2.2. Comparison of Selected Fundus Lenses

	Hruby lens	*Hand-held condensing lens*	*Universal three-mirror lens*	*Krieger lens*
Field of view	Small	Largest	Large	Large
Image	Virtual, erect	Real, inverted reversed	Virtual, erect	Virtual, erect
Surface reflections	Many	Variable	Variable	Variable
Patient tolerance	Good	Good*	Variable	Variable
Stereopsis	Good	Excellent	Excellent	Excellent
Photodocumentation	Poor	Excellent	Very good	Very good

*Excellent with yellow retina protector glass.
Source: Modified from R Gutner, A Cavallerano, D Wong. Fundus biomicroscopy: A comparison of four methods. J Am Optom Assoc 1988;59:388–390.

image system provide an improved view through mild-to-moderate media opacities. However, the view of subtle changes at the vitreo-internal limiting membrane surface is not always easily observed with this system.

Fundus Biomicroscopy

Indirect biomicroscopy takes advantage of stereopsis, high illumination, variable magnification, and an adjustable light beam to examine the macular region using auxiliary lenses. Subtle maculopathies, especially those occurring in the foveal avascular zone (FAZ) or at the level of the RPE, can be observed readily using fundus biomicroscopic techniques. Diabetic retinopathy, choroidal neovascularization, macular edema, and macular holes are detected and evaluated more easily. The examination is best conducted through a dilated pupil to allow maximum stereopsis. A better view through media opacities and more uniform illumination of the image make this examination method superior for macular evaluation. Uniformly, there is a more consistent view of the vitreous cavity, especially the vitreoretinal interface in the macular area. Thickening of the macula from diffuse or cystoid edema, choroidal neovascularization, retinal neovascularization, microaneurysmal changes, exudates, and fine drusen are best visualized using the slit beam and increased magnification.

Several options are available for fundus lenses, including Hruby lenses, hand-held condensing lenses, and universal fundus contact lenses. Table 2.2 summarizes the attributes of several systems.

Hruby Lens

The Hruby precorneal lens is a conventional device common to all biomicroscopes. Conveniently mounted, this

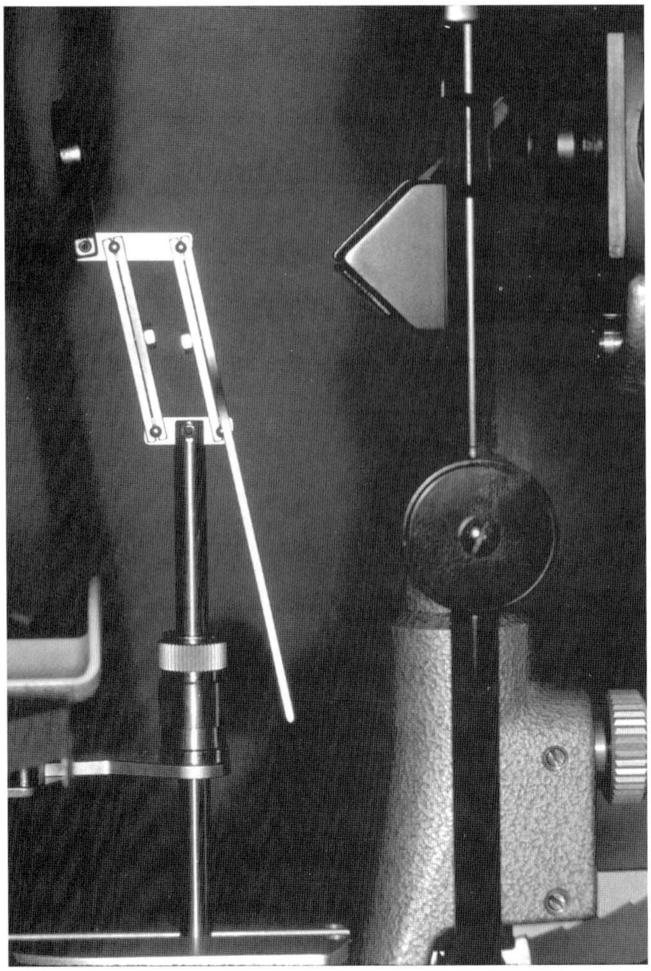

FIGURE 2.2. Typical slit lamp–mounted Hruby lens.

high-powered, –58.6 D, plano-concave lens permits evaluation of the posterior segment through the dilated pupil. With the plano surface facing the examiner, a magnified, erect stereoscopic image of the macula and foveal area is obtained. Limited by its design and the air interface between the lens surface and the patient's eye, this system suffers from reflectance, vignetting, small field of view, and variable image quality. Patient cooperation is a requisite, while maximal pupillary dilation and continual adjustment of the lens are needed to maintain a clear focus. However, the examiner can obtain a limited view of reasonable quality of the optic nerve, macula, fovea, and vitreoretinal interface using this system (Figure 2.2).

Hand-Held Condensing Lens

The recent emergence of a series of hand-held precorneal condensing lenses of various powers has made posterior segment examination more convenient. Multiple powers with different aperture diameters are available, including 60 D, 78 D, 90 D, and a variety of wide-angle lenses. The field of view is greatest with the wide-angle lenses, greater than 120 degrees, but magnification is greatest with the 60 D lens. Since this system creates a real inverted image located between the lens and the biomicroscope, the working distance needs to be increased by moving the biomicroscope back toward the examiner. The hand-held condensing lenses are versatile and may be used to examine the equatorial and mid-peripheral retina. Table 2.3 summarizes the features of each hand-held condensing lens type.

The hand-held condensing lens neutralizes the power of the cornea and converts the biomicroscope to a telescopic system. These high-powered lenses are symmetric, aspheric biconvex designs that minimize aberrations and provide a uniformly illuminated image of the posterior pole. A real, inverted aerial image is produced between the condensing lens and the slit lamp biomicroscope (Figure 2.3). A field of view reaching 65–70 degrees is possible and is limited only by the maximum width obtained with the slit beam of the biomicroscope. The optic disc and macular area can be examined precisely using the variable angulation of the slit beam. Subtle changes in the macula can be observed, and the hand-held lens is one of the best methods for detection of macular edema.

The highly stereoscopic, uniformly bright image this system produces makes it the method of choice for examining the macula and optic nerve. One drawback results from the brightness and diffusion of light throughout the RPE. Because of this, fine drusen and subtle changes of the internal limiting membrane and vitreoretinal interface may go undetected with this system. For this purpose, or if any question of diagnosis remains, a fundus contact lens is the recommended lens of choice.

Because hand-held condensing lenses do not contact the surface of the cornea, a topical anesthetic is not required. Subsequent procedures may be carried out without optical interference from intervening fluids. Photography is easily possible through these lenses as well. Although pupil dilation will yield a superior image, the 90 D lens, due to its optics, allows a view through a small or semidilated pupil. For example, this lens is preferred over the other sizes for patients who do not dilate well, i.e., patients with diabetes, chronic anterior uveitis, iris sphincter damage, or posterior synechiae, or glaucoma patients on chronic miotic therapy.

The hand-held condensing lenses are available in clear or yellow retina protector material for improved patient comfort. Some clinicians believe the yellow lens distorts the color appearance of the pathology, but noticeable patient comfort and less eye movement and blinking may afford a more accurate view of the details of the macula (Figure 2.4).

TABLE 2.3. Specifications for the +60 D, +78 D, +90 D, and Superfield NC Hand-Held Condensing Lenses

Specifications	*+90 D*	*+78 D*	*+60 D*	*Superfield NC*
Magnification (×)	0.73	0.88	1.1	0.71
Field of view (degrees)	63	61	58	120
Lens aperture (mm)	20.78	28.7	28.7	26
Working distance from cornea (mm)	6.5	7.0	11	6.5
Coating and glass	Clear crown or yellow retina protector material/filter	Clear crown or yellow retina protector material/filter	Clear crown or yellow retina protector material/filter	High-index lanthunum glass

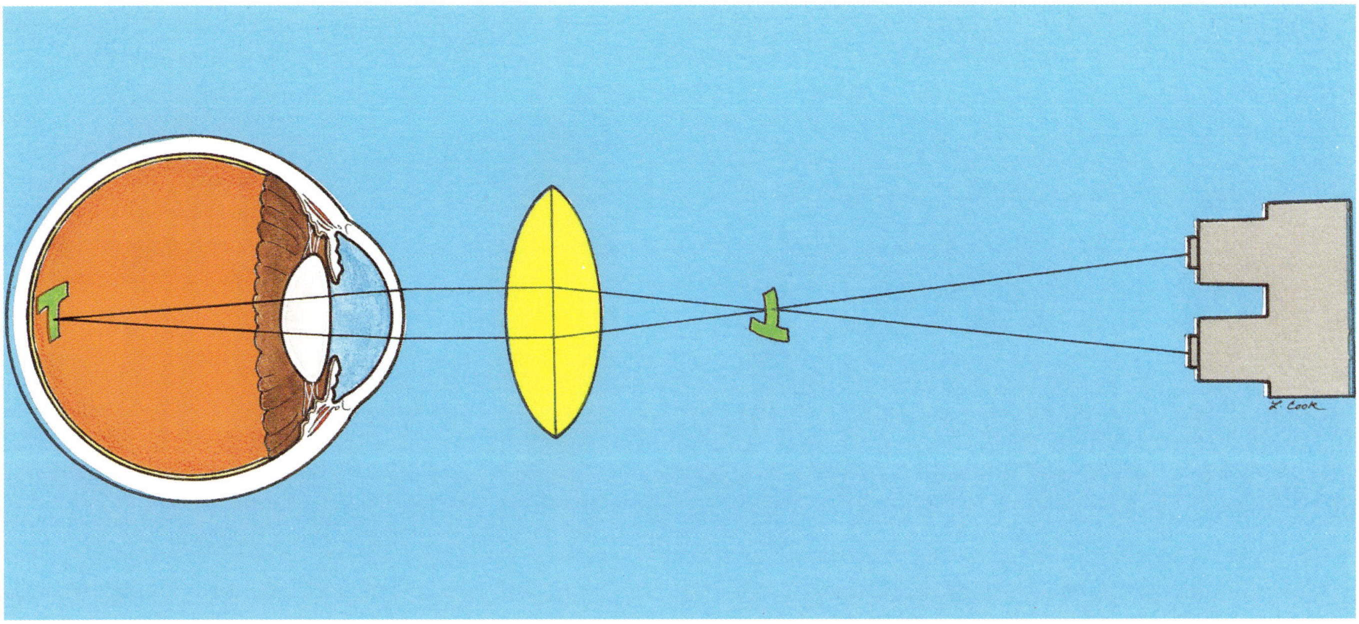

FIGURE 2.3. The optics of formation of a real inverted image with the hand-held condensing lens used for fundus biomicroscopy.

Universal Fundus Contact Lens (Including the Goldmann Lens)

Numerous fundus contact lenses are available for direct examination of the macula. These lenses are available in a variety of sizes and configurations and are sometimes used for examination of other regions of the retina, including the periphery. In general, it is best to have a lens design that is versatile and can be used for complete vitreous as well as retinal observation.

The fundus contact lens yields a virtual, erect, stereoscopic, high-quality image. The universal contact lens has a central power of 64 D and may be used to examine the entire posterior pole region. Since there is no air interface, the image is relatively free from distortion and aberration. The superiority of the image makes this the method of choice for examining subtle changes in the macular region. Magnification, illumination, and slit beam width may be adjusted to meet the examination requirements.

Pupil dilation is required for maximum image quality. A topical anesthetic is instilled, and the lens is placed directly on the corneal surface using an intervening fluid. Conventional gonioscopic solutions of varying viscosities are available for this purpose. Viscous solutions may lead to corneal disruption from preservatives and may blur the patient's vision and make fundus photography or other fundus examination techniques difficult. The gonioscopic solution should be irrigated from the patient's eye immediately after removal of the lens (Figure 2.5).

Preserved solutions may be toxic to the ocular surface if the lens is in place on the cornea for a lengthy period of time. This reaction is characterized by overall conjunctival hyperemia and chemosis and a diffuse superficial punctate keratitis involving the entire corneal surface. To avoid this, and for the sake of con-

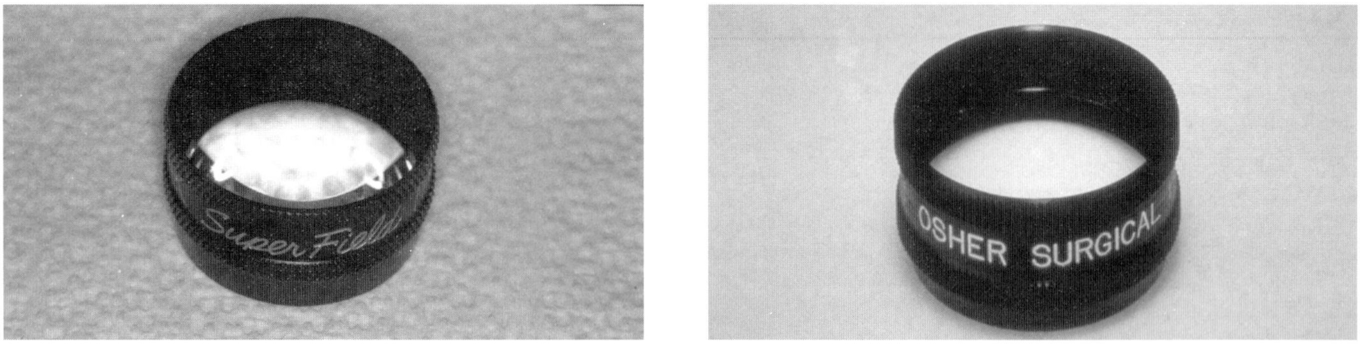

A B

FIGURE 2.4. Examples of the various hand-held condensing lenses used for fundus biomicroscopy. A. Volk Super Field lens. B. Osher Pan-Fundus lens.

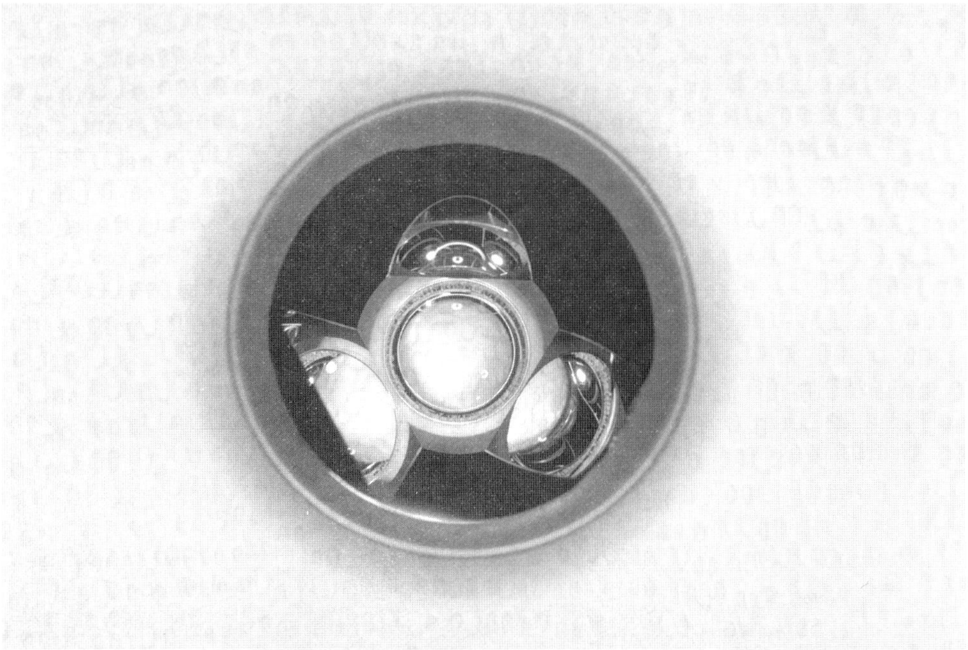

FIGURE 2.5. The universal fundus contact lens with a central lens and equatorial and peripheral retinal mirrors. The lens is also equipped with a mirror inclined at a 59-degree angle for use during gonioscopy.

venience, it is suggested that a single dose, a 1-ml drop of cellulose-based ocular lubricant, be used as an intervening fluid. The volume is adequate to fill the ocular surface of most lenses, the solution is nontoxic to the ocular surface, and postremoval irrigation is not required. However, there is less lens adherence to the cornea due to less viscosity, making bubbles more common (Figure 2.6).

Other lenses are available through Ocular Instruments (Bellevue, WA) and Volk Optics (Mentor, OH), including the Hruby contact lens, the Krieger lens, and a series of wide-angle lenses that have some utility for macular examination but are better suited for a panoramic view of the retina. All of these lenses have a convex front surface. Popular versions include the Quadraspheric lens, the panfunduscopic lens, and the Mainster lens. Many other lenses are available for fundus examination, and some of these may be used for laser photocoagulation as well.

Excellent photographic results of the disc, surrounding vessels, and especially the macula may be obtained with the hand-held condensing lenses and a photo-slit lamp. For macular disease, especially the subtle variety, it is often beneficial to take stereoscopic photographs so that they may be studied later using stereoscopic viewers. The uniform illumination of the biconvex plus lenses yields superior quality photographs of well-defined areas of the macula. The universal three-mirror and Hruby lenses do not yield as satisfactory photographic results for documentation and evaluation, but the photographs are probably adequate for patient demonstration.

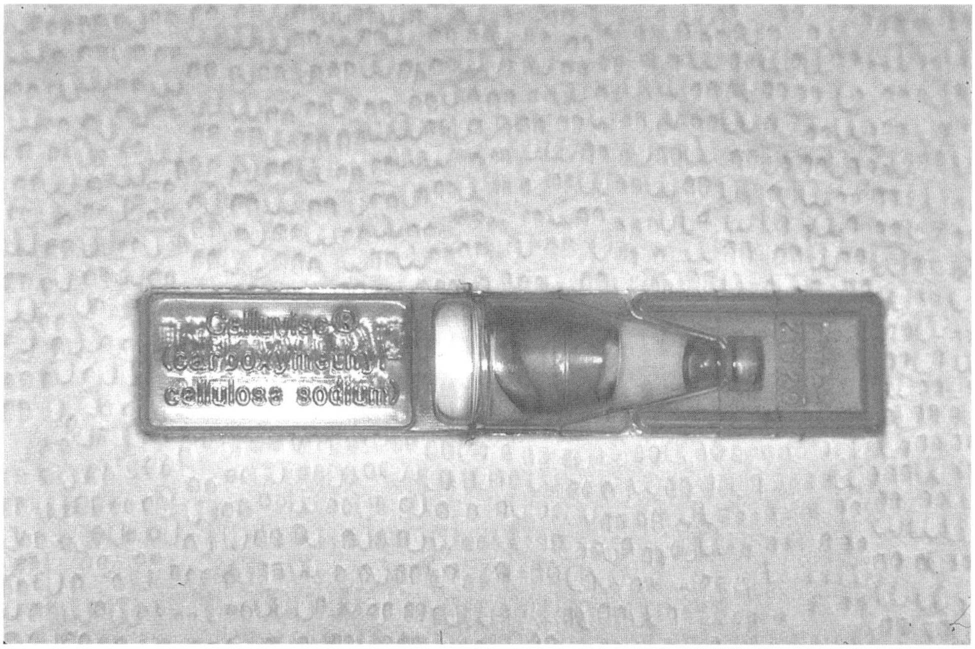

FIGURE 2.6. Single-dose ampule containing 1 ml of cellulose-based lubricant suitable for use as an intervening fluid with fundus contact lenses.

SUGGESTED READING

Barker FM. Vitreoretinal biomicroscopy: A comparison of techniques. J Am Optom Assoc 1987;58:985–992.

Cavallerano A, Gutner R. Fundus biomicroscopy: A comparison of hand-held condensing lenses. Clin Eye Vis Care 1990;2:28–31.

Cavallerano A, Gutner R, Garston M. Fundus biomicroscopy techniques. J Am Optom Assoc 1986;57:755–758.

Cavallerano A, Gutner RK, Semes LP. Enhanced fundus biomicroscopy. J Am Optom Assoc 1994;65:231–234.

Fingeret M, Casser L, Woodcome HT. Direct Ophthalmoscopy. In M Fingeret, L Casser, HT Woodcome (eds), Atlas of Primary Eyecare Procedures. East Norwalk, CT: Appleton & Lange, 1990;186–189.

Griffith T, Semes L, Cutter G. Patient preference between clear and yellow lenses for binocular indirect ophthalmoscopy. Clin Eye Vis Care 1989;1:163–165.

Gutner R, Cavallerano A, Wong D. Fundus biomicroscopy: A comparison of four methods. J Am Optom Assoc 1988;59:388–390.

Houston G. Fundus photography using the Volk 90-D lens. So J Optom 1988;6:13–15.

Potter J, Semes L, Cavallerano A, Garston M. Binocular Indirect Ophthalmoscopy. Boston: Butterworth, 1988.

Semes L. Direct Ophthalmoscopy. In JB Eskridge, J Amos, JD Bartlett (eds), Clinical Procedures in Optometry. Philadelphia: Lippincott, 1991;238–241.

CHAPTER

3 Psychophysical Testing

Leonard J. Oshinskie and
Anthony A. Cavallerano

Both subjective and objective tests are used in assessing macular disease. The initial diagnosis, monitoring of progression or regression of macular disease, and the decision to treat often depend on the cumulative profiles generated by these tests. Certain tests, such as visual acuity, are used in every case, whereas others, such as electrodiagnostic testing, are required only occasionally. The following section describes the psychophysical tests, discusses indications for their use, and explains interpretation as it relates to macular disease.

VISUAL ACUITY

Despite a number of psychophysical tests available for evaluating vision, visual acuity remains the most commonly used method for the initial assessment and monitoring of central visual function. The standard, projected Snellen chart is the most commonly used method of assessing visual acuity and often gives the clinician the first indication of macular disease.

Interpretation of visual acuity must always be correlated with the clinical appearance of the macula, as well as other indicators of macular function, before making a definitive diagnosis. If the fovea is not directly involved in the disease process, visual acuity can remain unchanged in the presence of significant disease elsewhere in the macular region. For example, some diabetic patients with clinically significant macular edema or patients with an active extrafoveal chorioretinitis may have normal visual acuity. Careful evaluation using fundus biomicroscopy will help detect such conditions.

Conversely, in some macular conditions visual acuity may be decreased when ophthalmoscopically the macula appears relatively normal. These include:

Congenital conditions
- Early stages of Stargardt's disease
- Ocular albinism
- Leber's congenital amaurosis
- Cone degeneration/dystrophy

Acquired conditions
- Diabetic retinopathy, including clinically significant macular edema and capillary nonperfusion
- Diffuse macular edema
- Cystoid macular edema
- Resolved central/branch retinal artery occlusion
- Macular holes (full and partial thickness or lamellar)
- Early epiretinal membrane
- Solar maculopathy
- Small subretinal neovascular membrane with associated sensory or RPE detachment
- Idiopathic central serous choroidopathy
- Drug-induced maculopathy

In these cases, other tests of macular function such as contrast sensitivity, color vision, Amsler grid testing, central threshold visual fields, or fluorescein angiography may be abnormal.

The process of obtaining a visual acuity provides other information that may be indicative of macular disease, such as the speed of patient response, eccentric viewing, comments from the patient that he or she only sees characters when "looking to the side" of the character, and no improvement in visual acuity when a pinhole is used.

In addition to the initial evaluation of macular status, visual acuity plays an important role in monitoring disease progression. The traditional Snellen chart suffers

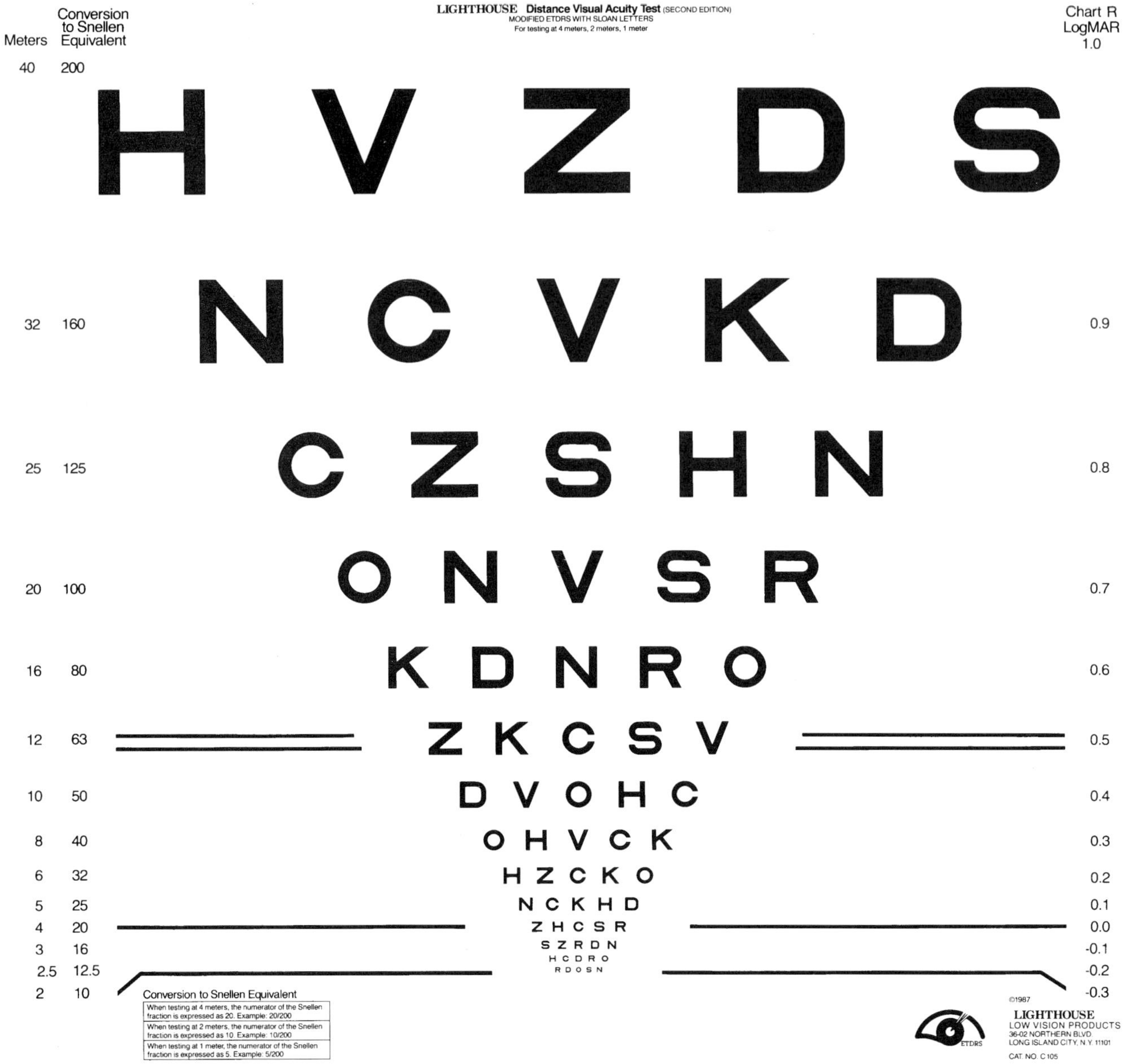

FIGURE 3.1. Early Treatment Diabetic Retinopathy Study visual acuity chart. Acuity may be recorded traditionally as Snellen fraction or in a notation known as logMAR, an abbreviation for logarithm of the minimum angle of resolution. Since the stroke of a 20/200 letter subtends 10 minutes of arc (or in logarithmic terms 10 °1), it is given a logMAR value of 1.0. The stroke of a 20/20 letter subtends 1 minute of arc (logarithmically expressed as 10°) and is therefore assigned a logMAR notation of 0.0. While the logMAR notation is often used by researchers for statistical purposes, clinicians may simply record the value and use it, as with Snellen fractions, to determine if vision is decreased compared with the normal logMAR of 0.0. (Courtesy of The Lighthouse Inc., 36-02 Northern Blvd., Long Island City, NY 11101.)

from specific limitations that may hinder the clinician's ability to detect the insidious changes of advancing macular disease. Many of these problems have been overcome by more recently designed charts pioneered by Bailey and Lovie as well as Ferris. These printed charts, frequently used in research protocols, like the Early Treatment Diabetic Retinopathy Study chart (Figure 3.1), provide optotypes that decrease geometrically by approximately 20% (0.1 log units) in size between each line. These additional increments between lines eliminate the traditional large jump in optotype size, such as between 20/200 and 20/100 characters, and allow detection of smaller increments of vision change. These charts provide the patient with the same number of optotypes to identify at any acuity level. The spacing between letters is uniform to maintain a constant contour interaction between lines. These charts are limited to only 10 letters of the alphabet, selected because they are nearly equally recognizable.

There are some disadvantages in using these charts. It is difficult to isolate a single line of letters, and there is a possibility that patients may identify letters when the first eye is tested and then recite them from memory when the second eye is measured. This latter problem is overcome by using charts with different letter sequences so that one is used for the right eye and another for the left eye. A standard, uniform illumination is necessary to maintain consistency in testing. This requires measurement of illumination using a light meter at various points on the chart; adjustments of the light source are necessary to ensure uniformity and eliminate glare.

Consistency in testing parameters may help ensure that changes will be detected in any patient being followed for subtle changes in visual acuity, such as a patient taking hydroxychloroquine or a diabetic person with macular edema. When monitoring the status of a macular condition, the consistency and ability to detect small changes in vision provided by the newer charts are important measurement requirements.

If visual acuity is not improvable by refraction and the ocular media is clear, additional testing is indicated to rule out macular disease; this commonly includes fundus biomicroscopy.

Additional information regarding the nature and locus of vision loss may be obtained with color vision testing, contrast sensitivity testing, the photostress test, the Amsler grid, and perimetry of the central 10 degrees with spacing between testing points of 2 degrees or less.

Psychophysical testing must be performed prior to exposing the macula to the bleaching effects of a bright light source used in biomicroscopy or ophthalmoscopy. If these procedures have already been completed, the patient must be given ample time to recover. If the patient is suspected of having subtle macular disease on the basis of these tests, fluorescein angiography may be necessary to confirm a specific diagnosis.

Easily overlooked diseases of the optic nerve or other nonmacular causes of vision loss should be considered if macular disease is not obvious. The nonmacular causes of vision loss are legion and include some of the following conditions:

Cornea/tear film
- Precorneal tear film dysfunction
- Early keratoconus/irregular astigmatism
- Corneal dystrophy with resulting stromal edema

Crystalline lens
- Capsular opacities following extracapsular cataract extraction

Vitreous
- Posterior vitreous detachment overlying fovea
- Internal limiting membrane wrinkling (early epiretinal membrane formation)

Optic nerve
- Amblyopia secondary to congenital optic nerve head abnormalities such as optic nerve head hypoplasia
- Demyelinating disease
- Nutritional amblyopia

Cerebral cortex
- Cerebrovascular accident with visual field defect or alexia

Other causes
- Drug-induced vision loss
- Hysteria/malingering
- Monofixation syndrome
- Small-angle esotropia

COLOR VISION TESTING

Color vision testing can provide an important early clinical indication of the onset of insidious macular disease. The test should always be performed monocularly through the best corrected near prescription with appropriate illumination. Dyschromatopsia may precede or accompany other changes in vision, such as visual acuity or visual field defects in patients with maculopathy. When detected, dyschromatopsia affects the blue-yellow (B-Y) range in the initial stages of the disease, but may expand to include the red-green (R-G) region. Finally, achromatopsia will be evident if macular disease is extensive.

Indications for Color Vision Testing in Macular Disease

When the clinician suspects maculopathy due to decreased visual acuity or visual field, color vision testing is essential to elicit or confirm a diagnosis and to determine appropriate management. Regardless of the method, color vision should be tested monocularly because the asymmetry in color vision suggests acquired versus congenital dyschromatopsia. In fact, baseline R-G testing for all patients should be conducted at their initial visit using pseudoisochromatic plates to rule out inherited congenital defects that might affect occupational or vocational requirements.

Color vision testing may also assist in the differential diagnosis of vision loss from macular disease versus optic nerve disease. R-G defects are often indicative of optic nerve disease, whereas B-Y defects are usually suggestive of early retinal dysfunction. This observation is known as *Kollner's rule*; exceptions to this rule are discussed in the next section. For example, dyschromatopsia of the B-Y type in diabetes may indicate clinically significant macular edema, a condition that often requires treatment.

Another example of patients at risk for maculopathy are those using retinotoxic drugs such as digoxin, chloroquine, tamoxifen, or one of the phenothiazines. Toxic retinopathy resulting from drug use is uncommon due to a better understanding of dose-related effects. Commonly used drugs known to cause dyschromatopsia are listed in Table 3.1.

Color vision testing is useful in diabetic persons to detect color vision defects that might interfere with the use of blood glucose monitoring systems. Several of these systems rely on color comparisons to judge the blood glucose reading. Dyschromatopsia may cause errors in reading the blood glucose levels, a misinterpretation that may result in using the incorrect amount of insulin.

Methods of Color Vision Testing

The commonly used Ishihara pseudoisochromatic plates are designed to detect R-G defects and therefore are not sensitive enough to detect some forms of early maculopathy. For definitive testing, a color arrangement test such as the Farnsworth-Munsell 100-hue test is highly sensitive for detecting mild deficiencies, but it is time consuming to administer. The Farnsworth dichotamous standard D-15 test takes approximately 2–3 minutes per eye and detects congenital R-G as well as moderate-to-severe acquired color defects. Some individuals have suggested methods for improving the sensitivity of the D-15 test using quantitative methods. Desaturated versions of the test have also been shown to increase the sensitivity of this test. Other color vision tests that have the ability to test for B-Y defects include the Sahlgren Saturation test, the Lanthony Desaturated Panel D-15 test, the Lanthony New Color test, the American Optical H-R-R Plates, the F2 Tritan Plates, and the Igaku-Shoin Plates, Part II.

A suggested protocol for clinical screening for color vision in a case of suspected macular disease includes pseudoisochromatic plates (11-plate model) that are sensitive for R-G defects and a test such as the desaturated D-15 or Sahlgren Saturation test to test for B-Y deficiencies.

To avoid false-positive errors, all these tests should be done monocularly and with proper illumination, near correction in place, and standardized conditions.

Interpretation of Color Vision Testing

A bilateral, symmetric R-G defect usually indicates congenital dyschromatopsia, which by definition is not associated with disease, occurs almost entirely in male subjects (95%), and remains stable. Patients are often initially unaware of their color deficiency and usually have no other abnormalities of the visual system such as visual field defects, a relative afferent pupillary defect, or decreased visual acuity.

TABLE 3.1. Commonly Used Drugs Causing Dyschromatopsia

Drug	*Type of dyschromatopsia*
Aspirin	Transient R-G
Chloramphenicol	R-G
Chloroquine	R-G
Digitalis glycosides	R-G and B-Y
Erythromycin	B-Y
Ethambutol	R-G
Ethyl alcohol	R-G
Ibuprofen	R-G
Oral contraceptives	B-Y and R-G
Phenothiazines	B-Y and R-G
Sulfonamides	R-G
Tamoxifen	B-Y

R-G = red-green; B-Y = blue-yellow.
Source: Adapted from ML Fischer. Clinical color vision testing as a diagnostic tool. Prob Optom 1991;3:94–119.

Various results of D-15 testing are shown in Figure 3.2. Many patients with acquired dyschromatopsia secondary to macular disease will have errors that tend to parallel the tritan axis, errors that cannot be classified as B-Y or R-G but that still should be considered evidence of disease.

Some patients with normal color vision will make a few random errors with the desaturated version, resulting in false-positive errors. Since nuclear sclerosis and age both cause defects in the B-Y range, they can confound interpretation of color vision defects detected with either version of the D-15 test. Congenital dyschromatopsia of the B-Y type is almost nonexistent, so when a patient presents with this type of color vision deficiency it is assumed to be due to a disease process until proven otherwise.

Although a B-Y defect usually suggests retinal disease, some types of optic nerve disease, including glaucoma, anterior ischemic optic neuropathy, dominantly inherited optic atrophy, and chronic papilledema, also cause B-Y defects. This observation is contrary to Kollner's rule, which states that B-Y defects are generally associated with retinal disease and R-G defects with optic nerve disease. Obviously optic nerve disease must be ruled out when a B-Y defect is found before the results are useful in the diagnosis of macular disease.

Any asymmetry of color vision, including the R-G or B-Y type, should arouse suspicion of disease. A comparison of color vision asymmetry may be obtained by alternately covering one eye and then the other while showing the patient a pseudoisochromatic plate. It is always possible for a patient to have an acquired color deficiency superimposed on a preexisting, inherited defi-

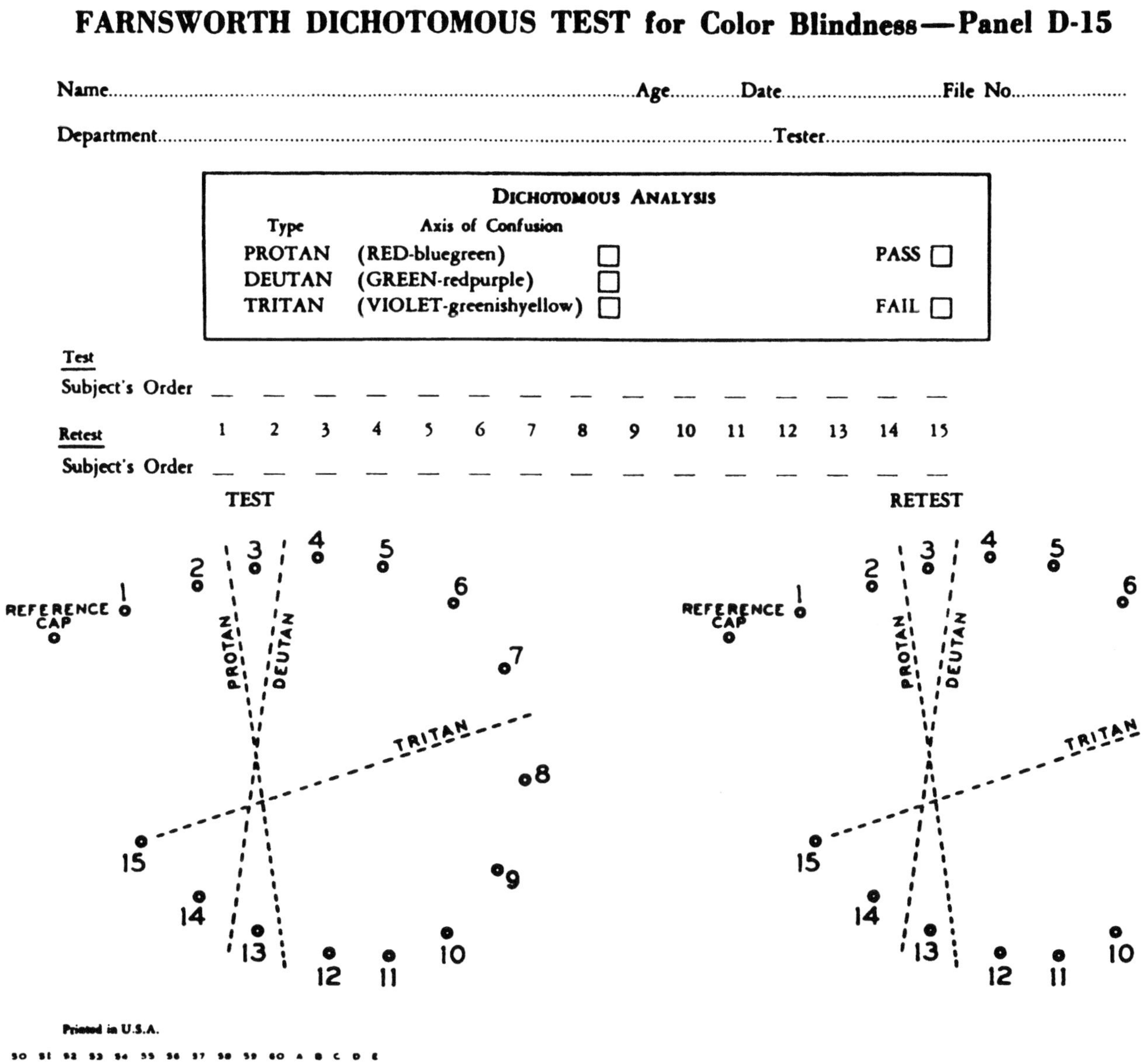

FARNSWORTH DICHOTOMOUS TEST for Color Blindness—Panel D-15

Name........................ Age........ Date........................ File No....................

Department.. Tester..

Dichotomous Analysis

Type	Axis of Confusion		
PROTAN	(RED-bluegreen)	☐	PASS ☐
DEUTAN	(GREEN-redpurple)	☐	
TRITAN	(VIOLET-greenishyellow)	☐	FAIL ☐

Test
Subject's Order _ _ _ _ _ _ _ _ _ _ _ _ _ _ _

Retest 1 2 3 4 5 6 7 8 9 10 11 12 13 14 15
Subject's Order _ _ _ _ _ _ _ _ _ _ _ _ _ _ _

Printed in U.S.A.

50 51 52 53 54 55 56 57 58 59 60 A B C D E

A

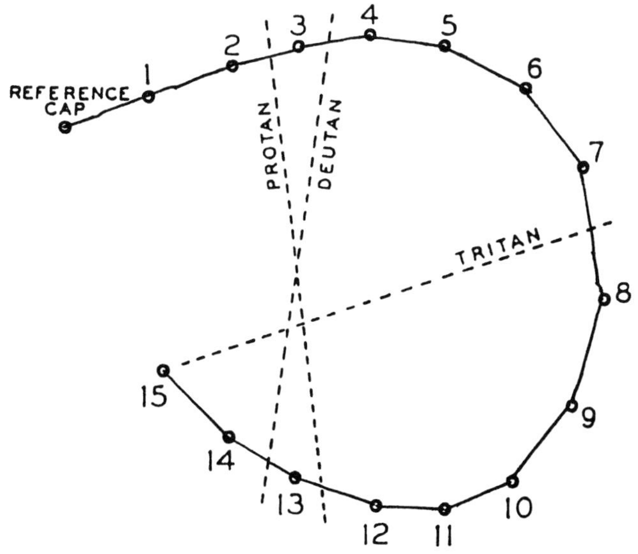

B

Figure 3.2. A. Scoring for the Farnsworth Dichotomous Test for Color Blindness, Panel D-15. B. Normal score of the Farnsworth dichotomous panel D-15 tests. *(continued)*

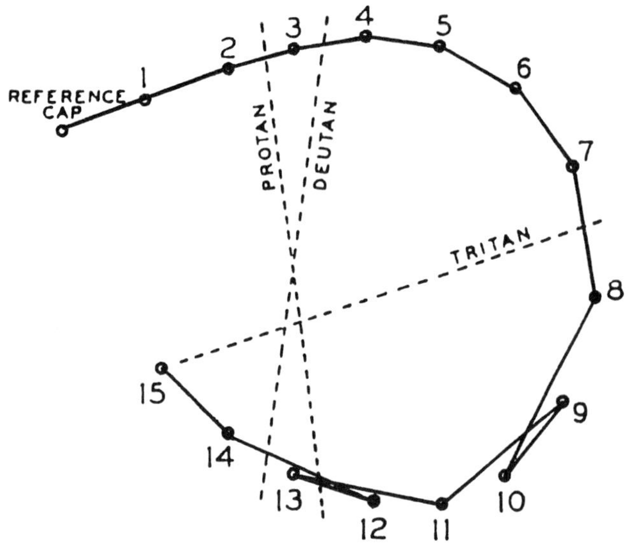

C

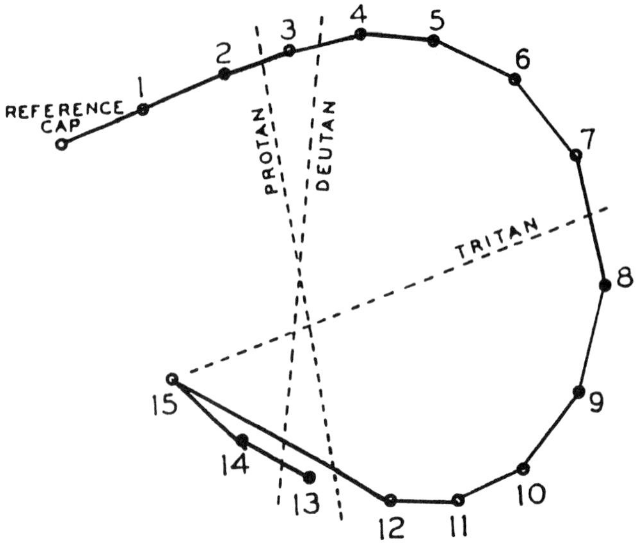

D

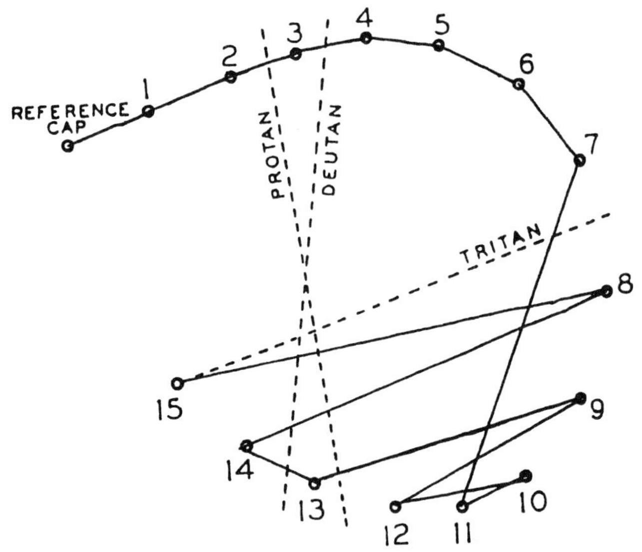

E

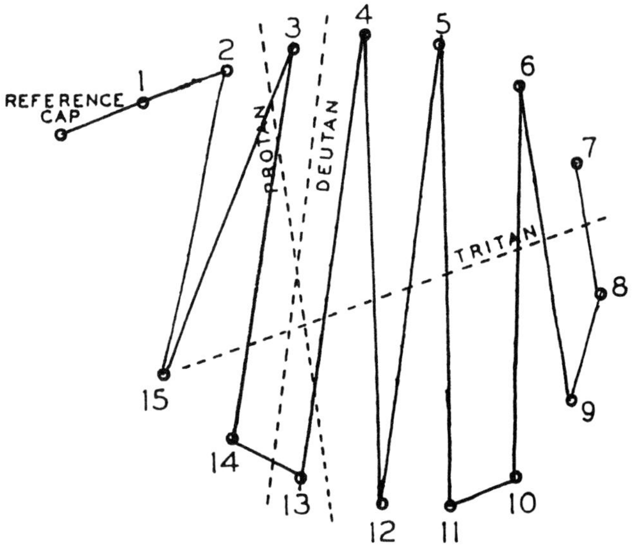

F

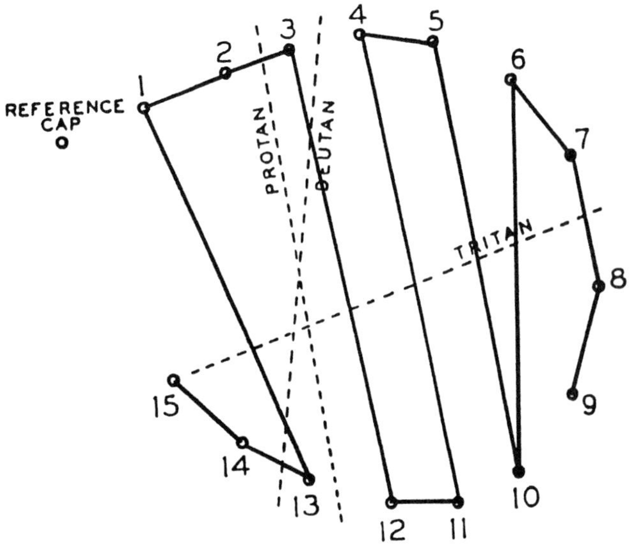

G

Figure 3.2. *(continued)* Examples of minor failing errors using the standard Farnsworth Dichotomous Panel D-15. C. Two "one-place" errors. D. One "two-place" error. E. Illustrates the desaturated D-15 scoring of a diabetic patient with macular edema and dyschromatopsia paralleling the B-Y axis. Scoring of the standard Panel D-15 typical of a congenital deutanope (F) and protanope (G), respectively. (Scoring form copyright © 1947 by The Psychological Corporation. Reproduced by permission. All rights reserved. A, B, and C redrawn with permission from AJ Adams, RR Rodic, R Husted, R Stamper. Spectral sensitivity and color discrimination changes in glaucoma and glaucoma-suspect patients. Invest Ophthalmol Vis Sci 1982;23:516–524.)

ciency since congenital dyschromatopsia is relatively common. Additionally, while an acquired R-G deficiency is often a sign of optic nerve disease, several macular conditions, including Stargardt's disease and primary cone dystrophy, have been reported to cause an R-G defect in their later stages; B-Y defects are found in the early stages of these maculopathies. Interpretations of results for several standard color vision tests are summarized in Table 3.2.

Color vision can provide the clinician with important information regarding the status of the macula. Monocular color vision testing should be performed routinely if early macular disease is suspected in the absence of objective clinical signs.

TABLE 3.2. Interpretation of Color Vision Testing

Pseudoisochromatic plates
Most patients with congenital dyschromatopsia will miss many plates, e.g., >15 on 38-plate Ishihara test, >8 on 11-plate test
Patients with acquired R-G deficiency due to early macular disease may miss a few plates, e.g., <5 on a 38-plate test
Patients with optic nerve disease may miss more plates than patients with early retinal disease
Color arranging tests (such as the D-15)
Normal patients may make one or two "one-place errors"
Patients with retinal disease may have many (three or more) one-place or multi-place errors. Look for errors that tend to parallel the tritan axis (see Figure 3.2)
Patients with optic neuropathy make errors in R-G testing and tend to score better as a group than patients with retinal disease

R-G = red-green.

SPATIAL CONTRAST SENSITIVITY TESTING

Contrast sensitivity is an exacting, subjective psychophysical method of assessing visual function. This test can be useful in detecting early macular disease, especially when visual acuity is essentially normal as documented by the Snellen chart.

The concept of using spatial contrast sensitivity testing (SCST) to evaluate vision was first considered in the 1700s, but this method of psychophysical testing has only recently gained wide use in clinical practice. This section limits the discussion of SCST to the evaluation of macular disease.

Several methods of SCST are employed for detecting and monitoring macular disease, using either gratings or letters. Gratings are generated photographically or electronically by the use of lasers. Grating-based tests vary both contrast (difference in luminance between the dark bars and the lighter background) and spatial frequency (the number of pairs of gratings per degree of visual angle) in order to evaluate visual function.

Waveform generators electronically create gratings of various spatial frequencies and contrast, which are viewed on a cathode ray tube. These instruments have demonstrated spatial contrast sensitivity loss at various frequencies in research studies to assess macular disease; however, due to their expense and the requirement for multiple time-consuming responses, these instruments are not as popular in the clinical setting as other methods of SCST.

Laser interferometers that project a grating onto the retina are also used in SCST. These devices are attached to a slit lamp to facilitate aiming the grating through the pupil and media opacities to determine potential acuity, and thus macular status, prior to cataract surgery.

Photographically produced grating-based charts are easily used in a clinical setting and are relatively inexpensive compared with the previously mentioned devices. Recording the responses to these tests creates a spatial contrast sensitivity curve that is compared to normative data (Figure 3.3). Spatial frequency values of 1.5 and 3 cycles per degree (cpd) are considered low spatial frequency, 6 cpd as mid-frequency, and 12 and 18 cpd as high frequency. Since high spatial frequency gratings subtend a small visual angle, the patient's performance at this end of the spatial contrast sensitivity curve generally corresponds to good visual acuity. For example, a patient with 20/20 visual acuity would be expected to have a normal value along the spatial contrast sensitivity curve at 18 cpd with these tests. If visual acuity is good, but SCST is abnormal at high spatial frequencies, early macular disease may be present.

The Vision Contrast Testing System (VCTS-6500) by Vistech Consultants, Inc. (Dayton, OH) provides a progressive decrease in contrast of sinusoidal gratings for five spatial frequencies (1.5, 3.0, 6.0, 12.0, and 18.0 cpd) and is illuminated externally (Figure 3.4).

The CSV-1000, by Vector Vision (Dayton, OH), provides similar gratings in four spatial frequencies (3.0, 6.0, 12.0, and 18.0 cpd) used in a forced choice manner with internal illumination that is automatically calibrated (Figure 3.5). With these tests as well as letter-based tests, it is always important to use the specified testing distance and illumination to allow a comparison with normative reference values and to ensure consistency from one testing period to another.

Other methods of SCST that use changes in contrast of gratings or grating-like test patterns include the Arden plates, the Melbourne Edge Test, and the Cambridge Contrast Test.

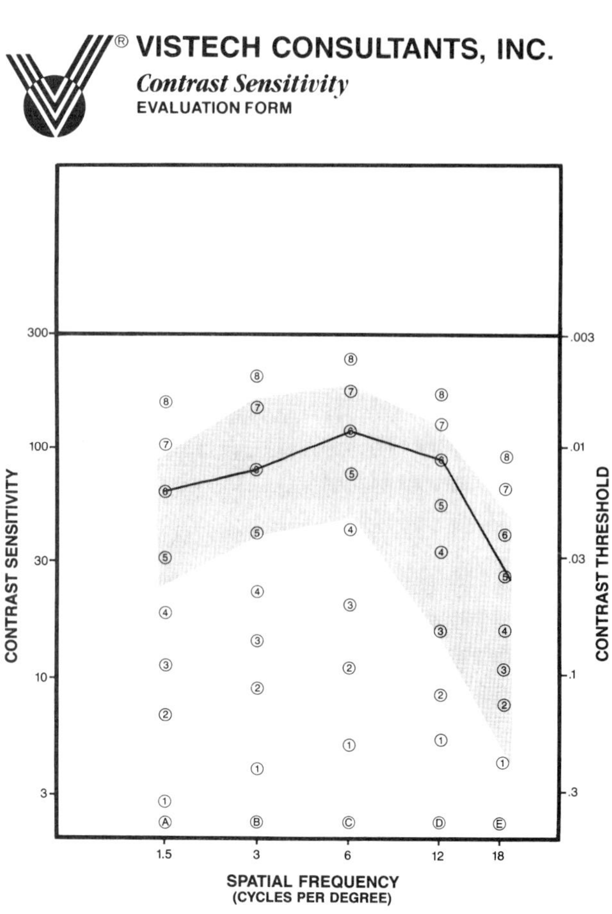

A

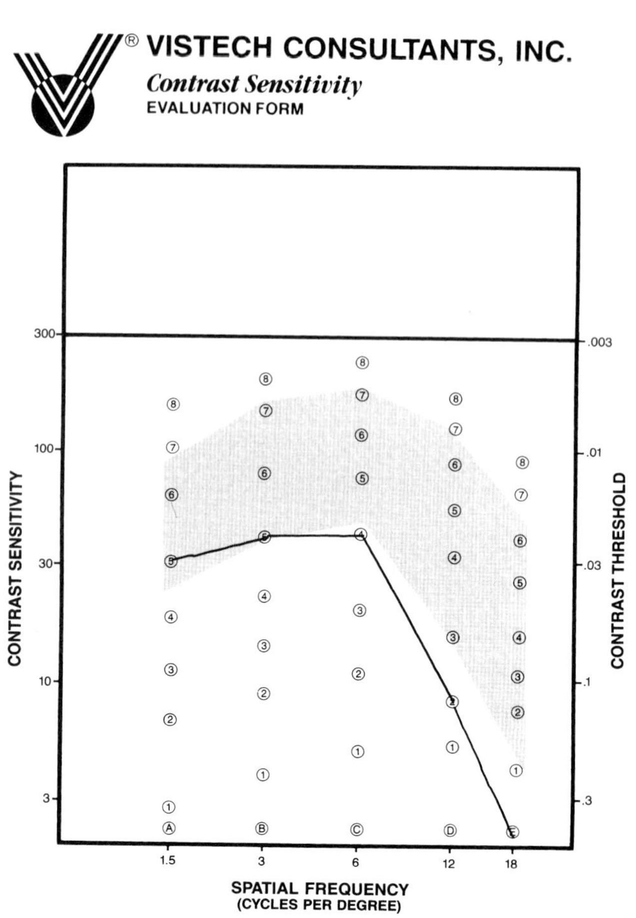

B

FIGURE 3.3. Spatial contrast sensitivity function curve using Vistech Visual Contrast Testing System (VCTS-6500). A. The curve for a normal eye with a visual acuity of 20/20. B. The curve shown for the left eye illustrates the high frequency loss of a diabetic patient with early macular edema and 20/25 visual acuity. (Courtesy of Vistech Consultants, Inc., 4162 Little York Rd., Dayton, OH 45414.)

Letter-based charts used in SCST are fundamentally familiar to patients, relatively inexpensive, and easy to use in a clinical setting. Letter-based tests, generated photographically or electronically, use either one chart that varies contrast with a constant optotype size or several charts that vary both optotype size and contrast.

The Pelli-Robson chart uses Sloan design optotypes of a uniform, low spatial frequency size (approximately 1 cpd) arranged in groups of three letters of decreasing contrast ranging from almost 100% (0.00 log contrast sensitivity) to 0.56% (2.25 log contrast sensitivity) (Figure 3.6). Results are scored according to the log contrast sensitivity, with normal values considered to be 1.80 or greater for patients younger than 50 years and 1.65 or greater for older patients. A significant change in SCST with this method is 0.30 log units (two groups of letters).

Regan's method uses several Snellen-like charts with various contrast levels ranging from 95–3% and contains characters of graduated size from 20/200–20/10. Like Regan's chart, high and low contrast Bailey-Lovie charts vary optotype size and contrast to measure spatial contrast sensitivity.

When using SCST in the evaluation of macular disease, the clinician must consider the confounding effects of refractive error, age, media opacities, and optic nerve and neurologic disease in both the initial interpretation and the monitoring of results. Since these factors can cause losses in SCST in the same spatial frequencies as macular disease, when present they complicate the interpretation of SCST considerably and therefore limit its usefulness in evaluation of macular disease. A brief discussion of these confounding effects follows.

Interpretation of Spatial Contrast Sensitivity Testing Results

Optical blur from refractive error causes loss at all frequencies in grating-based tests, although the loss is greater at the higher frequencies. Results of SCST obtained using the Pelli-Robson chart are not affected by optical blur as much as the Vistech chart. Obviously, all

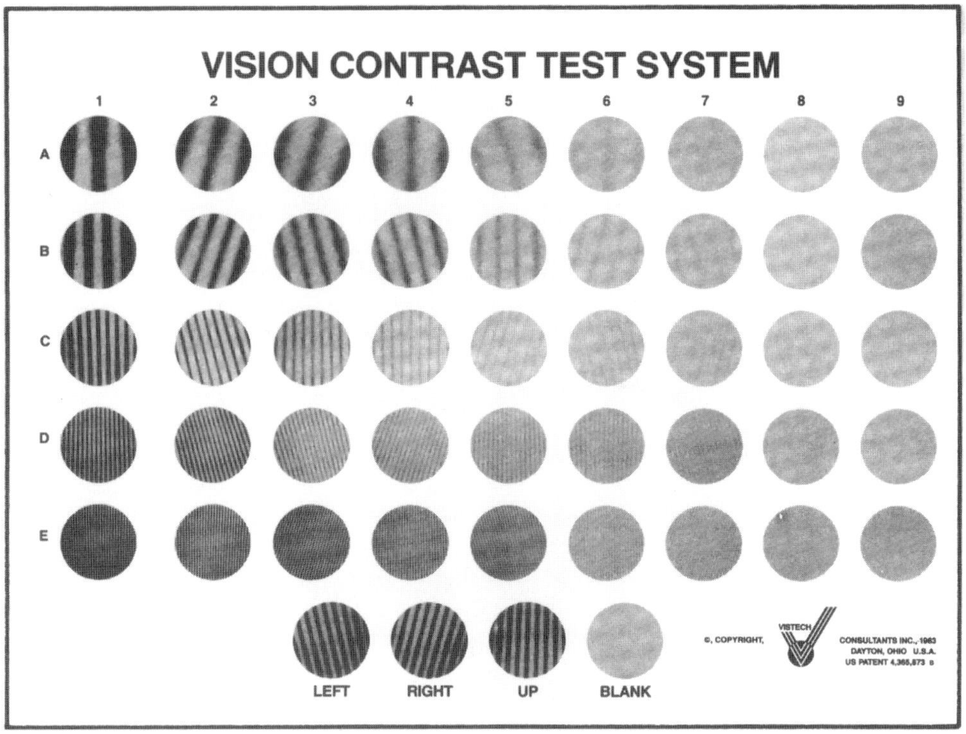

FIGURE 3.4. Vision Contrast Test System. (Courtesy of Vistech Consultants, Inc., 4162 Little York Rd., Dayton, OH 45414.)

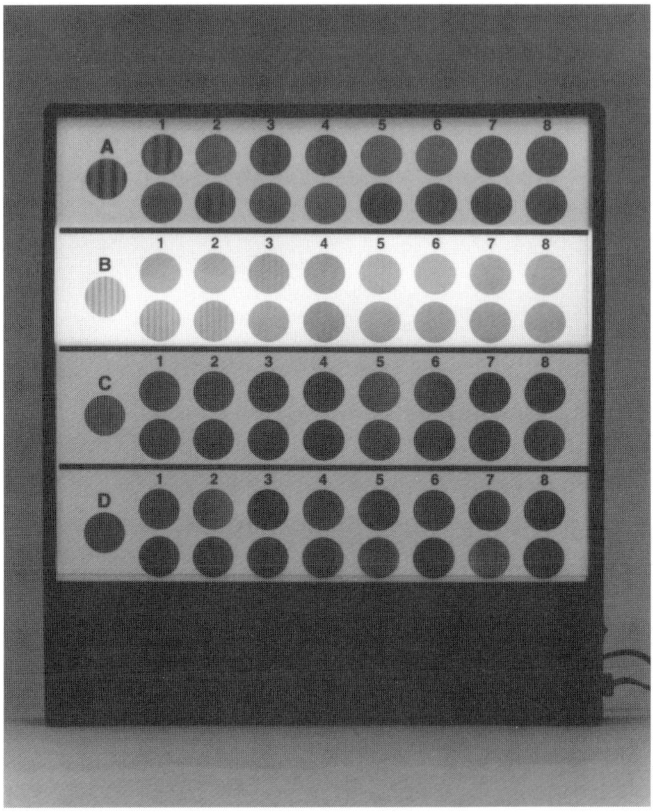

FIGURE 3.5. The CSV-1000 by Vector Vision. (Courtesy of Vector Vision, Dayton, OH.)

patients should be evaluated with the optimal refractive correction in place.

Most studies indicate that increasing age causes decreased sensitivity, especially at mid and high spatial frequencies. This decline has been observed in patients as early as age 45.

Cataracts have been reported to cause losses at various levels of spatial frequency. Some reports suggest spatial contrast sensitivity loss correlates with the type and grade of opacity, with early cataracts causing losses at mid to high frequencies. Early lens opacities seem to have little significant effect on letter-based tests.

Amblyopia is associated with loss of contrast sensitivity at all frequencies, although some amblyopic patients have loss only at high frequencies. Loss of contrast sensitivity in the low and middle frequencies leads to a suspicion of disease along the visual pathways, although all frequencies can be affected in these processes. Visual pathway disorders also cause lower values with letter-based SCST.

If these confounding ocular conditions are eliminated as a cause of decreased spatial contrast sensitivity, then an abnormal SCST may indicate macular disease. In general, patients with disease involving the fovea primarily show a greater loss at higher spatial frequencies with grating-based tests. More widespread macular disease generally demonstrates loss at intermediate and high frequencies. In diffuse or advanced macular disease, the degree of contrast sensitivity loss usually decreases across

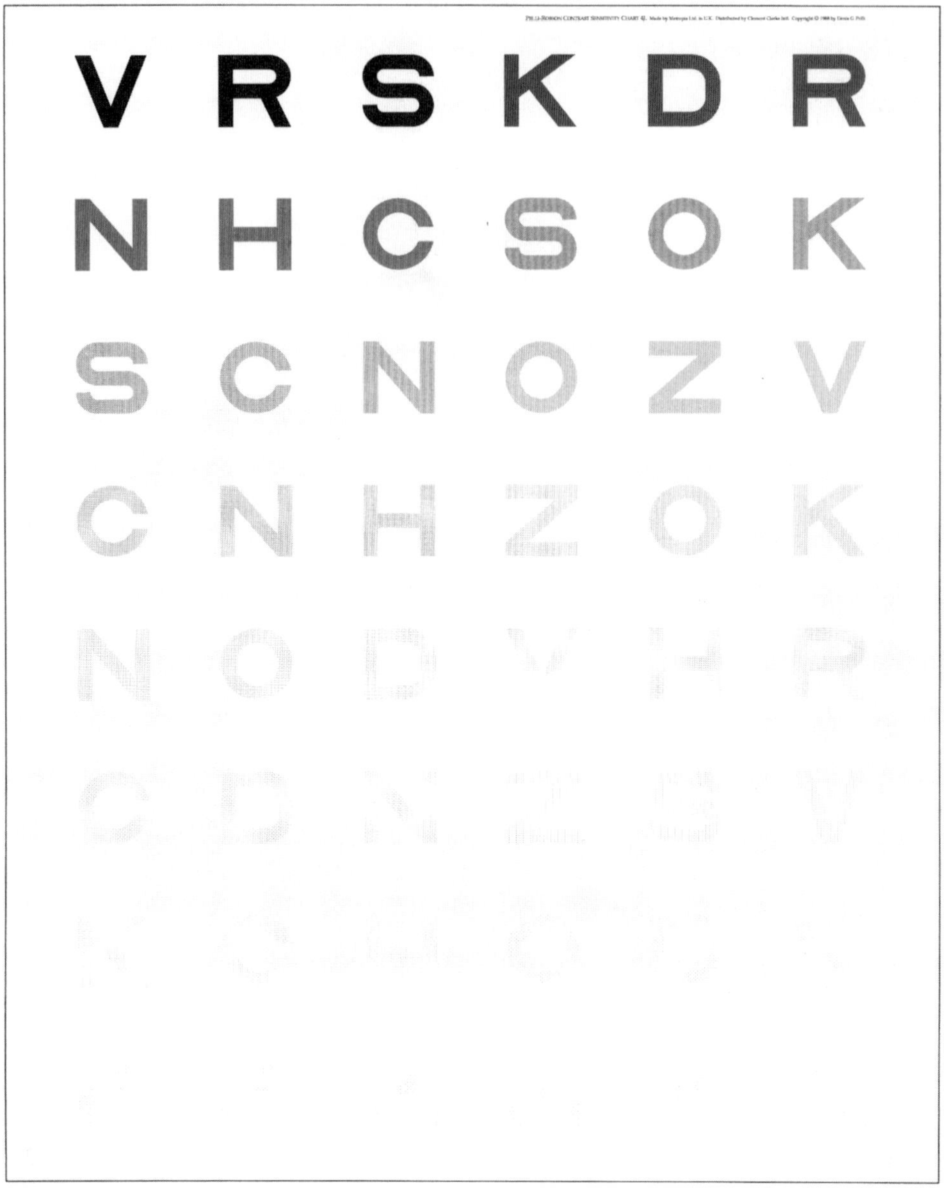

FIGURE 3.6. The Pelli-Robson Contrast Sensitivity Chart. (Courtesy of Clement Clarke, Inc., 3128 E. 17th St., Columbus, OH 43219.)

all frequencies and often correlates with the relatively greater loss of visual acuity.

Studies of patients with diabetic retinopathy using grating-based tests show that SCST is often abnormal at high spatial frequencies even before visual acuity begins to decline significantly (<20/30). Normal SCST results do not, however, rule out retinopathy since approximately 40–70% of patients in these studies with retinopathy had normal SCST results. Therefore, the sensitivity of SCST (ability of a test to detect disease when present) is low for diabetic retinopathy if visual acuity is good.

Published results of SCST studies using letter-based charts in patients with specific macular diseases, such as diabetic retinopathy and idiopathic central serous choroidpathy, suggest that 40–50% of these patients have abnormal scores when tested with the low-contrast letters. Therefore, like grating-based tests, sensitivity is less than ideal. Patients with age-related macular degeneration demonstrate loss with middle- and low-contrast letters compared with age-matched normal subjects. A study of patients with macular drusen and 20/20 visual acuity showed grating SCST to be affected at high frequencies compared with controls.

In general, SCST is not a test that will establish a specific diagnosis in macular disease. The value of SCST as a screening device in macular disease has been questioned by some and advocated by others. It may be useful for testing selected patients with risk factors or symptoms consistent with early, treatable macular disease. One example is in diabetic patients with clinically significant macular edema, with the understanding that the sensitivity of SCST is low for diabetic patients as a group. Used as an adjunct in detecting early or subtle macular disease, a loss in SCST occurring at mid to high frequencies directs the clinician to consider other diagnostic modalities, including fundus contact lens examination, central automated visual fields, or fundus fluorescein angiography.

SCST may have the most value in demonstrating the progression or regression of visual loss in patients with macular disease. For example, if a diabetic patient who is being followed regularly develops clinically significant macular edema, but the subjective visual acuity has not changed, SCST may be used to show the patient how his or her vision has changed and may be helpful in educating the patient that laser therapy is indicated.

SUGGESTED READING

Visual Acuity

Bailey IL, Lovie JE. New design principles for visual acuity letters charts. Am J Optom Physiol Optics 1976;53:740–745.

Ferris FL, Kassoff A, Bailey I. New visual acuity charts for clinical research. Am J Ophthalmol 1982;94:91–96.

Ferris FL, Sperduto RD. Standardized illumination for visual acuity testing in clinical research. Am J Ophthalmol 1982;94:97–98.

Johnston AW. Making Sense of the M, N and Log MAR Systems of Specifying Visual Acuity. In R London (ed), Problems in Optometry. Philadelphia: Lippincott, 1991.

Sherman J, Richter S, Epstein A. The differential diagnosis of visual disorders in patients presenting with marked symptoms but no observable ocular abnormality. Am J Optom Physiol Optics 1980;57:516–522.

Color Vision

Adams AJ, Rodic R, Husted R, Stamper R. Spectral sensitivity and color discrimination in glaucoma and glaucoma-suspect patients. Invest Ophthalmol Vis Sci 1982;23:516–524.

Bowman KJ, Collins MJ, Henry CJ. The Effect of Age on Performance on the Panel D-15 and Desaturated D-15: A Quantitative Evaluation. In G Verriest (ed), Colour Vision Deficiencies VII. The Hague: Dr. W Junk Publishers, 1984;227–231.

Fischer ML. Clinical Color Vision Testing as a Diagnostic Tool. In R London (ed), Problems in Optometry. Philadelphia: Lippincott, 1991.

Frisen L. Clinical Tests of Vision. New York: Raven, 1990.

Frisen L, Kalm H. Sahlgren's saturation test for detecting and grading acquired dyschromatopsia. Am J Ophthalmol 1981;92:252–258.

Hart WH. Acquired dyschromatopsias. Surv Ophthalmol 1987;32:10–31.

Lanthony P. The new color test. Doc Ophthalmol 1978;46:191–199.

Vingrys AJ, King-Smith PE. A quantitative scoring technique for panel tests of color vision. Invest Ophthalmol Vis Sci 1988;29:50–63.

Spatial Contract Sensitivity

Adamsons I, Rubin GS, Vitale S, et al. The effect of early cataracts on glare and contrast sensitivity. Arch Ophthalmol 1992;110:1081–1086.

Cavallerano JD, Aiello LM. Glare and Contrast Sensitivity for Clinicians. New York: Springer, 1990.

Derefeldt G, Lennerstrand G, Lundh B. Age variations in normal contrast sensitivity. Acta Ophthalmol 1979;57:679–690.

Elliott DB, Sanderson K, Conkey A. The reliability of the Pelli-Robson contrast sensitivity chart. Ophthalmic Physiol Optics 1990;10:21–24.

Elliott DB, Whitaker D. How useful are contrast sensitivity charts in optometric practice? Case reports. Optom Vis Sci 1992;69:378–385.

Greeves A, Cloe BL. Assessment of contrast sensitivity of patients with macular disease using reduced contrast near visual acuity charts. Ophthalmol Physiol Optics 1988;8:371–377.

Kleiner RC, Enger C, Alexander MF, Fine SL. Contrast sensitivity in age-related macular degeneration. Arch Ophthalmol 1988;106:55–57.

Lasa MS, Datiles MB III, Podgor MJ, Magno BV. Contrast and glare sensitivity. Ophthalmology 1992;99:1045–1049.

Marmor MF, Gawande A. Effect of visual blur on contrast sensitivity. Ophthalmology 1988;95:139–143.

Regan D, Neima D. Low-contrast letter charts as a test of visual function. Ophthalmology 1983;90:1192–1200.

Sjostrand J. Contrast sensitivity in macular disease using a small-field and large-field TV system. Acta Ophthalmol 1979;57:832–846.

Sjostrand J, Frisen L. Contrast sensitivity in macular disease. Acta Ophthalmol 1977;55:507–513.

Sokol S, Moskowitz A, Skarf B, et al. Contrast sensitivity in diabetics with and without background retinopathy. Arch Ophthalmol 1985;103:51–54.

Wolkstein M, Atkin A, Bodis-Wollner I. Contrast sensitivity in retinal disease. Ophthalmology 1980;87:1140–1149.

CHAPTER

4

Additional Tests of Macular Function

Anthony A. Cavallerano and Leonard J. Oshinskie

Assessment of macular function should include subjective testing of retinal sensitivity. The Amsler grid, threshold visual fields, and potential acuity testing (for evaluation of the unseen macula) provide the clinician with important adjunctive clinical information. Despite their subjectivity, these tests are relatively simple to perform and provide useful information regarding the status of the macula. The results derived from these tests, however, must be correlated with the clinical appearance of the macula.

AMSLER GRID

The Amsler grid and similar test grids are the mainstay for assessing and monitoring macular function in both the office and home. The ability to detect dysmorphopsia may be vital when first suspecting a choroidal neovascular membrane. Similarly, a scotoma may be an early sign of macular dysfunction, for example, in diabetic patients or those taking hydroxychloroquine, a retinotoxic drug taken by patients for arthritis or systemic lupus erythematosus.

Amsler grid macular testing is a qualitative method for assessing central vision. It is a rapid, concise, but nonspecific method for testing the central fovea to 10 degrees of vision surrounding the fixation point. Several other grid types are available, including a red grid, the threshold Amsler grid (TAG), and an Amsler grid with smaller boxes that subtend 1 degree within the central degrees. This functional test is used to detect distortion and scotomas in the central visual area. Amsler grid assessment is indicated whenever there is suspected macular disease or if there is unexplained central vision loss. It is the standard of care for in-office and home monitoring of visual function in a variety of acute and longstanding macular disorders, including age-related macular degeneration (AMD), diabetic retinopathy, and patients at risk for developing choroidal neovascular membrane from any cause.

Amsler charts are provided in a loose-leaf bound format and consist of seven charts with a variety of grids and targets. Charts 1–3 are the most commonly used in clinical practice. Chart number 1 (Figure 4.1), the familiar grid pattern, is the most widely used and consists of a 20-degree by 20-degree grid of white lines on a black background with a central fixation point. Each of the lines is separated by 5 mm and subtends a visual angle of 1 degree when held 30–35 cm from the patient. The test should be administered monocularly through the near correction and prior to instilling topical agents or directing a bright light source into the patient's eye.

Chart number 3 is a red grid and is useful in testing patients suspected of having chloroquine maculopathy, toxic maculopathy, nutritional amblyopia, alcohol-related vitamin B deficiency, or diabetic macular edema. The red target is considered to be slightly more sensitive in detecting early lesions affecting the retinal pigment epithelium (RPE) in the macular area.

Acute or chronically progressive macular disease resulting in central visual disturbance can often be detected using the Amsler grid. The patient is instructed to look for distorted, cloudy, wavy, or missing areas in the Amsler chart while monocularly fixing on the central white dot with the best near correction. Interpretation of the test results is immediate. It should be noted that the absence of a defect in the Amsler grid does not exclude the presence of a lesion. However, being a functional test, a defect does indicate an incompetence in the retinal and choroidal architecture and vasculature. The Amsler grid test also detects optic nerve and visual pathway defects in neurologic disease. The Amsler grid test is difficult for patients with severe loss of central fixation, but chart

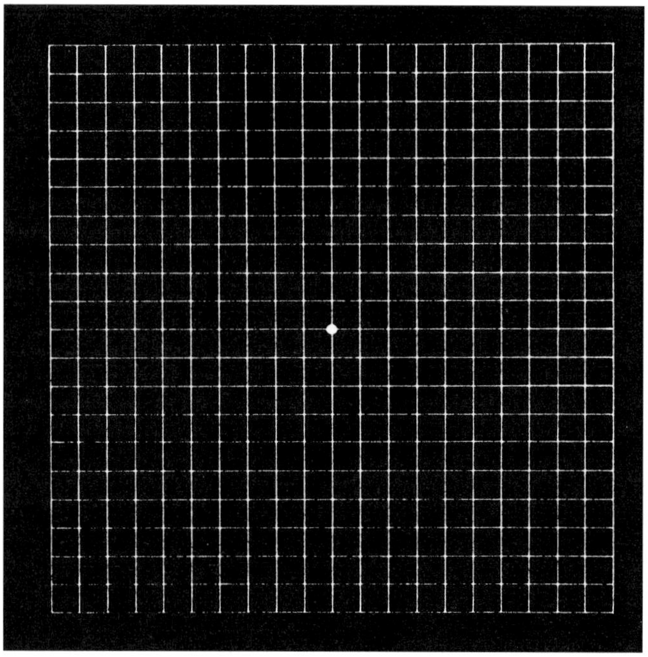

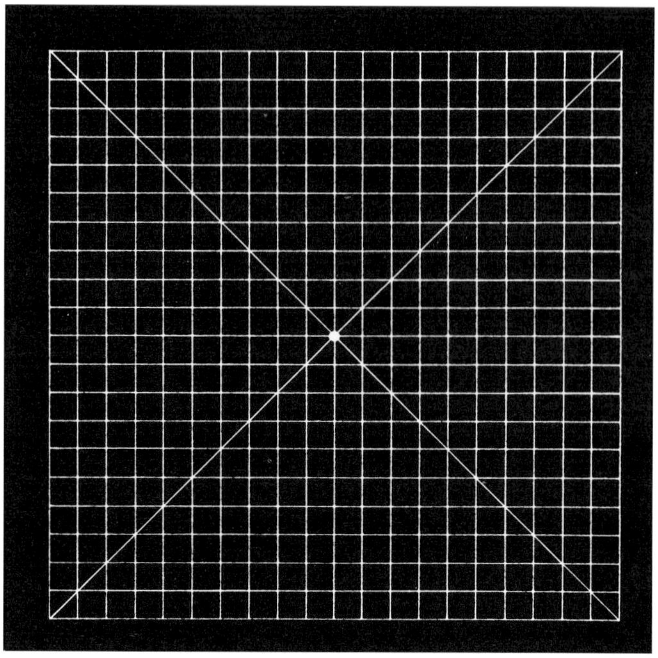

FIGURE 4.1. Chart numbers 1 (left) and 2 (right) of the Amsler grid test.

number 2 (see Figure 4.1) may be employed to promote central fixation in the patient with a central scotoma.

Scotomas apparent on the Amsler grid testing without confirmed retinal disease warrant a careful evaluation of the prechiasmal optic nerve if unilateral and the postchiasmal visual pathway if bilateral (hemianopic, quadrantic, and so forth) (Figure 4.2). False-positive results may be encountered with dense media opacities or significant vitreous floaters. Patients with poor fixation, nystagmus, or amblyopia may respond inconsistently.

In addition to assessing macular function, Amsler charts may be used to detect diseases of the optic nerve, retinal nerve fiber layer, and any retinal or choroidal anomaly falling within 10 degrees of fixation.

Indications for Amsler Grid Testing

The Amsler grid test is indicated for any patient with unexplained visual loss, even when the macula appears normal by direct examination. Amsler grid testing is also indicated in monitoring patients taking systemic medications known to affect central macular function (Table 4.1). A patient at risk from any condition causing choroidal neovascularization, including AMD, presumed ocular histoplasmosis syndrome, myopic degeneration, traumatic rupture of Bruch's membrane, or any lesion that disrupts the Bruch's membrane, photoreceptor, or RPE complex, is a candidate for Amsler grid testing, as are diabetic patients at risk for clinically significant macular edema. Other uses include postoperative evaluation of the macula, especially if cystoid macular edema is suspected, and follow-up for retinal vascular disease or any fundus condition where macular edema is possible. Additionally, a patient with macular disease should test the fellow eye regularly.

Yannuzzi Card

This version of the Amsler grid is designed to be dispensed to the patient for home use. The method of use and interpretation is identical to that of the conventional Amsler test. This version of the test is of playing card size and is laminated and has a matte finish to reduce glare. It is composed of 16×10, 0.5 mm squares with an angle subtense of 1 degree at 30 cm. The reverse side of the chart contains explicit instructions for patient use (Figure 4.3).

Some caveats and admonitions to the patients should be discussed when the card is dispensed. The patient should be reminded to put the card in a conspicuous place, such as on a mirror, where it can be used regularly, because if placed in a wallet or purse it will likely go unobserved. The patient should be given instructions on the frequency of use, and she or he should be reminded to view the card monocularly through the near correction.

Additionally, functional testing may be carried out by the patient on a regular basis using other less sophisticated means. For example, the patient with retinal disease should be instructed to evaluate the vision of each eye separately by covering one eye and checking his or her overall vision daily. The patient may also use tile in

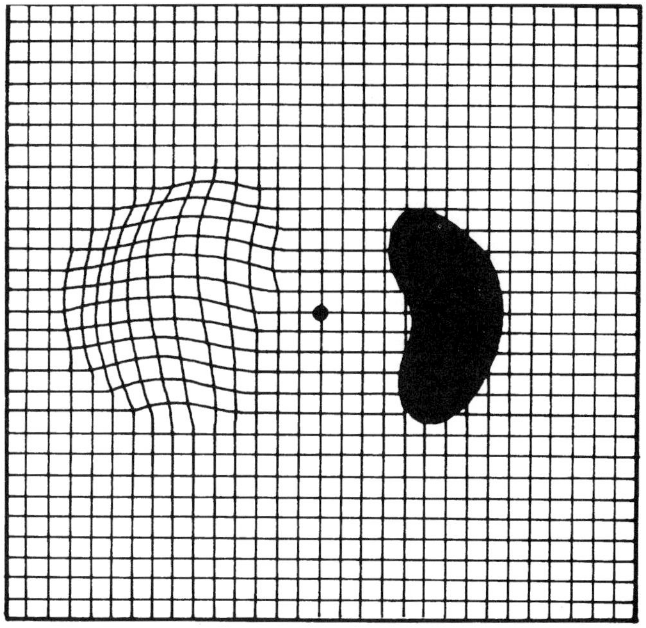

FIGURE 4.2. The test chart as it appears to a patient with dysmorphopsia (left side of fixation) and a scotoma (right side of fixation).

TABLE 4.1. Medications Allegedly Causing Amsler Grid Changes Due to Alteration in Macular Integrity

Allopurinol
Beta-blockers (topical)
Canthaxanthin
Carbonic anhydrase inhibitors (acetazolamide, methazolamide)
Chloroquine
Epinephrine and derivatives (topical)
Hexamethonium
Hydroxychloroquine
Iodine and iodide compounds (including radioactive compounds)
Nonsteroidal anti-inflammatory agents (indomethacin, naproxen)
Niacin, niacinamide
Quinine
Tamoxifen

Source: Modified from FT Fraunfelder. Drug-Induced Ocular Side Effects and Drug Interactions. Philadelphia: Lea & Febiger, 1989.

a bathroom or venetian blinds or door frames (monocular view) to detect dysmorphopsia or scotomas in the distance, and newsprint is useful for testing near function.

Threshold Amsler Grid

Since the standard Amsler grid is a suprathreshold test, a variation of it has been designed to be more sensitive. The TAG has been found to be more sensitive for detecting subtle, relative scotomas compared with the standard grid. It is probably not better, however, than the standard grid in detecting dysmorphopsia.

TAG testing makes use of polarized filters to obtain threshold and reduced contrast by creating a low level of luminance. The grid is observed against a black background, and the patient records any defects on a tear-off sheet.

Diamond Chart

This modified version of the standard Amsler grid is designed to obtain more repeatable information in patients with AMD. The chart consists of bold, black, vertical or horizontal lines similar to some Amsler grids. The background is white, and a red diamond is situated 10 cm from the central fixation dot. The function of the diamond is to promote and ensure central fixation on the dot. When correctly held at 40 cm, the diamond should fall within the patient's physiologic blind spot and therefore be invisible, thus ensuring proper fixation (Figure 4.4).

AUTOMATED PERIMETRY AND VISUAL FIELDS

The tangent screen is a useful adjunct to Amsler grid testing and permits examination of a greater extent of the central visual field. The test is considered reliable but sometimes is difficult for the patient with severe central fixation loss; if difficulty occurs, the clinician can design a more visible target.

Automated perimeters have test strategies specially designed to test the central 5 or 10 degrees of the macula. The test points for these programs are spaced at 2 degrees instead of the standard 4–6 degree separation found with 25 or 30 degree fields. The closer placement of test targets makes it more likely to detect small scotomas. The programmed test measures the threshold and presents additional targets within this central area. With projection perimeters, the stimulus size, color, and presentation time may be altered to perform customized macular tests. Test strategies available for macular function include the Interzeag M2X and the Humphrey Zeiss 10-2 (Figure 4.5).

Some field devices, for example, present 45 points within the central 4-degree area, and there are 36 additional test points between 5 and 10 degrees in the M2X macular program. There is a resolution of 0.7

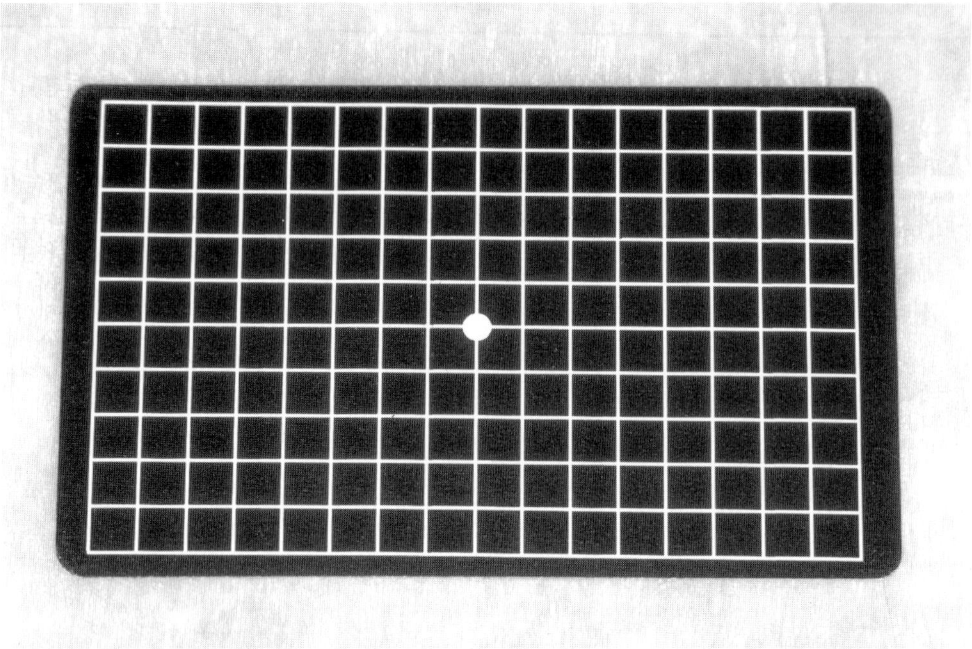

FIGURE 4.3. The Yannuzzi card for home use.

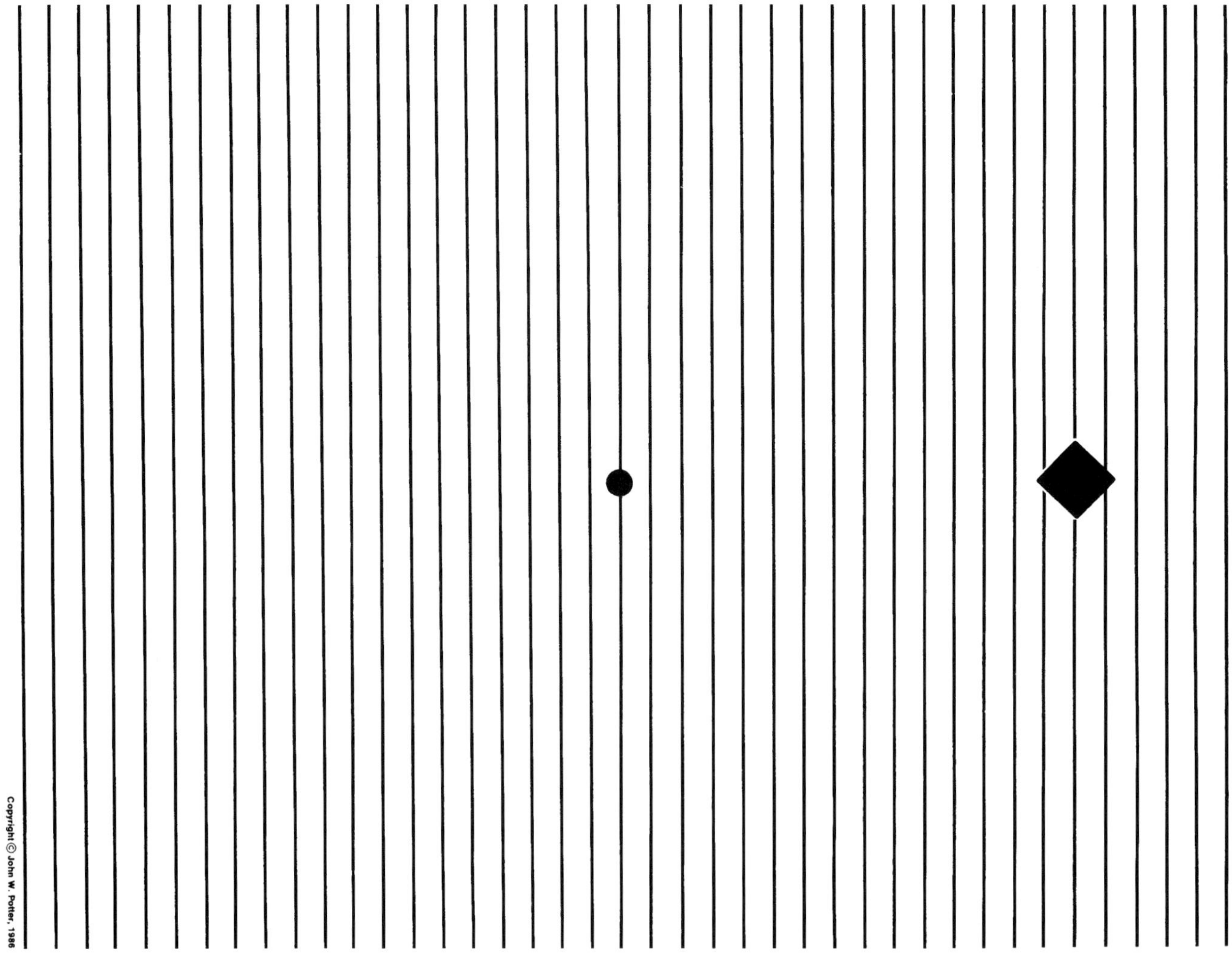

FIGURE 4.4. The vertical line diamond chart. (Reprinted with permission of John W. Potter, 1988.)

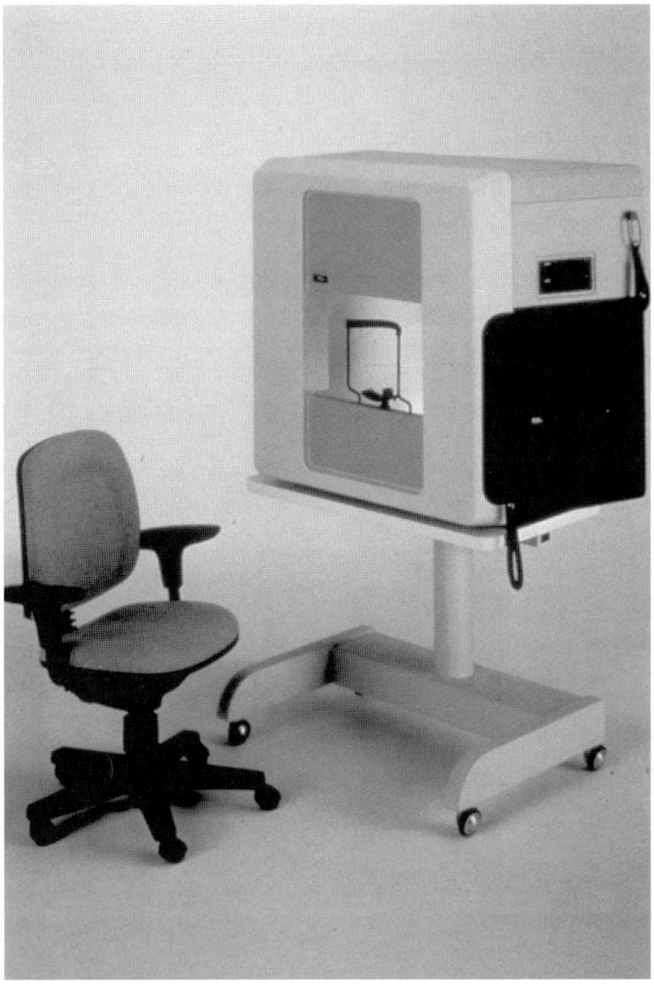

FIGURE 4.5. Humphrey Field Analyzer. (Courtesy of Humphrey Zeiss, San Leandro, CA.)

degrees in the fovea, and full thresholding is available to 1 dB accuracy.

The time and expense of automated perimetry, however, plus the patient learning curve, make this a less desirable method than the Amsler grid for evaluating macular function.

EXAMINATION OF THE UNSEEN MACULA

Media opacities may prevent a direct view of the macula in spite of pupil dilation and the use of stereoscopic fundus techniques. Cataract, vitreous hemorrhage, corneal edema, or posterior capsular haze may interfere with the examination of the macula. It is perplexing to differentiate visual loss from macular disease (and optic nerve abnormalities) from loss due to media opacities.

Methods of examination are available that will circumvent media opacities. Some unsophisticated methods include the pinhole test, the super pinhole, the swinging flashlight test, and the Blue Field Entoptoscope (Medical Instrument Research Associates, Waltham, MA). Entoptic imaging tests such as the Blue Field Entoptoscope are interesting adjuncts but are highly subjective and rely on patient observation to appreciate the entoptic phenomenon. Results from the Blue Field Entoptoscope are variable, and the test is also nonspecific.

Appreciation of the Purkinje vessel shadows and elicitation of the Haidinger's brush phenomenon and color discrimination have also been used. Electrophysiologic tests may be employed, but the results are limited and not specific to macular disease unless a focal electroretinogram is performed.

More direct and quantitative methods of measuring macular function and central acuity behind a media opacity are available. The most popular devices for this purpose include the Potential Acuity Meter (PAM; Mentor O&O, Norwell, MA) and the clinical interferometer. Potential acuity testing is useful for predicting macular acuity when contemplating cataract surgery or when a quick estimation of potential retinal acuity is necessary. These devices may be used to predict the level of visual function following cataract surgery, or they may be used to estimate macular function even if surgery is not being considered.

The PAM makes use of the principle of passing a narrow beam of light through opacified media (Figure 4.6). This narrow beam is directed around lenticular opacities and an eye chart with black optotypes is focused on the retina, adjusting the instrument for the patient's refractive error. This system makes use of Snellen's letters or numbers and is thus more familiar to the patient than other targets, for example, contrast sensitivity figures. However, the PAM is less reliable through dense cataracts, posterior subcapsular cataracts, and in the presence of macular edema.

As noted previously, the other device that provides a useful estimate of macular acuity behind media opacities is the clinical interferometer. A number of devices are currently available that direct two coherent beams of light in a three-dimensional or fringe pattern on the retina, including the Lotmar Visometer (Haag-Streit, Inc., Waldwick, NJ) (Figure 4.7). In these tests, the patient is asked to identify the orientation or direction of the patterns. The system penetrates denser media opacities compared with the PAM, and patient interpretation is independent of refractive error. Problems occur with vitreous hemorrhage or end-stage glaucoma, both of which may cause false-negative results with both the PAM and interferometers.

A patient with macular disease may not be a good candidate for surgery if macular function is reduced. Potential acuity testing is important for predicting visu-

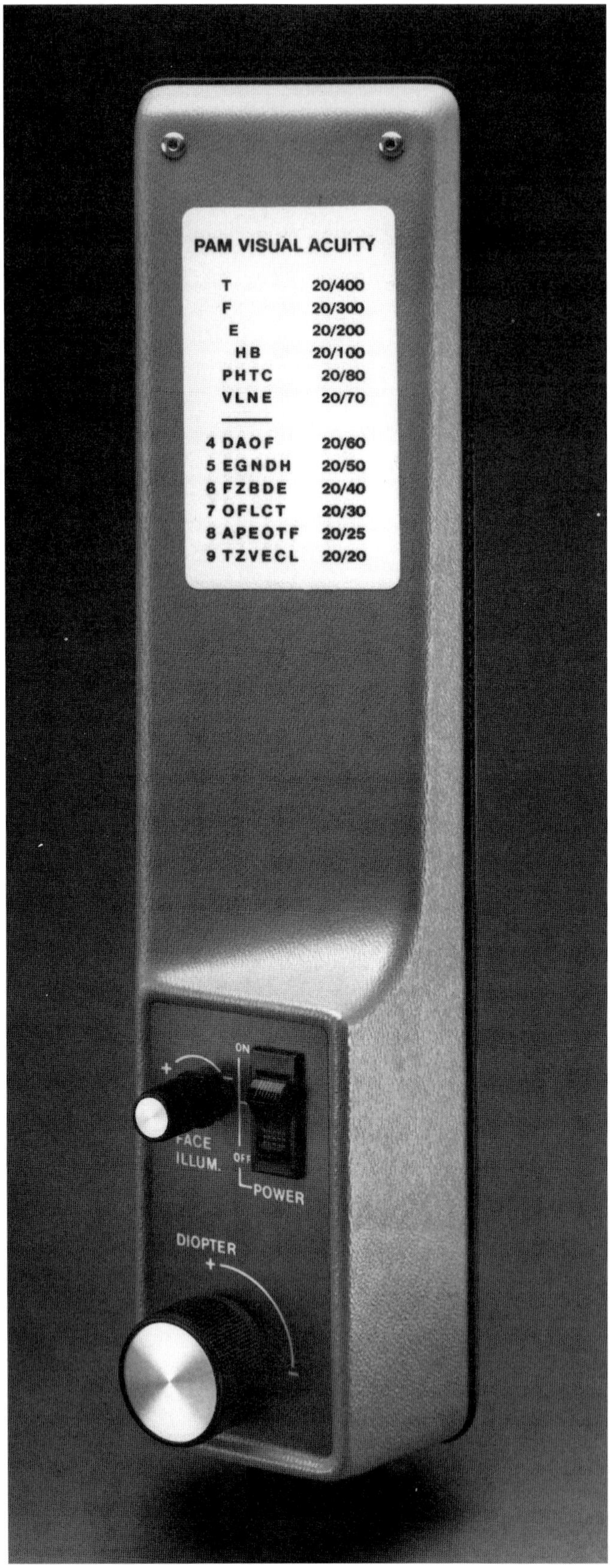

FIGURE 4.6. The Potential Acuity Meter (PAM) with Snellen acuity chart optotypes used for patient testing. (Courtesy of Mentor O&O, Norwell, MA.)

al function following cataract surgery, posterior capsulotomy, or penetrating keratoplasty.

Interpretation of Results

Potential acuity testing yields the minimal achievable level of acuity attainable with surgery. If potential acuity is 20/40 or better, or three lines better than the best vision obtainable by refraction, then it is likely that the patient's visual deficit is media-related. Dense cataracts, including cortical and posterior subcapsular opacities, will likely yield falsely poor vision. Problems also occur with advanced glaucoma and vitreous hemorrhage, where falsely poor vision is predicted.

Limitations that may affect the results of potential acuity testing include:

- Poor pupil dilation
- Dense, diffuse media
- Poor patient posture, fixation, or cooperation
- Nystagmus
- Senility
- Fatigue
- Language barrier

False-positive findings, i.e., better acuity than the patient is likely to achieve, result from macular edema from any cause, including early postoperative macular edema, exudative AMD, and serous retinal detachment. Other causes of false-positive results include:

- Cystoid macular edema
- Serous detachment of the RPE
- Geographic atrophy of the RPE
- Visual field defect through fixation
- Recently reattached retina
- Macular hole
- Amblyopia
- Corneal irregularities

Ophthalmoscopically visible posterior polar disease exonerates the media opacities as the cause for the reduced visual function. If the posterior pole can be visualized by light ophthalmoscopy or fundus biomicroscopy and there is no macular edema or corneal irregularity, the clinician should consider a foveal lesion, glaucoma, optic neuropathy, or a neurologic field defect as the cause of decreased visual acuity.

PHOTOSTRESS TEST

The photostress recovery test estimates macular function by measuring the recovery time after timed exposure to a bright light source. In performing the photostress test, an intense light is directed into one eye for 10 or more seconds while the other eye is occluded. If the photore-

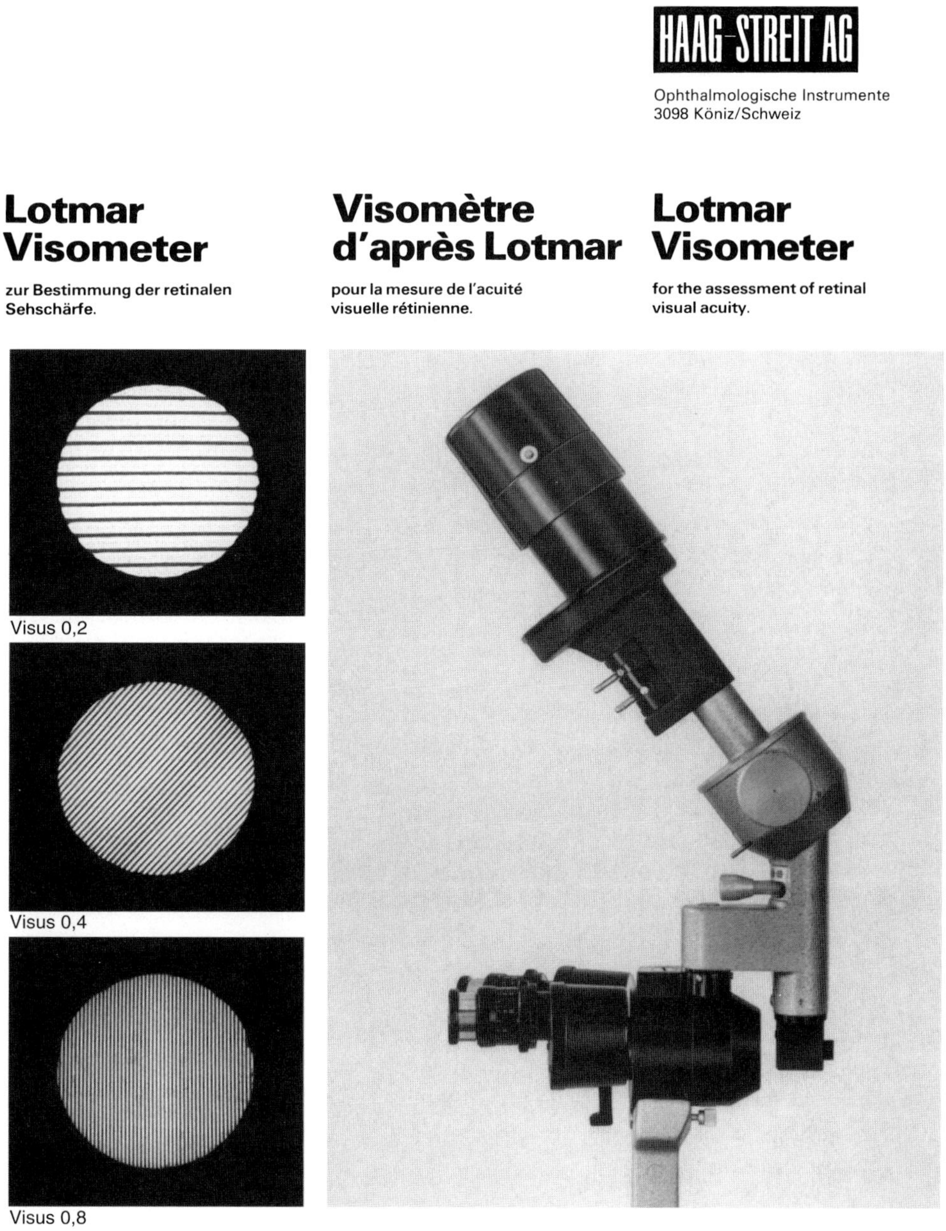

FIGURE 4.7. The Lotmar Visometer mounted on a slit lamp and examples of test patterns visualized by the patient. (Courtesy of Haag-Streit, Inc., Waldwick, NJ.)

ceptors or the adjacent supporting cell layers, namely the RPE or choriocapillaris, are compromised, visual acuity recovers more slowly in the affected eye. While various light sources may be employed, it is important to use a source that is consistent in its intensity and to establish normal recovery times for the particular procedure used. Typical light sources include a transilluminator, a strong penlight, or the light from a binocular indirect ophthalmoscope. A normal recovery time for a patient less than 40 years old viewing the line above the best corrected visual acuity is usually 40 seconds or less, although normal eyes of patients over 40 may take up to 60–70 seconds to recover. Disease should be suspected if recovery time exceeds 70 seconds in all age groups. Best corrected visual acuity less than 20/70 often decreases the validity of the photostress test.

The photostress test will not provide a definite diagnosis for macular disease but often gives an indication that subtle disease exists. It also helps to compare macular function between eyes or may be used to monitor changes in macular disease from one visit to the next. Macular edema from any cause, including diabetic macular edema or central serous retinopathy, has been reported to cause a significant delay in recovery time. A delay in recovery time also occurs in macular disease if the photoreceptors, RPE, or choroid are disrupted.

The photostress test may be used to differentiate vision loss due to macular disease from other causes, such as optic nerve disease. Recovery should only be prolonged if macular disease is present. Some reports indicate, however, that recovery times were prolonged in patients with chronic open-angle glaucoma (70.47 seconds) compared with a control group (41.97 seconds). Vision loss in bright outdoor light may suggest carotid artery occlusive disease as a cause for prolonged recovery times.

The photostress test is indicated in the following situations:

- In patients with vision loss and subtle or no clinically visible lesion
- In the differential diagnosis of optic nerve versus retinal disease
- To monitor progression or regression of vision loss
- In patients with diabetes or other conditions associated with macular edema

SUMMARY

Assessment of macular function is an important component of primary care of retinal disease. The ease of use and accessibility of Amsler charts make this the method of choice. However, additional tests may be performed when indicated and, although not specific, will provide the clinician with important information regarding the status and progression of macular disease. These tests will also help the clinician distinguish vision loss in macular disease from vision loss resulting from other causes.

SUGGESTED READING

Amsler Grid Test. In M Fingeret, L Casser, HT Woodcome (eds), Atlas of Primary Eyecare Procedures. East Norwalk, CT: Appleton & Lange, 1990;218–221.

Cavallerano AA. Potential Acuity Testing. In JB Eskridge, JF Amos, JD Bartlett (eds), Clinical Procedures in Optometry. Philadelphia: Lippincott, 1991;470–481.

Furlan AJ, Whisnant JP, Kearns TP. Unilateral visual loss in bright light. Arch Neurol 1979;36:675–676.

Glaser JS, Savino PJ, Sumers KD, et al. The photostress recovery test in the clinical assessment of visual function. Am J Ophthalmol 1977;83:255–260.

Minkowski JS, Guyton DL. New methods for predicting visual acuity after cataract surgery. Ann Ophthalmol 184;16:511–516.

Patorgis C. Amsler Charts. In JB Eskridge, JF Amos, JD Bartlett (eds), Clinical Procedures in Optometry. Philadelphia: Lippincott, 1991;436–446.

Potter JW, Wild BW. A new self-assessment test for age-related macular degeneration patients. South J Optom 1986;4:482–486.

Severin SL, Tour RL, Kershaw RH. Macular function and the photostress test 2. Arch Ophthalmol 1967;77:163–167.

Sherman MD, Henkind P. Photostress recovery in chronic open angle glaucoma. Br J Ophthalmol 1988;72:641–645.

Wall M, May DR. Threshold Amsler grid testing in maculopathies. Ophthalmology 1987;94:1126–1133.

Wiebers DO, Swanson JW, Cascino TL, Whisnant JP, et al. Bilateral loss of vision in bright light. Stroke 1989;20:554–558.

Wu G, Swanson JW, Santos S, et al. The macular photostress test in diabetic retinopathy and age-related macular degeneration. Arch Ophthalmol 1990;108:1556–1558.

Yannuzzi LA. A modified Amsler grid. A self-assessment test for patients with macular disease. Ophthalmology 1982;89:157–159.

CHAPTER

5

Electrophysiologic Testing in Macular Disease

Leonard J. Oshinskie

An electroretinogram (ERG) measures the electrical response of the retina to a light stimulus and characterizes the functional state of constituent retinal cell layers (photoreceptors versus middle retinal layers) and populations (cones versus rods). Three types of ERG include the Ganzfeld ERG, focal ERG, and pattern ERG. The Ganzfeld ERG is probably the most commonly used and is helpful in evaluating cases that involve pan-retinal disease. It is also indicated for the evaluation of some forms of macular disease. The focal ERG has been specifically developed for evaluation of macular disease. The use of the pattern ERG in general clinical practice is still evolving.

GANZFELD ELECTRORETINOGRAM

The Ganzfeld ERG measures a retina-wide mass response through the use of light stimuli against a background illumination. Varying these testing parameters to stimulate a particular class of retinal cells preferentially generates a wave form referred to as the *receptor potential.* The two major components of the Ganzfeld ERG receptor potential are the negatively deflected a-wave and the positively deflected b-wave (Figure 5.1). The photoreceptors are believed to generate the a-wave, and the middle retinal elements, especially the Müller cells, the b-wave. If an eye is dark adapted and short blue or violet flashes are used as stimuli, then the a-wave represents a rod response. In the same general sense, the a-wave in the light-adapted eye indicates a cone response.

A standard for Ganzfeld clinical electrophysiology published by Marmor et al. establishes norms for the basic technology, clinical protocol, and stimuli standards for eliciting five standard responses. These five standard responses include the rod response from dark-adapted rods, the maximal response from dark-adapted cones and rods together, oscillatory potentials measured in the dark-adapted eye, the single flash cone response in the light-adapted eye, and finally, the flicker responses in the light-adapted eye.

FOCAL ELECTRORETINOGRAM

The focal ERG (FERG) assesses macular function, separate from the remainder of the retina, by using small flickering lights with an annular surround of higher retinal illuminance as stimuli. The small target and flicker at 30–40 Hz stimulate macular cones from which the FERG arises. The intent of the bright annular surround is to bleach the rods and rod pathways so that they make a minimal contribution to the FERG response.

PATTERN ELECTRORETINOGRAM

The pattern ERG (PERG) uses checkerboard patterns or other formed patterns as stimuli. The response to this stimuli is thought to arise mainly from the inner retinal layer (ganglion cells) or middle retinal layer (glial cells), depending on the stimulus size.

INDICATIONS FOR AN ELECTRORETINOGRAM IN MACULAR DISEASE

Ganzfeld ERG testing is rarely needed for definitive diagnosis of common, acquired macular disease in adults. Since the macula makes up only a small area of the retina, disease isolated to the macula will have only minimal effect on the Ganzfeld ERG response. Even under light-adapted conditions that minimize the response from

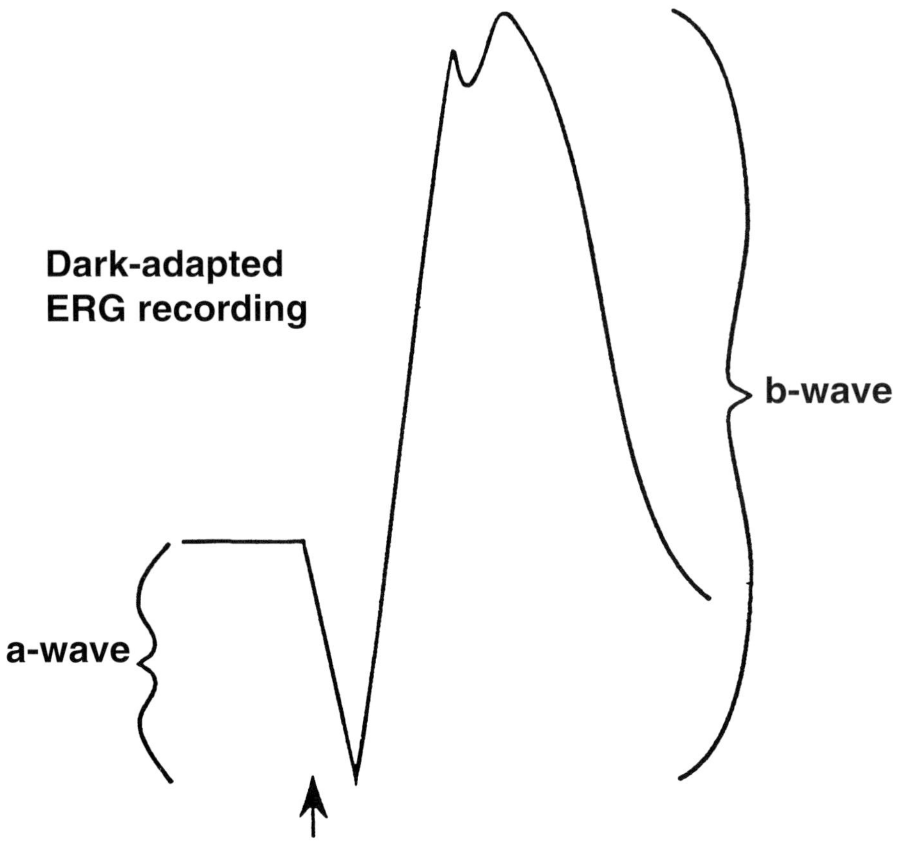

FIGURE 5.1. Examples of the two major components of the Ganzfeld electroretinogram (ERG) receptor potential: the negatively deflected a-wave and the positively deflected b-wave.

rods, the response is generated from all of the cones in the retina, not just those in the macula. Therefore, a normal light-adapted cone response using the Ganzeld ERG does not rule out maculopathy.

Diagnosis of specific retinal conditions, however, may be assisted in some patients whose macular lesions are suspected of being part of a diffuse retinal process. For example, some patients with retinitis pigmentosa, a generalized retinal degeneration, have decreased visual acuity and pigmentary changes in the macula mimicking other maculopathies, but will produce an extinguished or greatly diminished scotopic ERG.

Another useful application of ERG testing is in young patients with loss of central vision and no or little clinically evident maculopathy in order to help rule out conditions such as achromatopsia, cone dystrophies, X-linked retinoschisis, or Leber's congenital amaurosis.

Retinotoxic drugs that cause maculopathy, like chloroquine or phenothiazines at high, long-term doses, can diminish the ERG, making this diagnostic modality helpful in establishing a diagnosis of toxic retinopathy.

Used with other tests, the ERG can also help establish a diagnosis of functional (malingerer/hysterical) vision loss and help rule out retinal dysfunction as the cause of vision loss. A normal ERG result in a patient with decreased vision and no other obvious ocular abnormalities suggests a subtle optic neuropathy or a psychogenic process.

The Ganzfeld ERG has also been shown to have predictive value in determining which patients with central retinal vein occlusion will develop neovascular glaucoma and therefore require prophylactic laser photocoagulation. This method has not replaced fluorescein angiography, however, in determining the need for therapy.

Certain carriers of X-linked retinal disorders, such as X-linked cone dystrophy or retinitis pigmentosa, have been found to have abnormal ERGs. This indicates the value of ERG testing in family members of patients with these conditions.

Research employing the FERG suggests its appropriateness prior to cataract surgery to assess macular function, in predicting which patients with macular holes are likely to develop holes in the fellow eye, and in helping to establish a diagnosis in cases of unexplained vision loss in which the macula appears normal with fundus examination and fluorescein angiography. Although the FERG may be used to assess macular function prior to cataract surgery, other methods such as the potential acuity meter are more popular due to their clinical convenience. One limitation to this technique is that macular holes and cystoid macular edema can cause false-negative results.

INTERPRETATION

Most clinicians do not perform ERG in the office and must refer patients to an electrodiagnostic testing center. Since a normal ERG response varies at each testing site depending on the technique used to obtain the ERG, interpreting results without an accompanying letter of explanation from the electrodiagnostic testing center is difficult. However, being familiar with the basic patterns that certain disorders yield on the receptor potential wave form is important in understanding the ERG. The keys to diagnosis in interpreting the Ganzfeld ERG, in most cases, are (1) the amplitude of the a- and b-waves, and (2) the amplitude of the photopic compared with the scotopic ERG. Table 5.1 lists the conditions that affect these elements of the ERG.

TABLE 5.1. Electroretinogram Responses of Various Retinal Disorders

Extinguished electroretinogram
Retinitis pigmentosa
Ophthalmic artery occlusion
Unilateral retinitis pigmentosa secondary to worm infestation (diffuse unilateral subacute neuroretinitis)
Chorioretinitis
Metallosis
Retinal detachment
Drugs such as chloroquine and phenothiazines
Cancer-associated retinopathy
Reduced a- and b-wave electroretinogram
Some forms of retinitis pigmentosa and allied diseases
Congenital stationary night blindness with fundus albipunctatus or normal fundus
Phenothiazine use
Retinal detachment
Vitreous hemorrhage
Chorioretinitis
Normal a-wave and reduced b-wave electroretinogram
Congenital stationary night blindness with normal fundus, Oguchi's disease, high myopia, and nystagmus
Juvenile retinoschisis
Optic atrophy
Central retinal artery occlusion
Central retinal vein occlusion
Abnormal photopic (cone-generated) and normal scotopic (rod-generated) electroretinogram
Rod monochromatism
Progressive cone dystrophy

Source: Adapted from RE Carr, IM Siegel. Electrodiagnostic Testing of the Visual System: A Clinical Guide. Philadelphia: Davis, 1990.

ELECTROOCULOGRAPHY

Electrooculography (EOG) measures the difference in electrical potential between the cornea and retina during saccadic eye movements, first under conditions of dark adaptation and then with the patient light adapted. This potential depends principally on the integrity of the retinal pigment epithelium, with some contribution from the outer and middle retinal layers as well. The amplitude of the EOG is minimal in the dark and greatest with light stimulation. The amplitude of the light peak is divided by the amplitude of the dark peak to obtain a percentage known as the *Arden ratio*. A normal value is about 200%, with variations depending on sex and age.

Since general retinal degenerations cause a reduced EOG as well as a reduced ERG, ordering an EOG following an ERG usually does not provide additional information. Many retinal conditions have been reported to cause an abnormal EOG depending on the stage of development. However, an EOG is clinically indicated to assist diagnosis in cases of atypical Best's vitelliform macular dystrophy. In such cases, the ERG is normal and the EOG is greatly diminished. Butterfly dystrophy also causes an abnormal EOG and normal ERG. The EOG may have application in the diagnosis of other macular conditions such as cone dystrophy in which the EOG is usually normal and the ERG response from cones (photopic) is abnormal.

VISUAL-EVOKED POTENTIALS

The visual-evoked potential (VEP) measures the cortical response to light stimulation of the retina. The stimulus is usually a pattern such as a reversing checkerboard or a series of sine waves. The delayed latency of the VEP is used to help differentiate vision loss due to optic nerve disease versus other causes such as suspected macular disease. The amplitude of the pattern VEP response is more likely to be affected by macular disease than the flash VEP; however, its usefulness in evaluation of macular disease is limited because a condition anywhere along the visual system can influence the VEP response. If the macula is obviously diseased on clinical examination, the VEP provides little additional information.

Various electrical tests used in the diagnosis of visual loss are summarized in Table 5.2.

TABLE 5.2. Use of the Various Electrodiagnostic Tests in the Diagnosis of Visual Loss

	Standard ERG	*Focal ERG*	*Pattern ERG*	*Electrooculography light rise*	*Visual-evoked potential*
Macular disease	Normal	Abnormal	Reduced	Normal[a]	Abnormal[b]
Optic nerve disease	Normal	Normal	May be abnormal	Normal	Abnormal[b]
Higher center disease	Normal	Normal	Normal	Normal	Abnormal[b]
Hysteria or malingering	Normal	Normal	Normal	Normal	Normal
Generalized tapetoretinal degeneration	Abnormal	Variable	Variable	Abnormal	Abnormal[b]

[a]In vitelliform dystrophy of the macula (Best's disease) and butterfly dystrophy of the macula, this test is usually abnormal.
[b]Abnormality may be either a reduction in amplitude (as in early macular disease) or an increase in latency (as in some forms of optic nerve disease).
ERG = electroretinogram.
Source: Reprinted with permission from RE Carr, IM Siegel. Electrodiagnostic Testing of the Visual System: A Clinical Guide. Philadelphia: FA Davis, 1990.

SUGGESTED READING

Billson V, Billson FA. Macular electroretinograms and contrast sensitivity as sensitive detectors of early maculopathy. Doc Ophthalmol 1986;63:399–406.

Carr RE, Siegel IM. Electrodiagnostic Testing of the Visual System: A Clinical Guide. Philadelphia: FA Davis, 1990.

Fish GE, Birch DG. The focal electroretinogram in clinical assessment of macular disease. Ophthalmology 1989;96:109–114.

Heckenlively JR, Arden GB. Principles and Practice of Clinical Electrophysiology of Vision. St. Louis: Mosby, 1991.

Marmor MF, Arden GB, Nilsson SE, Zrenner E. Standard for clinical electroretinography. Arch Ophthalmol 1989;107:816–819.

Matthews GP, Sandberg MA, Berson EL. Foveal cone electroretinograms in patients with central visual loss of unexplained etiology. Arch Ophthalmol 1992;110:1568–1570.

Satabes R, Hirose T, McMeel JW. Electroretinography in the prognosis and classification of central retinal vein occlusion. Arch Ophthalmol 1983;101:232–235.

Weleber RG, Eisner A. Retinal Function and Physiological Studies. In DA Newsome (ed), Retinal Dystrophies and Degenerations. New York: Raven, 1988;21–69.

CHAPTER

6

Fundus Fluorescein Angiography

Michael T. Porter, Anthony A. Cavallerano, and Rodney K. Gutner

Fundus fluorescein angiography (FA) is an invasive clinical technique in which the intravenous injection of a fluorescent dye is immediately followed by serial fundus photography. This procedure is used to document retinal blood flow dynamics and to evaluate the integrity of the blood-retinal barriers. It is a valuable adjunct to stereoscopic fundus biomicroscopy and binocular indirect ophthalmoscopy and serves as a guide to laser photocoagulation surgery.

FA is an important tool used in the diagnosis and management of retinal diseases in general and specifically of macular disease. FA detects abnormalities of blood flow to the optic nerve, choroid, and retina. Abnormal fundus fluorescence results any time a lesion alters the retinal and choroidal architecture or renders the retinal or choroidal vasculature incompetent. FA clearly demonstrates the pathophysiology of retinal and choroidal vascular disease. Prior to the advent of this procedure, the histology of macular edema, retinal pigment epithelium (RPE) detachment, and choroidal neovascularization (CNV) could only be gauged by speculation.

Exudative macular degeneration, macular involvement with diabetic retinopathy, and vascular occlusive disease are three classes of disorders that warrant fluorescein studies to determine suitability for laser treatment. Fluorescein studies are also useful when contemplating laser surgery in patients with macular edema or CNV.

INDICATIONS FOR FLUORESCEIN ANGIOGRAPHY

Given its invasive nature, FA should be performed judiciously. The majority of retinal diseases can be managed successfully without the use of FA, and there is little justification for baseline angiograms in ophthalmic practice. Age-related macular degeneration (AMD) with modest visual acuity changes, little or no dysmorphopsia, and a macula devoid of CNV or exudation may not require fluorescein studies. Diabetic retinopathy with good visual acuity and without evidence of macular thickening or suspected neovascularization also would not require FA.

The four main categories of retinal and choroidal disease in which FA is most frequently indicated include macular disease, retinal vascular disease, optic nerve disease, and ocular tumors (Table 6.1). Within these main categories, AMD followed by diabetic retinopathy are the two most common indications for requesting FA. The angiogram can reveal retinal and choroidal changes not apparent by ophthalmoscopy alone. Fluorescein studies are strongly indicated in symptomatic patients with suspected CNV. Numerous dystrophic, degenerative, and inflammatory retinal diseases can compromise the Bruch's membrane–choriocapillaris complex, giving rise to choroidal neovascular membranes (CNVM). The most common conditions causing CNVM are AMD, presumed ocular histoplasmosis syndrome, degenerative myopia, angioid streaks, and choroidal tumors.

Diabetic persons with reduced visual acuity secondary to macular thickening are strong candidates for FA. If serious nonproliferative or preproliferative changes are evident, or if areas of ischemia are suspected, capillary nonperfusion is easily documented with FA. Capillary nonperfusion refers to either or both arterioles and venules that have reduced or restricted blood flow, usually resulting in retinal hypoxia and ischemia. FA is useful in the consideration and application of laser surgery in the treatment of macular edema and proliferative diabetic retinopathy.

TABLE 6.1. Indications for Fundus Fluorescein Angiography

Maculopathy in patients requiring laser photocoagulation
Suspected choroidal neovascularization from any cause (age-related macular degeneration, angioid streaks, presumed ocular histoplasmosis syndrome, myopic degeneration, etc.)
Idiopathic central serous choroidopathy
Cystoid macular edema
Retinal pigment epithelium detachment
Preretinal gliosis
Hereditary maculopathy
Circinate maculopathy
Retinal vascular disease
Diabetes—clinically significant macular edema; suspected capillary nonperfusion and retinal ischemia
Venous occlusive disease with macular edema or suspected retinal ischemia
Hypertensive retinopathy
Optic disc
Papilledema
Ischemic optic neuropathy
Drusen
Ocular tumors
Malignant melanoma
Metastases
Unexplained vision loss

PHYSICAL AND CHEMICAL PROPERTIES

Sodium fluorescein ($C_2OH_{10}O_5Na$), a vegetable dye, is an orange-red hydrocarbon powder. The primary component of the dye is resorcinol, a plant resin in the carrot family. In its clinical form, the solution takes on a characteristic yellow-red color and is available in vials of 5%, 10%, and 25% concentrations. The unique chemical and biophysical properties of fluorescein make it ideal for angiography. Fluorescein is considered pharmacologically inert, and eosin, erythrosin, and rose bengal dyes are derivatives of the basic chemical.

The low molecular weight of sodium fluorescein (376.27) allows it to diffuse out of capillaries, except those in the central nervous system including the retina. As a result, fluorescein permeates throughout extravascular spaces of the body, staining skin and mucous membranes within 60 seconds of injection. Consequently, many patients have a yellowish cutaneous discoloration that may persist for several hours after the injection of fluorescein. The dye is eliminated within 24–36 hours through metabolism within the liver and via the kidneys by glomerular filtration; the urine has a yellow-red discoloration during this period.

Following intravenous injection, sodium fluorescein binds to plasma proteins, mainly albumin. Estimates of the amount of bound fluorescein vary from 40–80%. This conjugation of sodium fluorescein and albumin may result in up to a 50% reduction of fluorescence. Fluorescein reportedly also binds to red blood cells. The decreased absorption and emission due to adjacent hemoglobin molecules also reduce the amount of fluorescence observed during angiography. This is in contrast to indocyanine green, an iodine derivative, which has binding capabilities of 95–98%.

The phenomenon of fluorescence is the ability of a compound to absorb light energy at one wavelength and subsequently re-emit light energy at a lower energy, higher wavelength. With the absorption of incident light, free electrons within the molecule are propelled to a higher or excited state called the *excitation phase.* These same electrons spontaneously (1^{-10} seconds) return to their initial energy level, emitting light in the visible spectrum (emission phase). When blue light (465–490 nm) is made incident upon sodium fluorescein in the blood, it fluoresces and emits yellow-green light (520–530 nm).

INSTRUMENTATION

Conventional Imaging Systems

High-quality angiograms are critical for accurate diagnosis and proper management of retinal disease, and therefore, a certified retinal angiographer or highly skilled ophthalmic photographer is essential. A fundus camera must be equipped with a fast recycling, high-intensity flash system, a motorized drive, and the appropriate excitation and barrier filters. In general, the filters are designed to transmit only desired frequencies of light and absorb or block all undesired wavelengths. The exciter (cobalt blue) filter transmits only blue light from the white flash of the camera to excite the fluorescein molecules in the retinal blood vessels. The barrier (yellow) filter permits only the fluorescent light re-emitted from the retina to expose the film. A high-speed black and white film, ISO 400, is ideal for high-quality negatives. Although color photographs can now be obtained during FA, most clinicians prefer high-contrast black and white film.

To ensure consistency in interpretation, photographs should be taken and read in a predetermined sequence. Convention calls for the patient's name, medical record or identification number, and date to be prominently displayed in the upper right-hand corner of the angiogram. The preinjection red-free photographs are the next in the sequence, reading from right to left, followed by the postinjection photographs. The transit, or

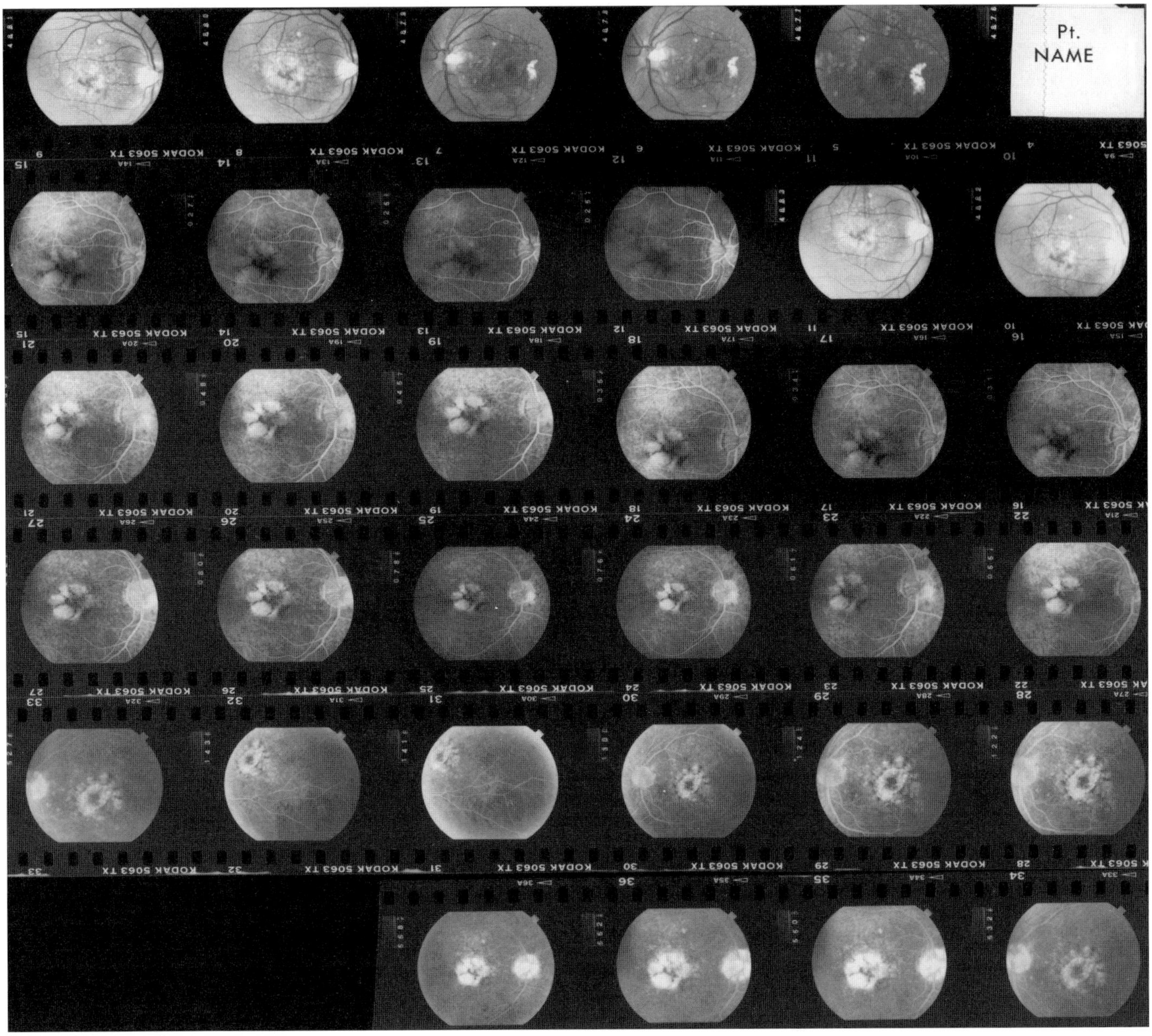

FIGURE 6.1. Fluorescein angiogram of a patient with cystic maculopathy. Patient's name in upper right-hand corner of the print is followed by red-free photographs and entire fluorescein transit. Late photos make up the last row of the angiogram.

sequence of photographs from the first to the last exposure, is followed through all of the phases of the angiograms, continuing to read from right to left on subsequent rows (Figure 6.1).

Negatives may be read directly or processed into positive transparencies or prints. The negatives offer superior resolution; however, the positive transparencies are most commonly read. Historically, a pair of +10.00 diopter (D) lenses were used to provide increased detail and stereopsis if available. Today, a +20 D indirect fundus lens or stereo viewer is commonly used.

Videodigital Imaging Systems

The introduction of state-of-the-art digital and video technology to FA has provided real-time imaging of retinal circulation. The development of this technology has the potential to influence the future of FA. A videodigital fluorescein system employs standard angiographic equipment, with the addition of a video camera, cassette recorder, central processing unit, digitizer, and video monitor. Enhanced resolution (1,280 × 1,024 lines) and improved monitors provide a sharp, clear image. An optical laser disk stores multiple images, and the system can be networked for transmission of images via telephone lines to other locations. An optional printer is used to produce page-size prints or transparencies from the digital source.

The advantages of videodigital angiography over serial photography are numerous. For the clinician, videodigital angiography provides a continuous visual display of the chorioretinal filling patterns and the evolution of normal and abnormal fluorescence. With pictures recorded at up to 30 frames per second, the use of stop frame and playback on the videocassette recorder offers enhanced analysis capabilities. The camera has zoom capabilities that allow for image magnification, and sharpening filters and contrast enhancement improve the image quality.

With digital systems, the angiographic results are available immediately and may be reviewed with the patient. Same-day emergency angiography and treatment is facilitated in cases of acute macular disease. The patients may also experience improved comfort as a result of the decreased illumination levels required by the video camera, absence of the flash, and a decreased dosage of sodium fluorescein (1 ml of 10% solution). The digital system is also a requisite for indocyanine green angiography (ICG), a format that is used to detect occult CNVM. The digitizer enables the system to quantify retinal blood flow parameters, measure areas of disease, and provide relief maps and area and line measurements. The digital imaging system also permits evaluation and analysis of the optic nerve head and is used for monitoring the status of the optic nerve and nerve fiber layer in glaucoma. The following list summarizes the features of digital imaging:

- Instant angiography
- Image enhancement
- Image manipulation
- Permanent storage on optical disks
- Superimposition of images providing immediate comparison
- Transmission of data over phone lines

The major disadvantages of video fluorescein angiography are the initial cost of the equipment and absence of direct stereo observation of the fundus. A lower degree of spatial resolution is also obtained with serial angiography. However, video systems are now available that enhance the image and superimpose multiple images, an advantage when comparing pretreatment and posttreatment lesions. Table 6.2 summarizes the advantages and disadvantages of videodigital fluorescein.

Currently, two systems are commercially available for digital angiography. The Topcon Corporation markets the IMAGEnet (Topcon, Paramus, NJ), and Ophthalmic Image Systems (OIS; WinStation 1024 Imaging Software, Ophthalmic Imaging Systems, Inc., Sacramento, CA) produces a digital imaging system. Both units are compatible with and adaptable to most types of fundus cameras.

TABLE 6.2. Advantages and Disadvantages of Videodigital Fluorescein Angiography

Advantages	*Disadvantages*
Increased patient comfort	Cost
Decreased illumination	Decreased spatial resolution
No flash	
Patient/doctor evaluation	
Lower dose of fluorescein	
Immediate real-time viewing	
Stop-frame review	
Quantitative evaluation of blood flow	

Confocal Laser Imaging Systems

There are two imaging systems that provide a high-quality digital image of the retina, optic nerve, and macula that do not require intravenous injection of fluorescein dye: the Scanning Laser Ophthalmoscope (SLO), manufactured by Rodenstock (Danbury, CT), and the Heidelberg Retinal Tomograph (HRT; Carlsbad, CA), distributed by Interzeag (Figure 6.2). Indications for use include examination of the macula, optic nerve head analysis, ocular tumor evaluation, and evaluation of retinal detachment. Both devices provide a high-quality, digitized image of the macula that can be stored on an optical laser disk. The image can be manipulated and used to compare the progression of lesions or to determine the success of treatment.

The HRT is a confocal laser scanning system adopted for fundus examination. A diode laser, with a wavelength of 670 nm, is used as a light source in conjunction with a scanning camera microscope. The HRT provides the clinician with a three-dimensional topographic view of the retinal surface. Because of the nature of the light source, pupillary dilation is not required. The camera focuses a scanning laser beam on the retina or optic nerve structure, and the resultant image is analyzed along the x-, y-, and z-axes. Immediate image formation provides a convenient method for instant appreciation and diagnosis. Clinical information can be stored on a computer disk, and there is no need for film processing or developing.

Stereometric imaging provides information regarding the integrity of the macula. The topography is color coded and a cross section of the image can be provided at any identifiable point.

Indocyanine Green Angiography

Fluorescein is an excellent dye for evaluating the retinal circulation. However, it is not as helpful in evaluating the choroidal circulation, an important requirement in identifying certain types of CNVM.

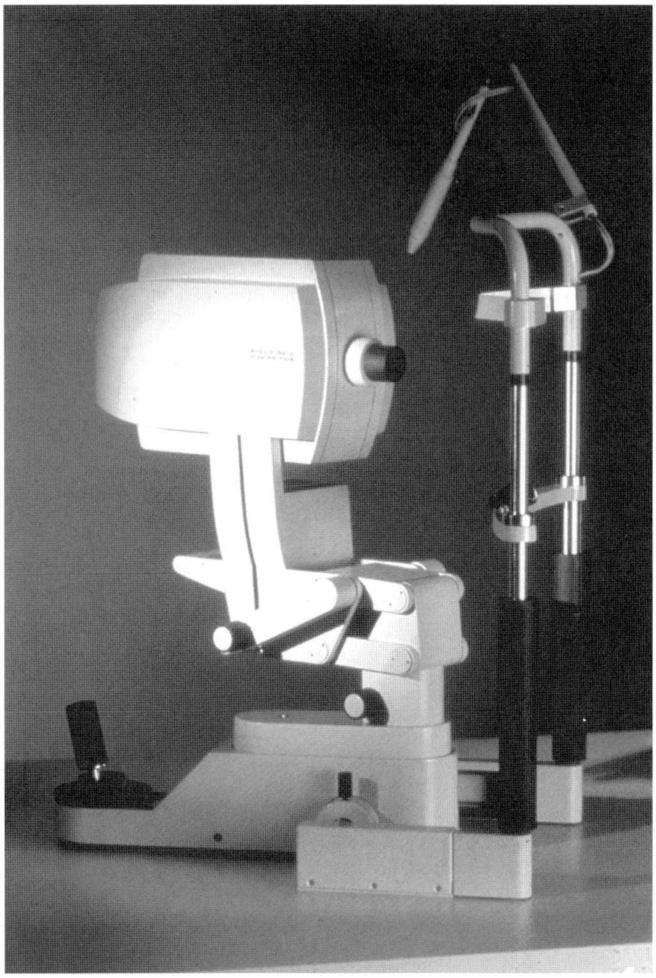

FIGURE 6.2. The Heidelberg Retinal Tomograph, a confocal laser device used to image the optic disc and macula. (Courtesy of Heidelberg Engineering, Carlsbad, CA.)

Choroidal fluorescence is diminished by media opacities, fundus pigmentation, hemorrhage, and exudate in abnormal retinal states, and rapid leakage from fenestrated choroidal capillaries. To effectively treat CNVM, there is a need for better identification and lineament of the membrane. ICG improves imaging capabilities of occult or ill-defined neovascular lesions, especially those located below a pigment epithelial detachment. Due to the highly recurrent nature of CNVM (50–60% recur), ICG is also useful in evaluating recurrent membranes after laser treatment.

ICG is a tricarbocyanine dye with a peak absorption at 805 nm and a fluorescence at 835 nm, and in the infrared range, penetration is not limited by ocular pigments such as melanin and xanthophyll. In fact, the choroid and RPE absorb almost 80% of light at 500 nm (blue-green); in the infrared range (800 nm), only half that amount is absorbed, thereby allowing for better penetration to the choroidal circulation.

ICG was originally approved for use in cardiac, hepatic, and ophthalmic investigative studies. One to 2 mg of ICG per kilogram of body weight is injected in solution form. The dye is relatively safe but should be avoided in patients who are allergic to shellfish or iodine. The dye has greater penetrance through blood, xanthophyll, and melanin. ICG also demonstrates decreased leakage from the choriocapillaris and therefore is not ideal for identification of well-defined CNVM. Although ICG has a fluorescence efficiency 1/25th that of fluorescein, the dye has greater protein-binding capabilities (98% compared with 40–80% for fluorescein). Since the dye is highly protein bound it does not leak from fenestrated choroidal capillaries. This characteristic allows ICG to sometimes convert occult or recurrent CNV to classic membranes, a phenomenon evident only in the late phase (30 minutes) of the angiogram. These properties make ICG ideal for the identification of occult, ill-defined, or oozing CNVMs. ICG is also useful for identifying membranes that recur at the borders of previously treated lesions.

It is estimated that 50% of CNVMs are undetected with conventional FA techniques. When used in conjunction with digital angiographic systems, ICG provides improved visualization of occult CNVM. Blood, turbid fluid, melanin, and xanthophyll may block the details of membranes with conventional FA. ICG leaks more slowly from new choroidal vessels, and in fact is apparent on the angiogram only in the late phase of the transit. This permits better visualization, since with fluorescein the flow of the dye is so rapid that the CNV may go undetected.

Since ICG fluoresces at a longer wavelength than fluorescein, an infrared light source is used to image the fundus. Transmission of the infrared wavelengths is enhanced by optical coatings on the lens elements of the fundus camera. Additionally, the diode laser, with a higher wavelength, can be used to treat CNV when used in conjunction with ICG, since ICG will absorb the higher wavelength energy. Although limited by power output, this laser allows for better penetration through blood and turbid fluid. The imaging capabilities of ICG and the use of the diode laser have exciting potential in the identification and treatment of occult or poorly defined macular lesions. However, ICG is not a substitute for FA and will not replace or supplant the conventional procedure with its high degree of resolution in studying the retinal vasculature. Rather, ICG offers the clinician an additional perspective when evaluating the choroidal circulation, especially in cases of suspected occult or recurrent CNVM.

TECHNIQUE

A summary of the technique and possible side effects of intravenous fluorescein should be reviewed with the patient prior to the procedure. Serious side effects are rare (Table 6.3), but a signed consent form is standard practice today. A complete medical profile should be obtained on each patient and should include a statement of the patient's general health and history of any allergies, adverse reactions to previous fluorescein injections, and evidence of pregnancy.

Prior to injecting fluorescein, the pupil is maximally dilated using the appropriate topical ophthalmic pharmaceutical agents. Color fundus photographs should be taken prior to performing the procedure, and baseline black and white red-free control photographs should be taken to eliminate confusion arising from autofluorescence, pseudofluorescence, and artifact. Autofluorescence is the emission of fluorescence and may be observed with optic nerve head drusen and astrocytic hamartoma in the absence of sodium fluorescein. Pseudofluorescence is a consequence of inappropriate barrier and exciter filter combinations, allowing blue light to expose the film prior to injection.

TABLE 6.3. Classification of Adverse Side Effects of Fluorescein Injection and Appropriate Management

Category	*Appropriate treatment*
Mild	
Nausea, vomiting	Time, reassurance, emesis basin
Extravasation of dye	Cold packs
Moderate	
Vasovagal response, syncope	Time, reassurance, smelling salts
Urticaria	Systemic antihistamine
Severe	
General	Vital signs, clear airway, cardiopulmonary resuscitation
Respiratory	Oxygen, pressor agents
Bronchospasm	Systemic steroids, antihistamine, epinephrine, aminophylline
Anaphylaxis	
Laryngeal edema	
Cardiac	Cardiopulmonary resuscitation
Cardiac arrest	
Myocardial infarction	
Shock	

INTERPRETATION OF THE FLUORESCEIN ANGIOGRAM

Anatomic and Histologic Considerations

A thorough understanding of retinal and choroidal anatomy, histology, and tissue response is a prerequisite to accurate interpretation of FA. The optic nerve and the choroidal vasculature are both supplied by the posterior ciliary arterial system. The choroidal network nourishes the macula, outer retinal layers, and the RPE.

FA provides spatial and temporal resolution of the retinal circulation. The RPE provides an excellent background for high-contrast imaging of the retinal capillaries. Once injected, fluorescein travels to the eye via the ophthalmic artery, which supplies the choroid through the posterior ciliary arteries and the retinal arterioles via the central retinal artery. The larger choroidal vessels and retinal vessels are impermeable to fluorescein. The retinal vessels serve as the inner blood-retinal barrier, whereas the RPE serves as the outer blood-retinal barrier. The choriocapillaris exhibits a fenestrated endothelium that is similar to capillary networks found outside of the central nervous system. These fenestrated blood vessels allow the exchange of large molecular weight compounds such as proteins and fluorescein (Figure 6.3). As the injected fluorescein permeates throughout the extravascular spaces of the choroid, it will funduscopically demonstrate a characteristic "ground-glass" appearance that becomes more diffuse as it radiates toward the ora serrata. In the young, healthy retina, the choroidal flush is obscured in the macular region due to the increased concentration of the RPE, choroidal melanocytes, and the presence of xanthophyll pigment. The extravascular fluorescein will eventually stain Bruch's membrane, the sclera, and the optic nerve, leaving a mild residual glow in the late phase of the angiogram (Figure 6.4).

The RPE is a monocellular layer of pigmented cells cemented together by tight junctions resulting in the outer blood-retinal barrier. Fluorescein is impermeable to the RPE in the young, healthy retina. However, RPE possesses the ability to migrate, proliferate, atrophy, and detach from either or both its adjacent Bruch's membrane and sensory retina. These changes can result in a compromise in the blood-retinal barrier and subsequent leakage of fluorescein into the neurosensory retina.

The retinal vasculature nourishes the inner sensory layers of the retina and, in contrast to the choriocapillaris, is nonfenestrated. The tight junctions within the nonfenestrated endothelial cells of the arterioles and venules provide the inner blood-retinal barrier that excludes extravascular fluid, including fluorescein, in a healthy eye. A defect in this barrier, for example, as found in retinal vascular disease, will result in extravascular fluorescein. Hyperpermeable, ischemic, and proliferative retinal vessels can be identified easily by FA.

The foveal avascular zone measures approximately 400–500 μ in diameter and is by definition devoid of any retinal vessels. This area of the retina is hypofluorescent compared with the surrounding retina due to the densely packed and more pigmented RPE and due to the accumulation of xanthophyll in the macular area.

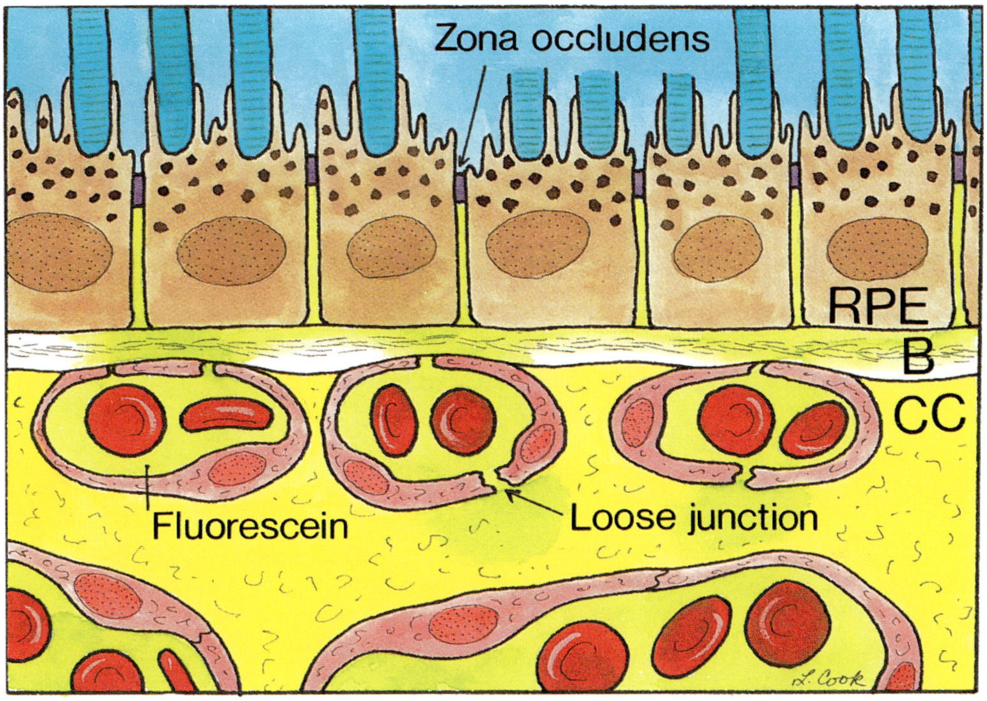

FIGURE 6.3. The retinal pigment epithelium (RPE), Bruch's membrane (B), choriocapillaris (CC) complex. The tight junctions of the retinal pigment epithelium (zona occludens) serve as the outer blood-retinal barrier, and the loose junctions of the choriocapillaris allow leakage of fluorescein dye into the extravascular space of the choroid. The larger choroidal vessels are nonfenestrated and do not leak fluorescein.

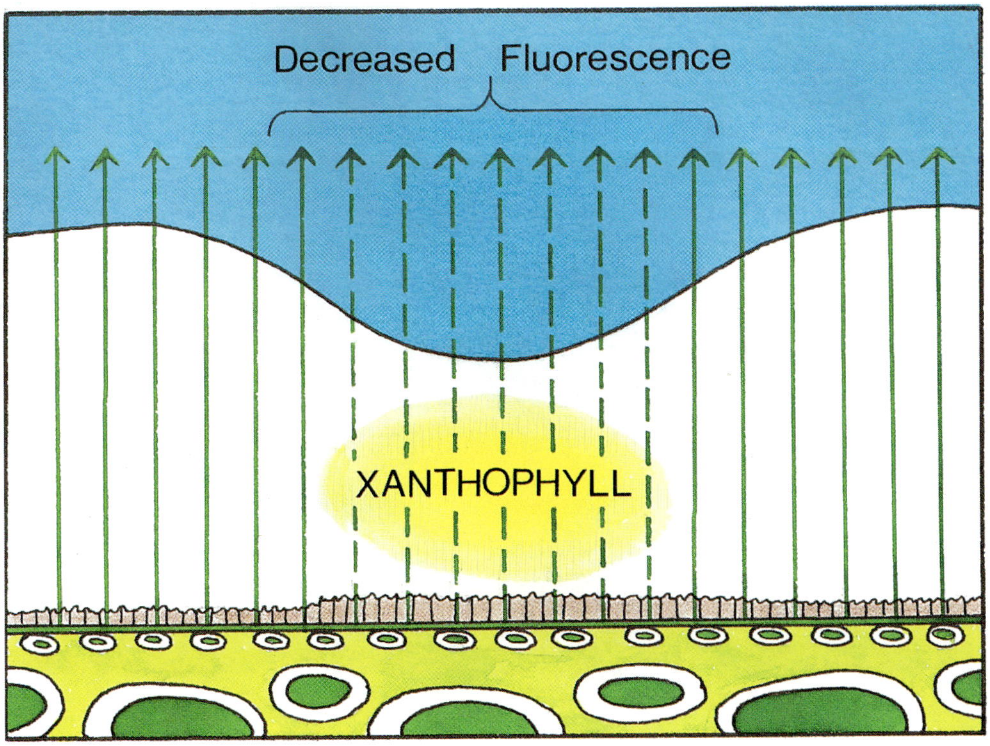

FIGURE 6.4. Fluorescein is evident in the extravascular space of the choroid. The increased concentration of xanthophyll and dense, columnar arrangement of the retinal pigment epithelial cells in the macula result in decreased fluorescence in this area compared with the surrounding retina.

Filling Patterns

Normal retinal blood velocity follows a parabolic curve in that the velocity of blood flow at the vessel wall is zero and increases exponentially toward the lumen center. This difference in blood velocity within the vessel creates discrete streaks or lamina that can be observed during FA. Although laminar flow is present in both retinal arteries and veins, only rarely can it be captured photographically in the retinal arteries because arterial filling occurs too fast (1–2 seconds). Laminar flow is first observed along the walls of retinal veins because the blood velocity is much slower in the veins. The fluorescein is initially directed toward the vessel endothelium or

TABLE 6.4. Summary of Normal Fluorescein Filling Phases

Phase	*Approximate time of appearance after injection*	*Characteristics*
Prearterial phase	8–12 seconds	Patchy choroidal glow
Choroidal phase		Macula void of fluorescence
		Cilioretinal artery filling
Arterial phase	10–13 seconds	Central retinal artery begins to fill; subsequent display of all retinal arterioles
Retinal filling		Arm to retina time calculated
Arteriovenous phase	12–15 seconds	Retinal venules and veins begin to fill
		Laminar flow in veins
		Definition to capillaries
Venous phase	13–17 seconds	Venous filling is now complete
Late arteriovenous phase		Intensity fades in choroid and arterioles
Late phase	10 minutes	Fluorescein not evident in choroidal or retinal vasculature
Recirculation phase	60 minutes	
Oral		Mild residual staining of choroid, sclera, and optic nerve

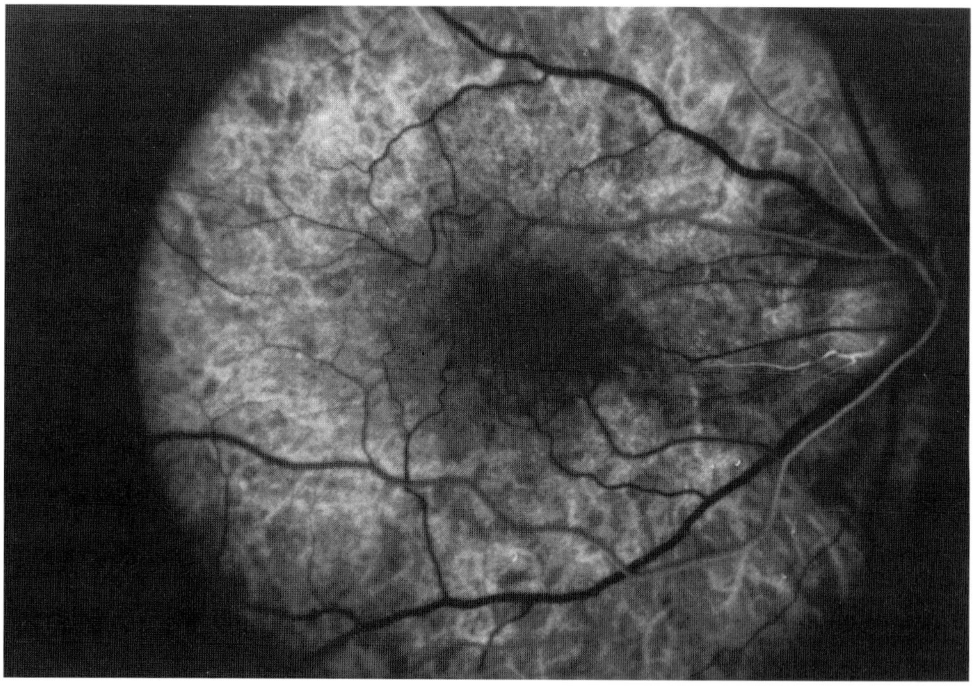

FIGURE 6.5. The choroidal flush phase of the angiogram of a right eye depicting the patchy glow of choroidal fluorescence and the "ground-glass" appearance. (Courtesy of J. Coppinger.)

wall as a result of the extensive capillary network emptying individually into the venous circulation.

The normal FA has a characteristic flow pattern (Table 6.4). The *prearterial* or *choroidal flush phase* marks the first appearance of fluorescein in the fundus (Figure 6.5). The filling of the larger choroidal vessels exhibits a patchy glow that becomes more diffuse with extravascular leakage. Cilioretinal arteries and the fine capillary network of the optic nerve will also fluoresce during this phase since they are fed by the posterior ciliary arteries (Figure 6.6). Diseases of the choroidal vasculature, RPE, and macula can be evaluated during this phase.

The *retinal arterial phase* occurs 1–2 seconds after the choroidal flush and is characterized by the filling of the central retinal artery and its superior and inferior branches, which appear white in contrast to the black venules (Figure 6.7). The arm-retina time (ART) is cal-

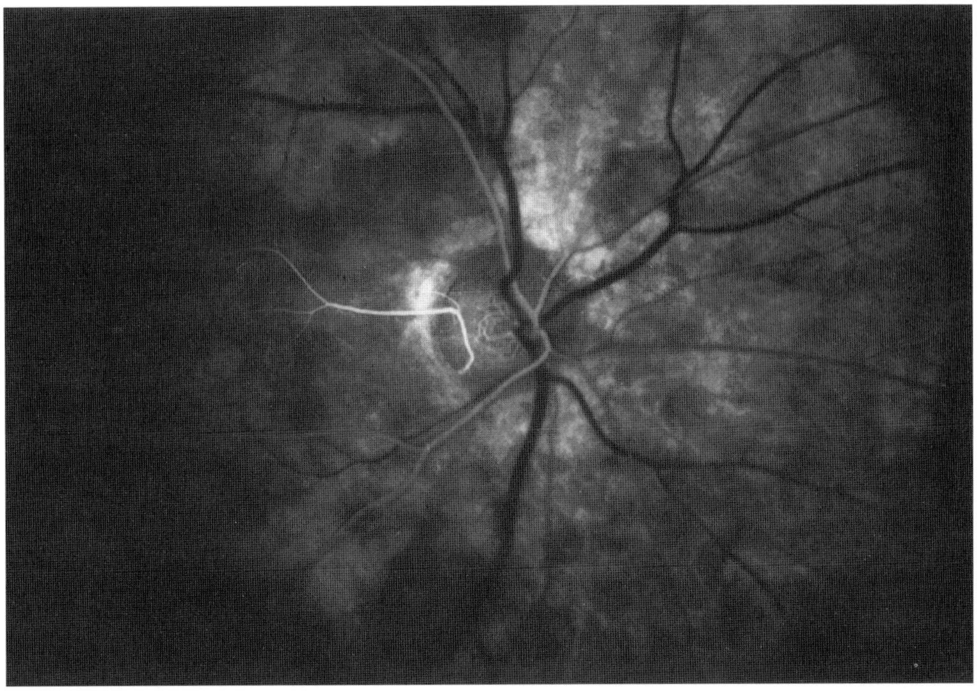

FIGURE 6.6. Choroidal flush with the fluorescent cilioretinal artery and fine capillaries on the optic nerve in the right eye fluorescing. (Courtesy of J. Coppinger.)

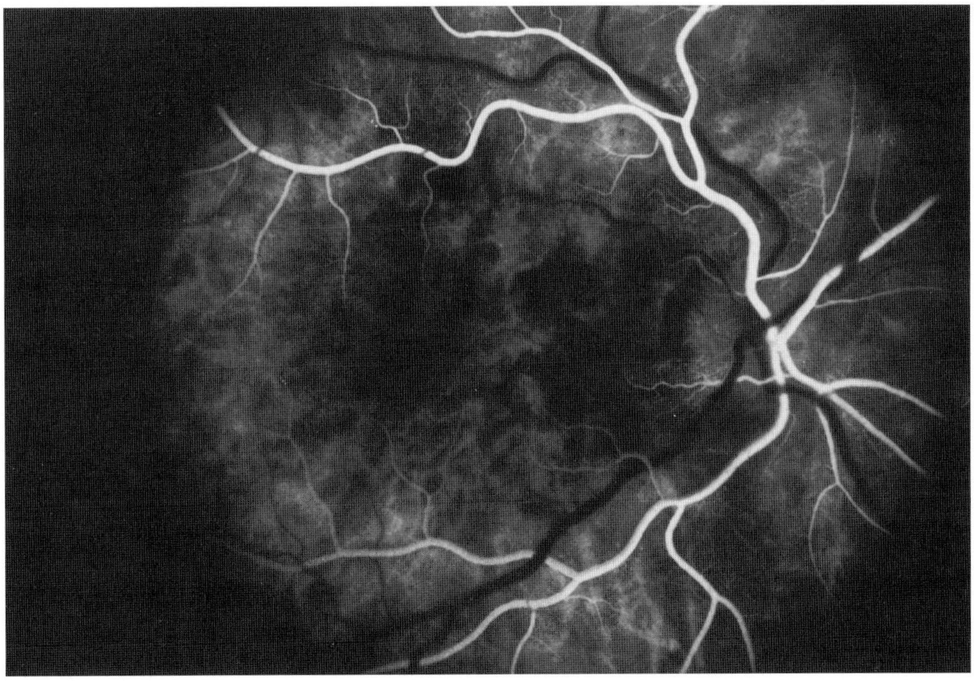

FIGURE 6.7. Angiographic appearance of arterial phase of the angiogram with complete filling of retinal arteries. (Courtesy of J. Coppinger.)

culated during this phase. The ART is the period between the injection of the dye into the antecubital vein and its first appearance in the retinal arteries. The mean ART is 11.2 ± 3.3 seconds and tends to be a shorter interval for children and young adults. A significant difference between eyes or a delay in one eye may indicate vascular insufficiency or occlusive disease.

The *arteriovenous phase* is marked by the appearance of fluorescein dye in the retinal veins emptying from the retinal arteries via the capillaries. Also referred to as the *midphase* or *transition phase*, it is characterized at first by the appearance of laminar flow (Figures 6.8 and 6.9). Visualization of capillaries is optimal during this phase, and therefore, capillary nonperfusion and leakage can be detected.

The *venous phase* is marked by a uniform fluorescence in retinal veins. Laminar flow has disappeared, yielding a more diffuse glow. Often referred to as the *late*

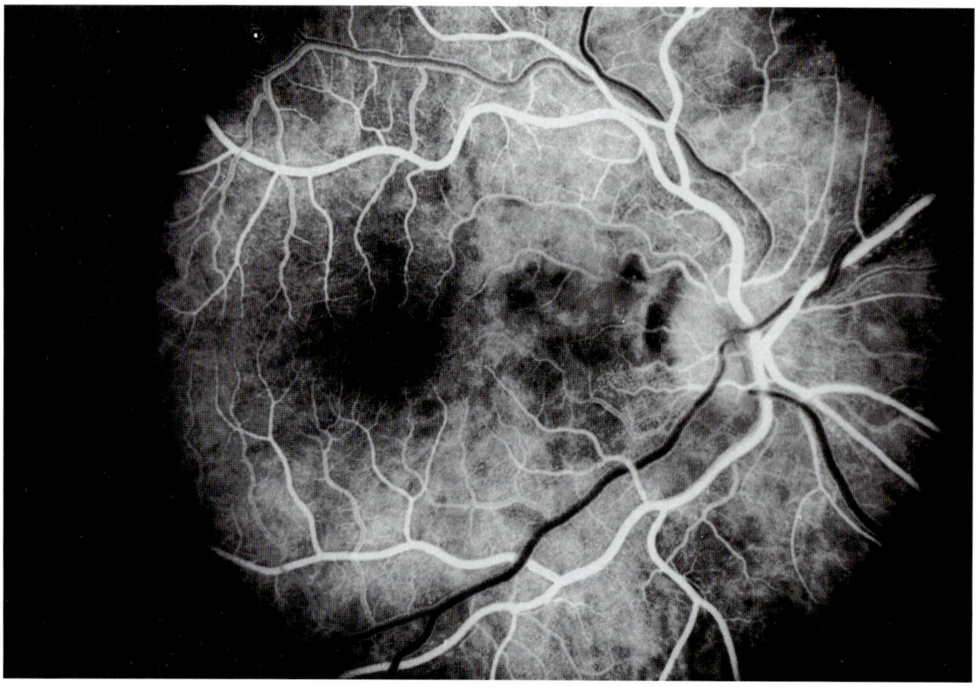

FIGURE 6.8. The appearance of fluorescence at the laminar wall of the vessels as seen through the camera filter. Laminar flow in the vein results from the greater force of blood flow through the retinal veins displacing fluorescein to the outer wall of the vessel. (Courtesy of J. Coppinger.)

arteriovenous phase, venous filling is now complete, with an overall decrease in the intensity of fluorescence in the choroidal and arterial vasculature (Figure 6.10).

In the *late* or *recirculation phase*, the normal angiogram is relatively devoid of any choroidal or retinal fluorescence. The retina appears dark; however, a mild residual glow may appear from the staining of the choroid, sclera, and optic nerve. Vascular leakage secondary to inflammatory disease or other retinal vascular disease is detected in the late phase (Figure 6.11).

It should be noted that the vitreous is clear and nonfluorescent in a normal FA. If neovascularization or inflammation is present, fluorescein molecules disperse into the gel and produce a fluffy appearing fluorescence.

INTERPRETATION OF THE ABNORMAL ANGIOGRAM

Interpretation of the FA is an important component in the management of retinal and choroidal disease, particularly those disorders involving the macula. The distribution of fluorescein dye and the filling patterns of the retinal and choroidal vessels can provide significant information regarding the integrity of the inner and outer blood-retinal barrier. This section discusses the methodology for reviewing the FA and proposes a protocol for interpreting the results when there is a compromise in the integrity of the retinal or choroidal vasculature.

Abnormal Fluorescence

A systematic approach should be employed when evaluating the angiogram. Initially, the positive or nega-

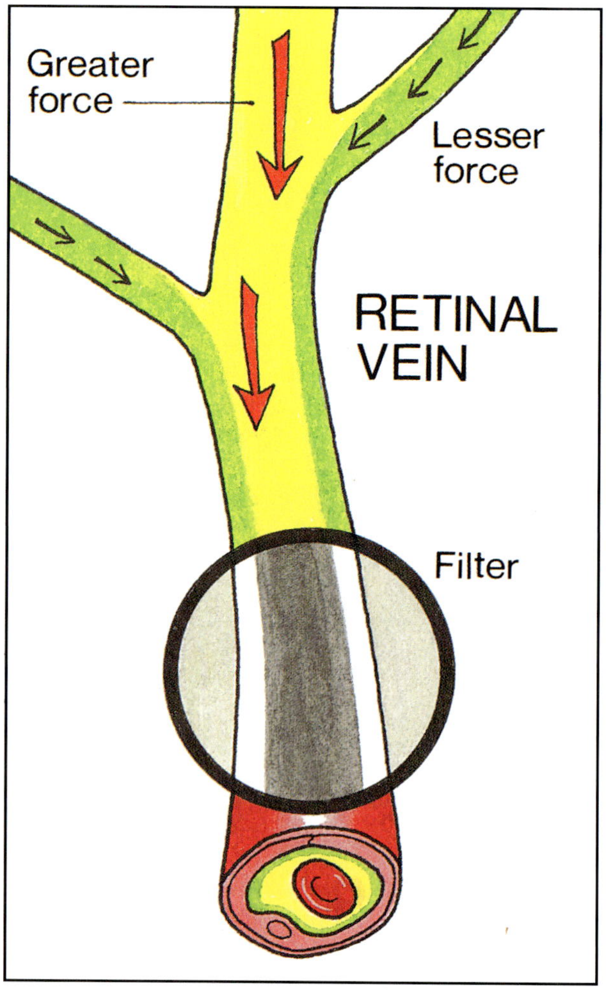

FIGURE 6.9. Angiographic appearance of the early laminar flow phase with distinct fluorescence of outer wall of the veins.

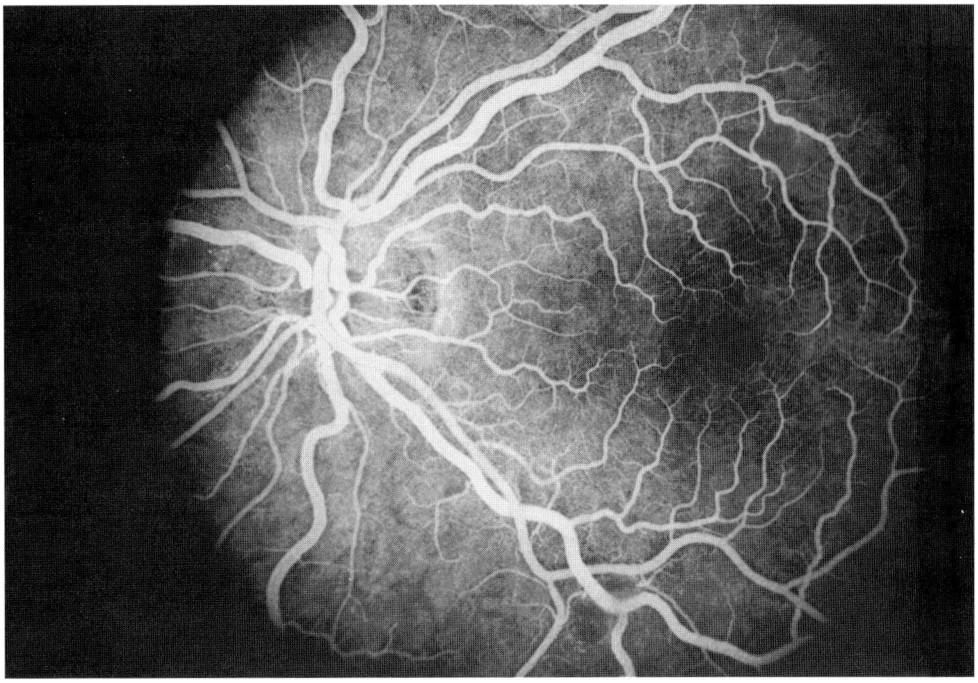

FIGURE 6.10. Later arteriovenous phase with both arteries and veins completely filled with fluorescein. (Courtesy of J. Coppinger.)

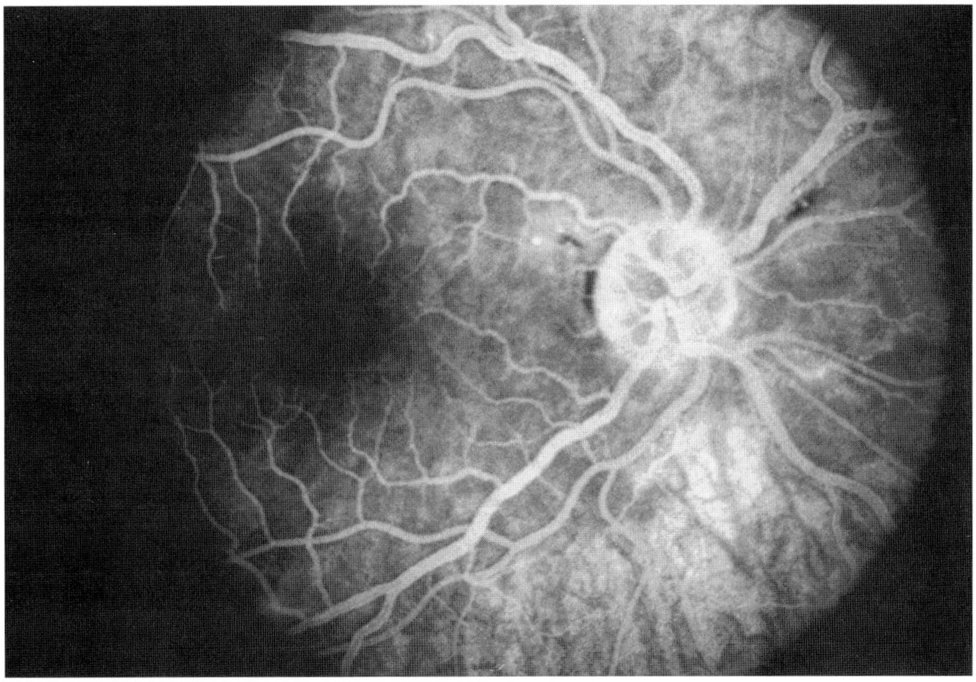

FIGURE 6.11. Late phase with fluorescein dye minimally evident in the retinal vessels while demonstrating staining of the choroid and sclera. (Courtesy of J. Coppinger.)

tive print should be compared with the red-free controls to determine the presence of pseudofluorescence or autofluorescence. Next, abnormal fluorescence may be categorized either as hyperfluorescence or hypofluorescence. Hyperfluorescence denotes an area of excessive fluorescence. Hypofluorescence implies a relative reduction or absence of normal fluorescence. Next, the anatomic location should be determined (i.e., media, retina), and changes in the size and intensity of the abnormal fluorescence should be noted as the angiogram progresses from the prearterial phase to the late phase. Finally, careful attention should be paid to any unique characteristics of the abnormal fluorescence that may be associated with a particular disease (Figure 6.12). A good example of this would be the "smoke-stack" appearance of the hyperfluorescence during the late phase of the angiogram associated with central serous choroidopathy.

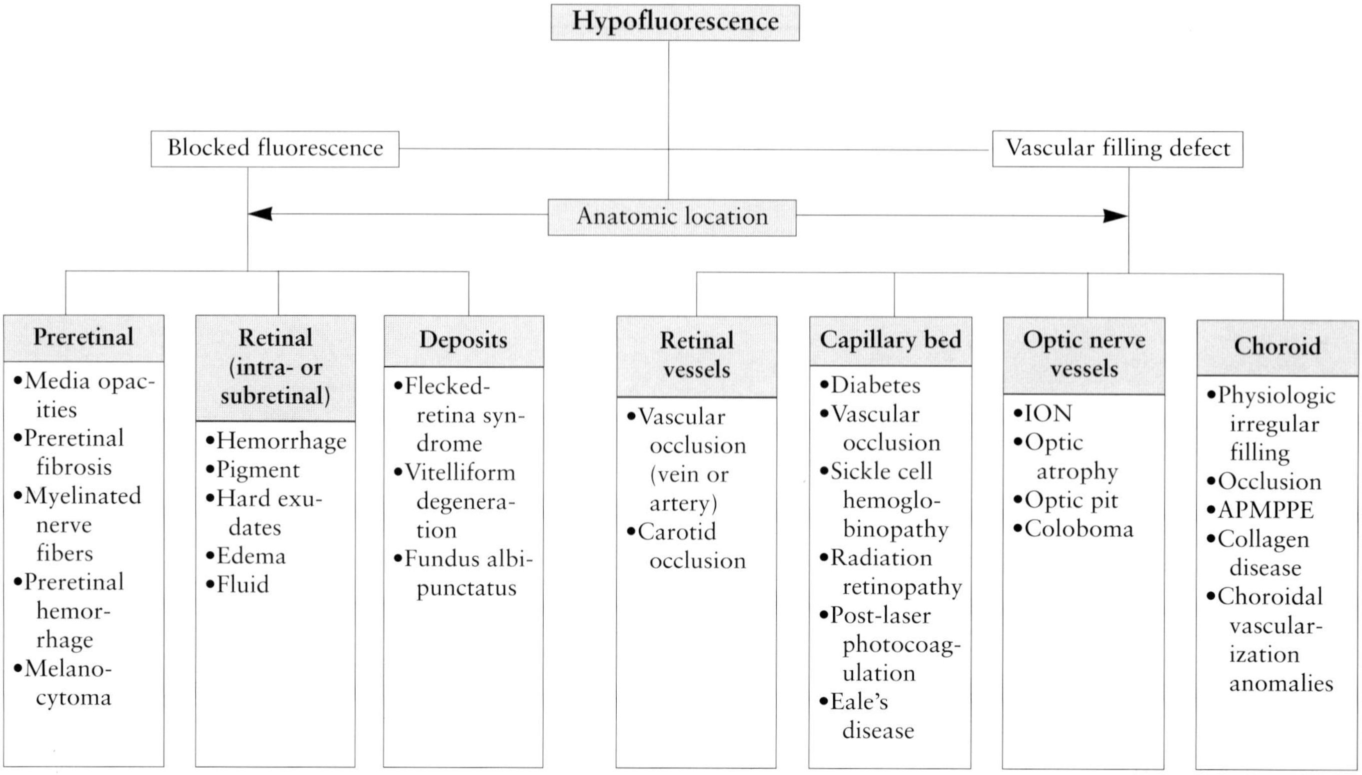

A

FIGURE 6.12. Representation of interpretation and anatomic location of angiographic abnormalities with (A) hypofluorescence and (B) hyperfluorescence. Anterior segment abnormalities can cause blocked fluorescence. ION = ischemic optic neuropathy; APMPPE = acute posterior multifocal placoid pigment epitheliopathy; RPE = retinal pigment epithelium; RD = retinal detachment; CNV = choroidal neovascularization; CME = cystoid macular edema; NSR = neurosensory retinal detachment. (Modified from H Schatz, TC Burton, LA Yannuzzi, MF Rabb. Interpretation of Fundus Fluorescein Angiography. St. Louis: Mosby, 1978.)

Hypofluorescence

Hypofluorescence is an absence or relative lack of fluorescence where fluorescein would normally be expected and is characterized by an abnormally dark area on the positive print or transparency. Vascular filling defects and blocked fluorescence are the two primary causes of hypofluorescence. The key to differentiating blocked fluorescence from a vascular defect is to compare the angiogram with the color fundus photograph. If the obstruction is visible in the clinical photograph and corresponds to the angiogram, it is considered blocked fluorescence. If no blocking material is apparent, then it may be considered a vascular filling defect. Blocked retinal fluorescence is produced by an opacification that will mask fluorescence emitted from the retinal vessels. The blocking material may be corneal or lenticular, an intraocular foreign body, hemorrhage, pigment, exudate, inflammatory cells, dystrophic remnants, or neoplasm. An opacification that blocks both the retina and choroid is located anterior to the retina. It is important to note that one exception to retinal material that does not cause blocking defects is cotton wool spots. Blockage of the choroid exclusively is situated below the retinal circulation. Vitreous hemorrhage, for example, blocks the entire retina, preretinal hemorrhage blocks the underlying retinal vasculature, and RPE hypertrophy blocks only choroidal fluorescence.

A vascular filling defect occurs if there is an absence of normal vasculature or an obstruction to normal blood flow to a corresponding area. Vascular filling defects can occur in both the retina and choroid, and the resulting hypofluorescence may be partial or complete. It is important to refer to the specific FA transit and the color photographs when attempting to determine an arterial, venous, or capillary origin of the hypofluorescence. Branch retinal vein occlusion is second only to diabetic retinopathy as the leading cause of retinal vascular disease and provides a good illustration of a vascular filling defect. Vision-threatening macular edema, vitreous hemorrhage, and neovascularization may occur depending on the site of occlusion, degree of ischemia, and the elapsed time of the occlusion. Ophthalmoscopically, the predominant signs include arteriovenous nicking, dilated and tortuous branch retinal veins, hemorrhage, and edema.

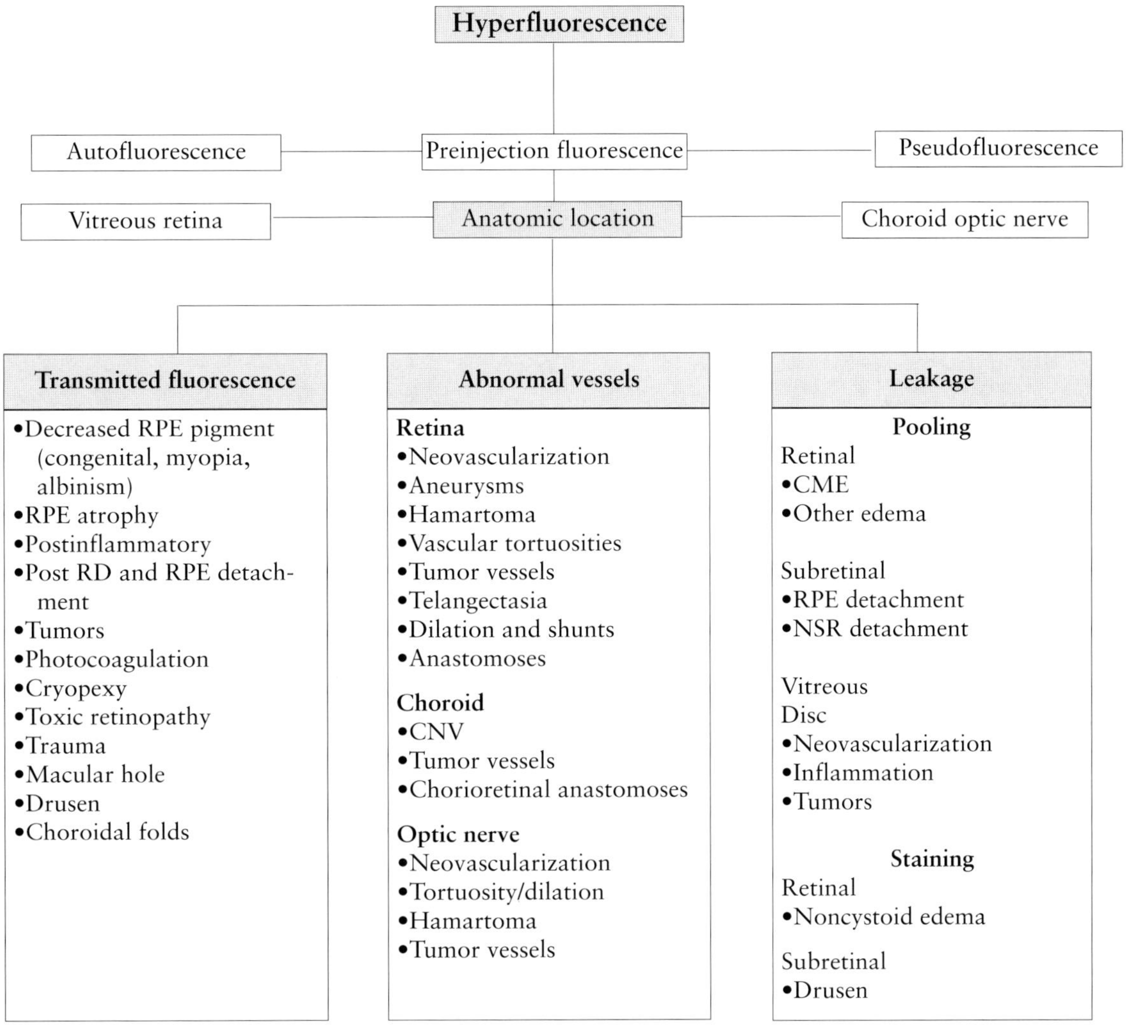

B

During FA, fluorescein dye in the vein distal to the occlusion may be sparse or absent during the arteriovenous and venous phases. As a result, the vein remains as a dark line silhouetted against the background choroidal flush.

Choroidal filling defects are the result of posterior ciliary artery obstruction or the absence of choroidal vasculature. Evidence of visible sclera ophthalmoscopically or on the color photographs is a significant finding. When the choroidal vasculature is absent, the white sclera is evident on the color photographs. Coloboma is an excellent example of congenital loss of choroidal tissue resulting in hypofluorescence. Cryotherapy, diathermy, and laser photocoagulation procedures used in the treatment of retinal disease destroy the choriocapillaris, also resulting in dark patches on the angiogram.

Hyperfluorescence

Hyperfluorescence is the appearance of fluorescein in an area where it would not be expected to accumulate. Hyperfluorescence is characterized by an abnormal light or bright area on the positive print or transparency. Possible causes of hyperfluorescence include abnormal pseudofluorescent or autofluorescent vessels, transmission defects, and vessel leakage. Transmission defects result in an increase in the choroidal fluorescence as a result of an RPE defect. The pigment epithelium acts as a barrier in preventing hyperfluorescence; the ability to block fluorescence is directly proportional to the concentration of pigment in the RPE. Transmission defects appear early in the prearterial phase, mirror the concentration of fluorescein in the choroid, and most importantly, do not increase in size or shape throughout the angiogram. Transmission defects are signs frequently associated with AMD. Sclerosis of the choriocapillaris and a loss of normal metabolic function of the overlying RPE can precipitate drusen and window defects. Drusen are small, nodular bodies that accumulate between the basement membrane of the RPE and Bruch's membrane. The pigment overlying the drusen may be absent or attenuated. These areas represent gaps or windows in the RPE that result in hyperfluorescence of the underlying choroidal vasculature.

FA is an ideal procedure for identifying abnormal vessels in the choroid, optic disc, and retina. Neovascular fronds, aneurysms, telangectasias, and vessels associated with tumors are the most common examples of abnormal vessels and are usually identified in the early prearterial or arterial phases of the angiogram. Diabetic retinopathy is an example of a disease that adversely affects the integrity of the small retinal vessels, frequently resulting in abnormal blood vessel formation. Intraretinal microvascular abnormalities (IRMA), microaneurysms, and neovascularization of the disc and neovascularization elsewhere are examples of abnormal vessels found in diabetic retinopathy. Their individual presence reflects the degree of retinal hypoxia, and therefore, the appearance of abnormal vessels is used to gauge and categorize the severity of retinopathy. Microaneurysms are focal outpouchings of capillary walls that frequently leak and can contribute to sight-threatening diabetic macula edema. They are often difficult to observe ophthalmoscopically but fluoresce brightly during the angiogram. Preproliferative diabetic retinopathy is characterized by the appearance of IRMA, venous beading, and cotton wool spots. IRMAs are dilated, irregular retinal vessels that shunt blood into hypoxic retinal areas. IRMAs usually do not leak or hemorrhage; however, ophthalmoscopically they may be difficult to distinguish from neovascular membranes. During FA, IRMAs hyperfluoresce brightly against the darker ischemic area they serve but do not leak or change in size throughout the entire FA.

Proliferative diabetic retinopathy is also characterized by abnormal vessels and neovascularization. These fragile vessels resulting from retinal ischemia bleed easily, causing vitreous hemorrhage and possible tractional retinal detachment. Neovascularization of the disc or neovascularization elsewhere may be difficult to identify by routine ophthalmoscopy but hyperfluoresce brightly and will leak fluorescein during FA.

Other causes of hyperfluorescence secondary to leakage of fluorescein can occur in the choroid, retina, optic nerve, and vitreous. Leakage usually appears in the early phases of the angiogram, but in contrast to transmission defects, it increases in size and shape in the later phases. In these cases, the fluorescein remaining in the late phase has penetrated the blood-retinal barrier, resulting in extravascular pooling or staining. Common examples of this phenomenon include idiopathic central serous choroidopathy, cystoid macular edema (CME), and CNV. In CNV, new blood vessels may grow into the subretinal space from the choroid and proliferate through breaks in Bruch's membrane. These fragile neovascular membranes frequently hemorrhage or leak, resulting in detachment of either or both the RPE and sensory retina. A resultant fibrous scar is responsible for the profound loss of central visual acuity. CNV is most commonly associated with exudative macular degeneration and presumed ocular histoplasmosis syndrome, and occurs less frequently with angioid streaks, myopic degeneration, idiopathic choroidal tumors, or traumatic choroidal ruptures. CNV can be difficult to identify definitively by direct fundus examination but may appear as a small greenish-gray subretinal area that can be surrounded by hemorrhage or exudate. FA more definitively reveals its characteristic lacy appearance in the early phase, which becomes more diffuse into the late phase as leakage occurs. Significant subretinal hemorrhage, often found in the late stages of CVN, will block the fluorescing membrane, resulting in an area of hypofluorescence.

FLUORESCEIN ANGIOGRAPHY AND LASER SURGERY

FA is an important tool when determining the suitability of laser treatment for retinal and choroidal disease. Due to the rapid rate of growth of CNVM, the angiogram should be performed within 48–72 hours of treatment. With diabetic retinopathy, including clinically significant macular edema and proliferative diabetic retinopathy, the angiogram should be obtained within 1–2 weeks of treatment.

The angiogram is viewed during laser surgery so that the surgeon can directly visualize the areas of the retina or choroid needing treatment. In most cases of macular disease, posttreatment angiograms are obtained 2–3 weeks after treatment for comparison.

Lasers used in the treatment of macular disease include the argon green, krypton yellow or red, or tunable dye laser, or the diode laser for occult neovascular membranes. Determining the appropriate laser depends on the nature of the disorder, the location of the lesion or lesions, and the status of the surrounding retina. Ophthalmic application of lasers in macular disease is discussed in Chapter 31.

SUMMARY

FA is an important adjunct in the management of macular disease. Although not considered a routine procedure, it is commonly performed to confirm a diagnosis and determine suitability for treatment of macular disorders, especially for CNV and diabetic macular edema.

The clinician is encouraged to obtain angiograms from his or her consultant and to review the findings to derive a better understanding of the etiopathogenesis of retinal and choroidal disease. The nature of the fluorescein study allows for interpretation and understanding of retinal tissue response and therefore a better predictive capability of visual performance and function for the patient.

CASE EXAMPLES

The following examples illustrate the angiographic features of select retinal and choroidal abnormalities. (Figures in this section reprinted with permission from MT Porter, AA Cavallerano, RK Gutner. Fundus fluorescein angiography—Part II: Interpretation of the abnormal angiogram. Clin Eye Vis Care 1993;5:131–138.)

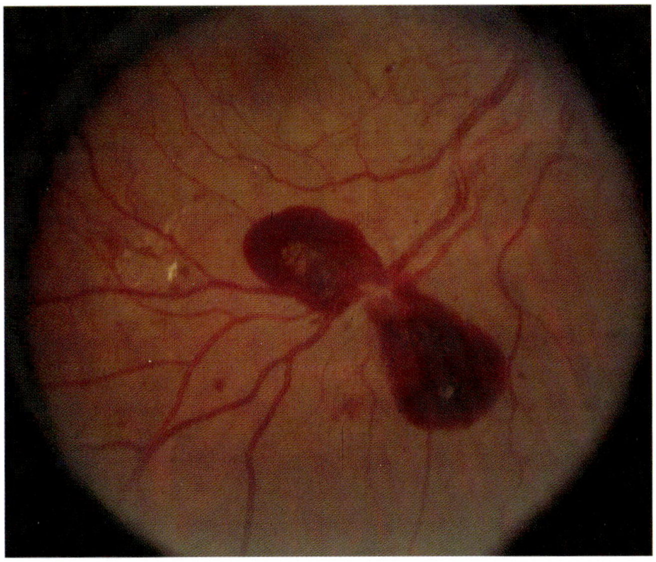

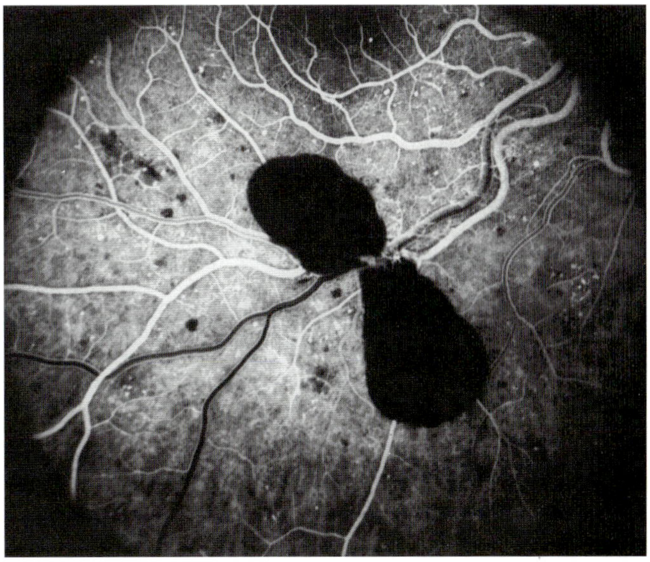

Example 1. Blocked Fluorescence

Diagnosis: Intraretinal hemorrhage in a diabetic patient
Color photograph: Hemorrhages—dot and blot
Exudates
Fluorescein angiogram: Laminar flow phase
Hypofluorescence—blockage from intraretinal hemorrhage

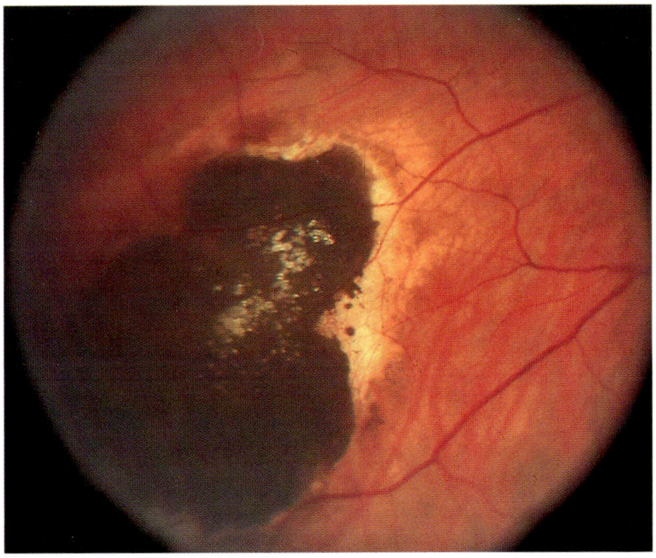

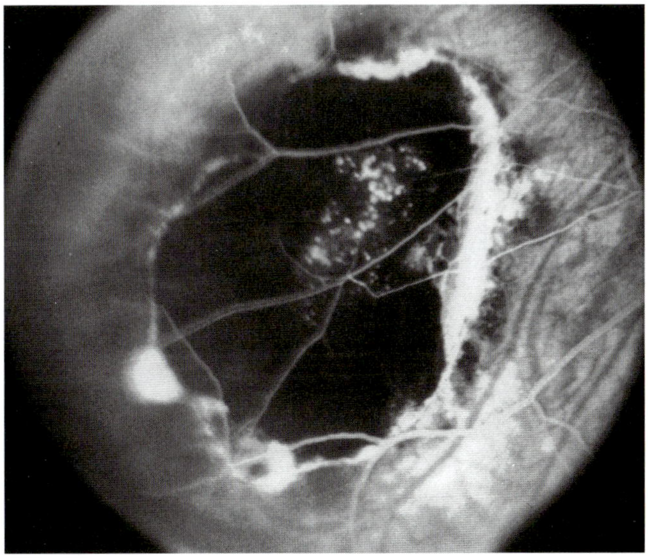

Example 2. Blocked Fluorescence

Diagnosis: Congenital RPE hypertrophy
Color photograph: RPE hypertrophy
Fluorescein angiogram: Late phase
Hypofluorescence—blockage at the RPE level

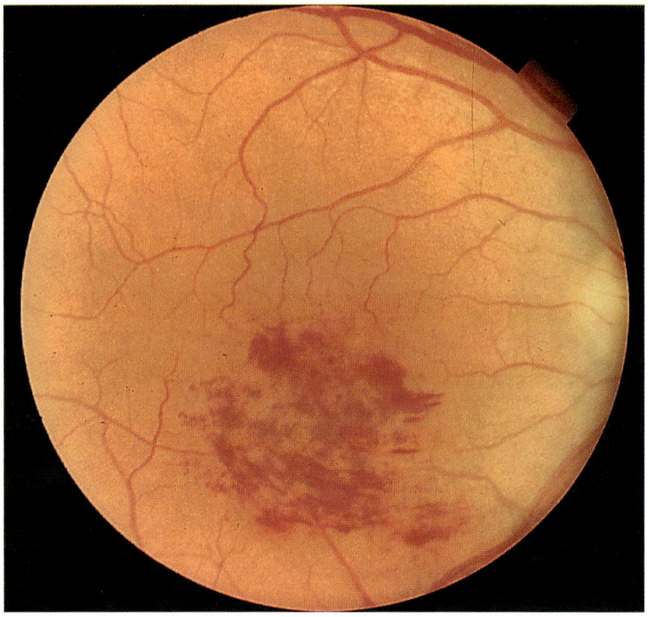
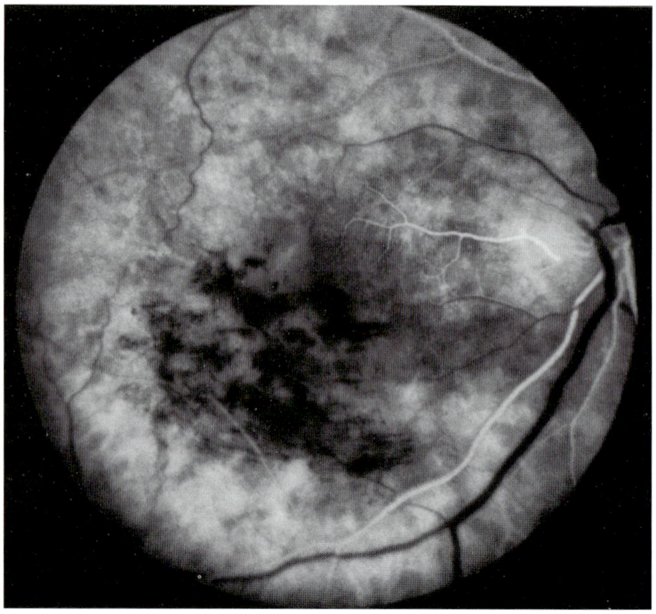

Example 3. Vascular Filling Defect

Diagnosis:	Macular branch vein occlusion in hypertensive patient
Color photograph:	Hemorrhages in the inferior macular field suggesting a macular branch vein occlusion
	Edema within the hemorrhagic area
Fluorescein angiogram:	Normal filling of choroid and retinal arterioles
	Delayed filling of venous system

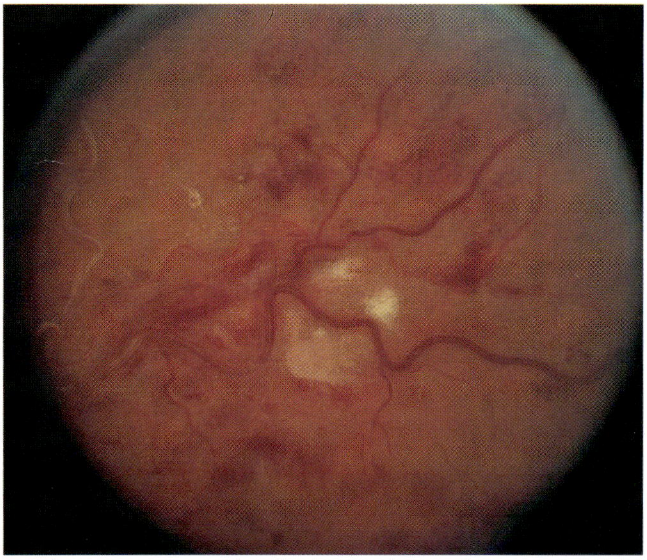
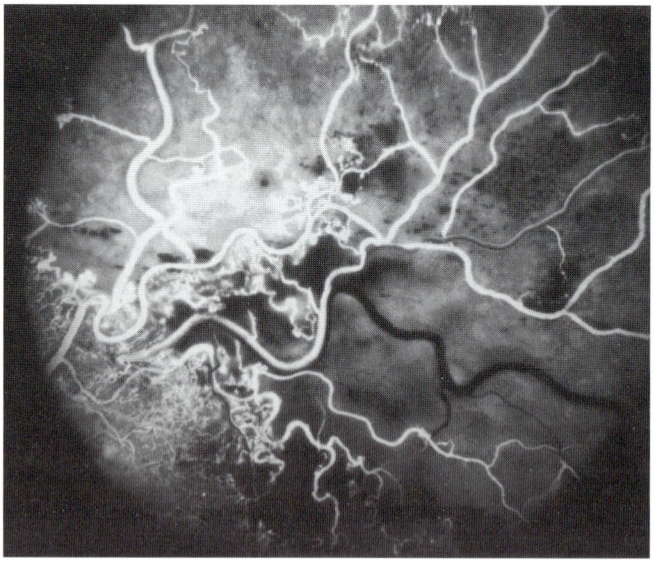

Example 4. Blocked Fluorescence From Capillary Nonperfusion

Diagnosis:	Old branch retinal vein occlusion
Color photograph:	Attenuation and tortuosity of retinal arteries
	Superficial and deep retinal hemorrhages
	Sclerosis of superior retinal artery
	Cotton wool spots
	Macular edema
Fluorescein angiogram:	Venous collaterals and intraretinal microvascular abnormalities
	Extensive areas of capillary nonperfusion causing hypofluorescence

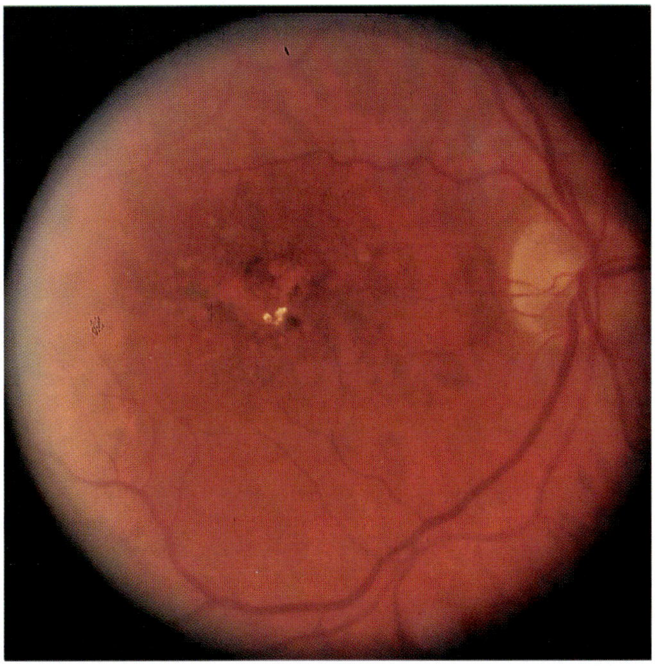

Example 5. Hyperfluorescence From Retinal Pigment Epithelium Migration and Dropout

Diagnosis:	Dry AMD
Color photograph:	RPE dropout and migration Scattered drusen
Fluorescein angiogram:	Early phase (left)—hyperfluorescence through transmission defect; drusen Late phase (right)—hyperfluorescence does not change throughout the transit

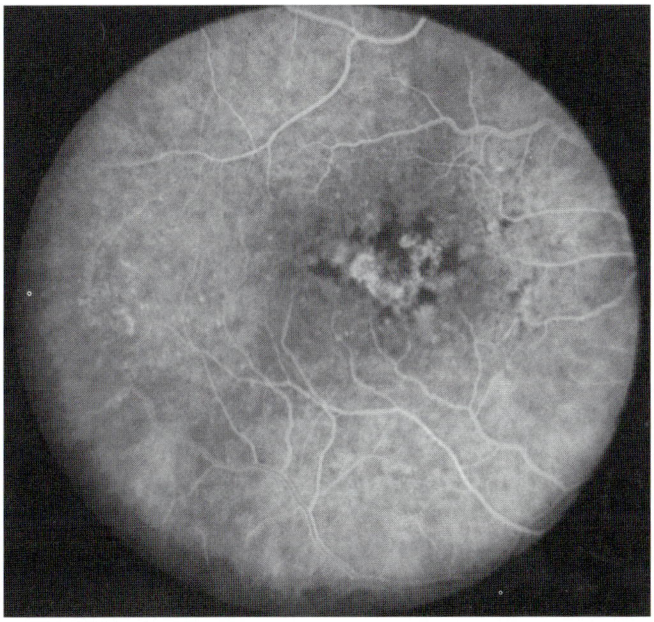

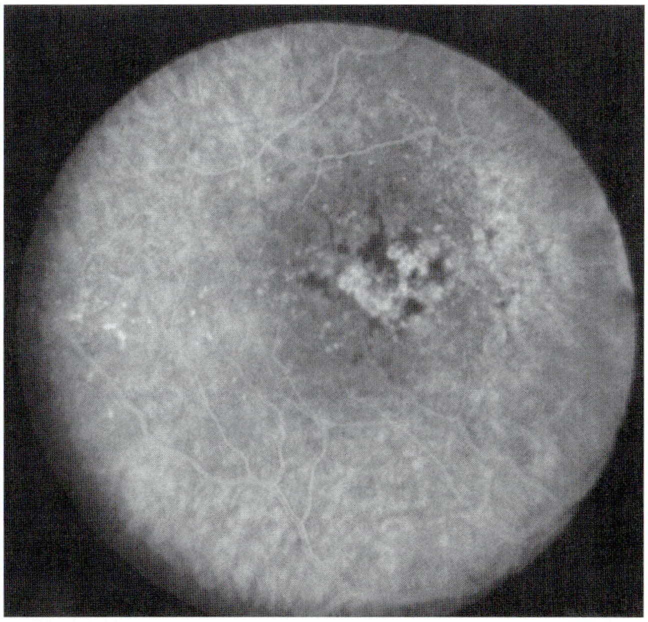

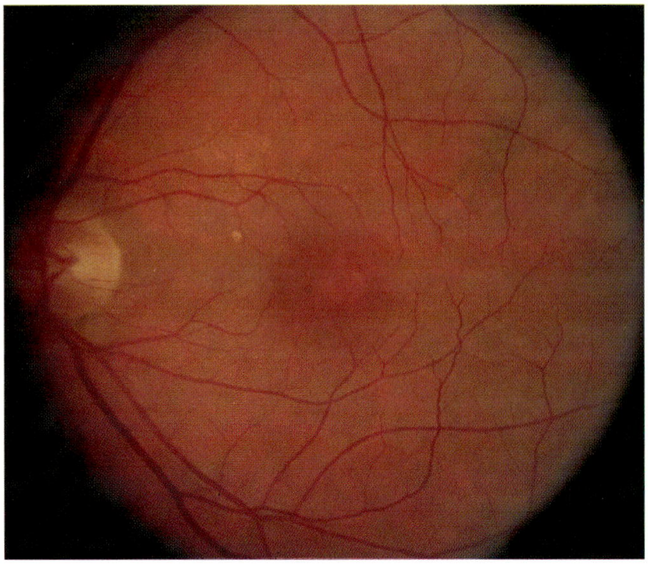
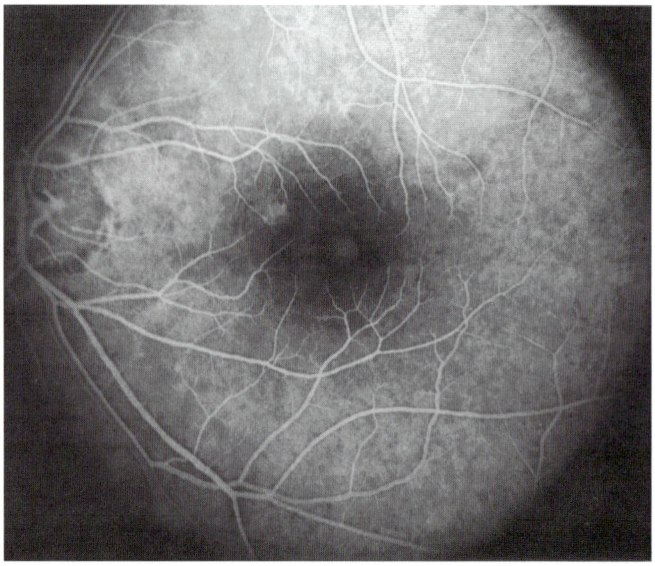

Example 6. Transmitted Fluorescence

Diagnosis:	Full-thickness macular hole in the left eye
Color photograph:	Full-thickness macular hole with cuff of edema
Fluorescein angiogram:	Arteriovenous phase Hyperfluorescence from transmission defect

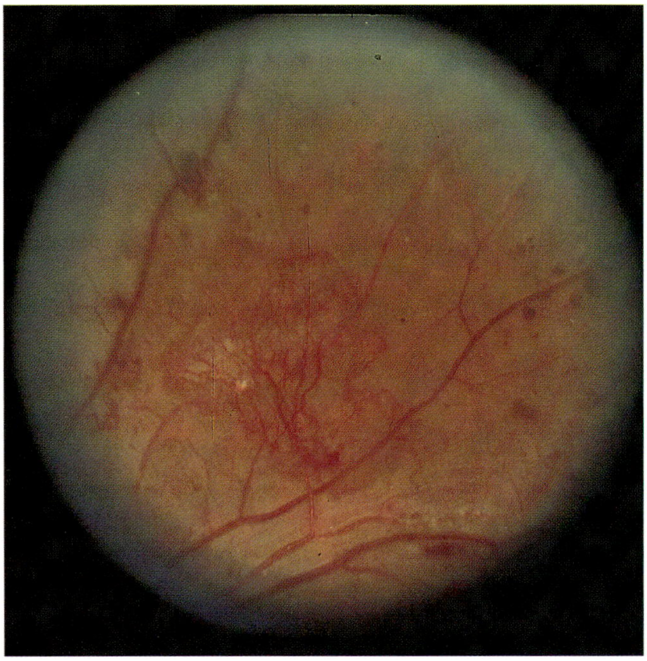
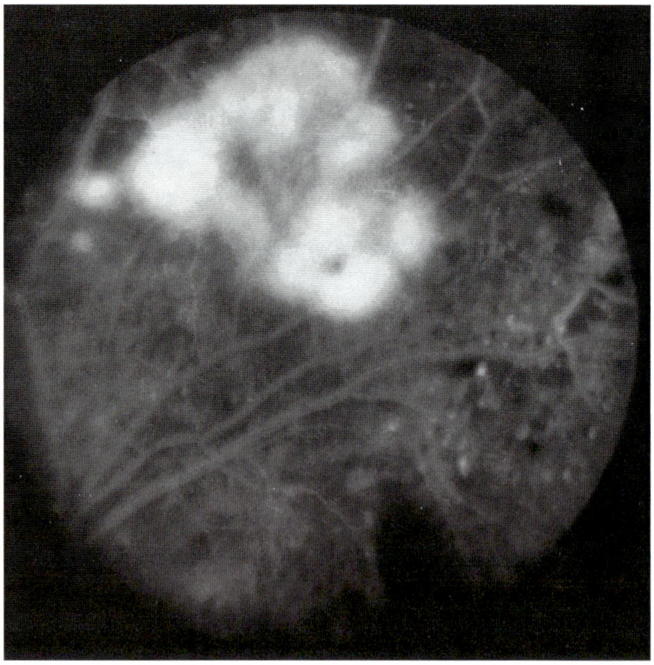

Example 7. Abnormal Vessels and Leakage Causing Hyperfluorescence

Diagnosis:	Proliferative diabetic retinopathy
Color photograph:	Dot and blot hemorrhages Rare exudate Neovascular frond
Fluorescein angiogram:	Late phase intense hyperfluorescence and leakage Blocked fluorescence from retinal hemorrhages

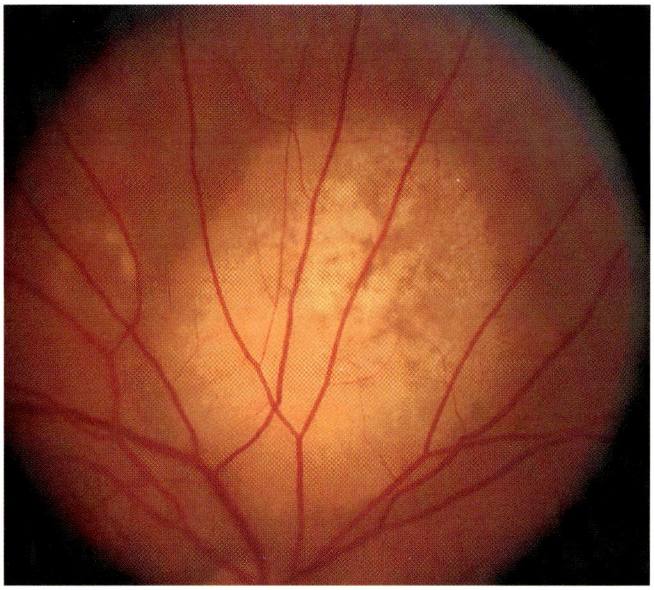

Example 8. Abnormal Tumor Vessels Causing Hyperfluorescence

Diagnosis: Metastatic carcinoma from liver

Color photograph: Elevated retina in macular area
Retinal striae along superior-temporal arcade
Pigmentary disturbance

Fluorescein angiogram: Laminar flow phase (upper left)—blocked choroidal fluorescence
Early venous phase (upper right)—hyperfluorescence over pigmentary disturbance
Arteriovenous phase (lower left)—increased hyperfluorescence from leakage overlying areas of blocked fluorescence
Later phase (lower right)—uniform hyperfluorescence over the entire lesion

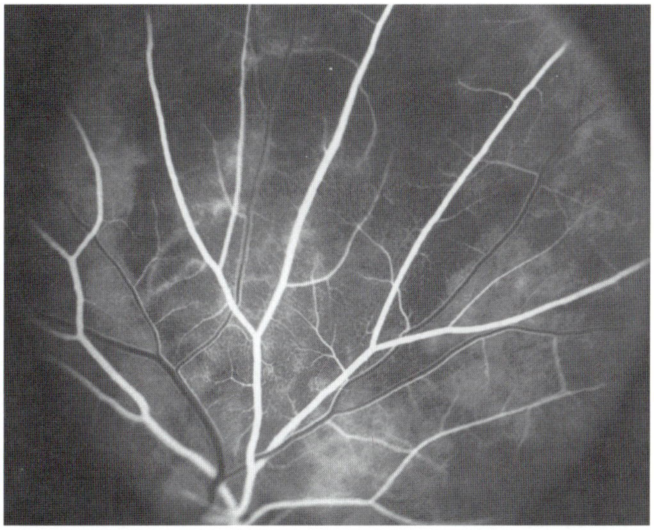

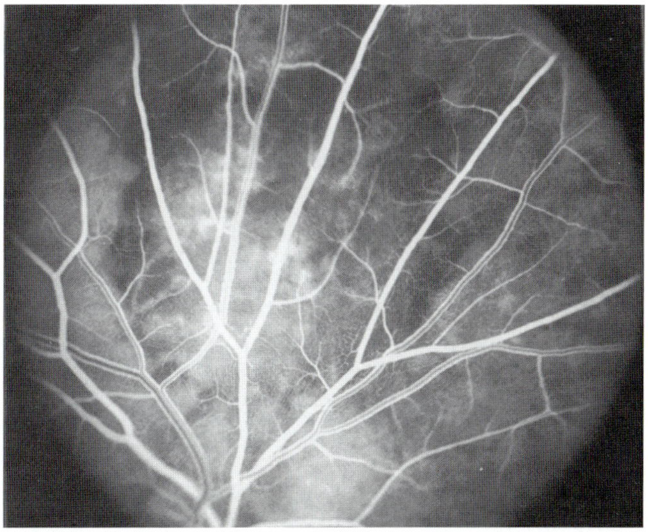

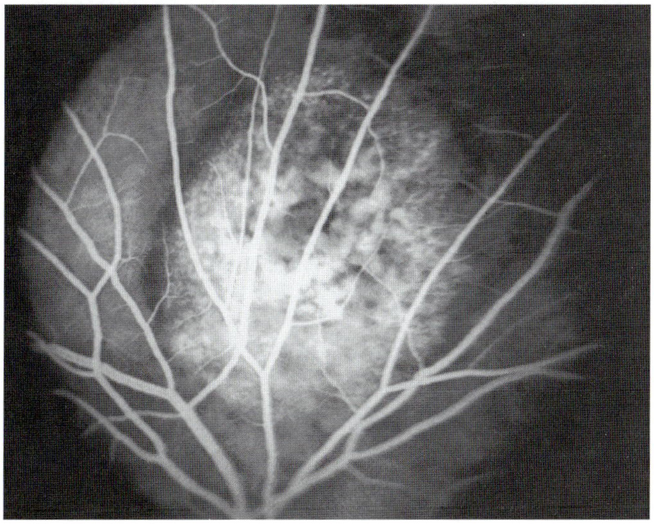

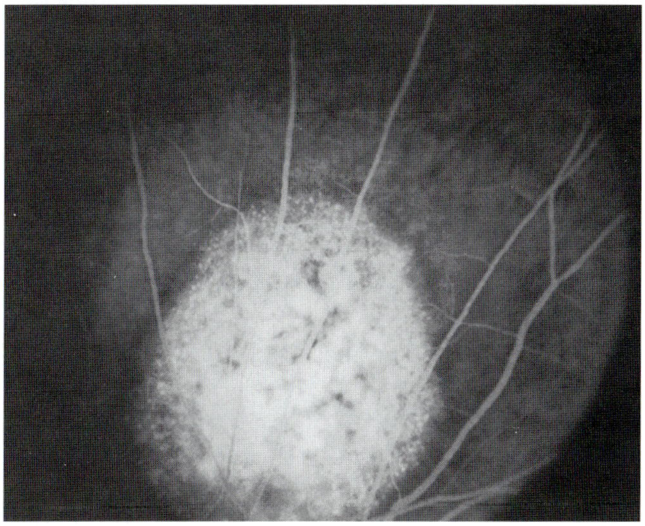

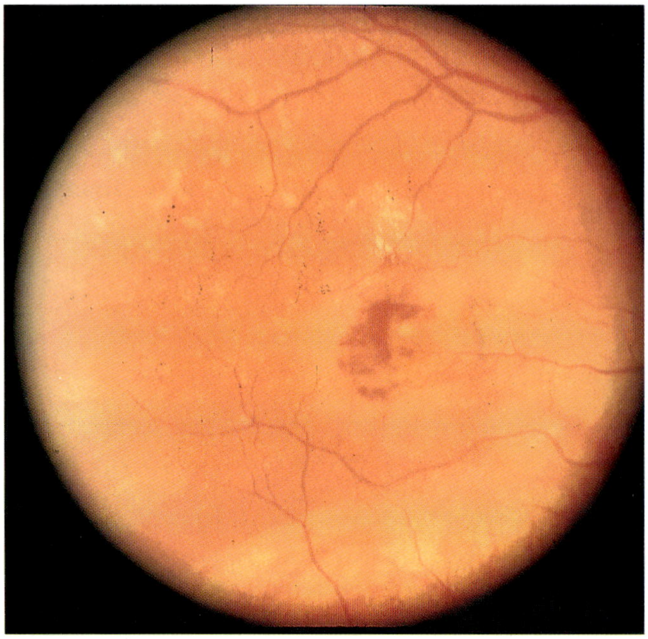

Example 9. Abnormal Choroidal Vessels Causing Hyperfluorescence

Diagnosis:	Exudative AMD
Color photograph:	CNVM Macular hemorrhage and exudate Small drusen
Fluorescein angiogram: (right)	Early arteriovenous phase (upper left)—blocked choroidal fluorescence Arteriovenous phase (upper right)—area corresponding to CNV demonstrates early, lacy hyperfluorescence Recirculation phase (lower left)—increased hyperfluorescence with adjacent and surrounding hyperfluorescence corresponding to pigment migration and hemorrhage Late phase (lower right)—hyperfluorescence with pooling and staining of fluorescein

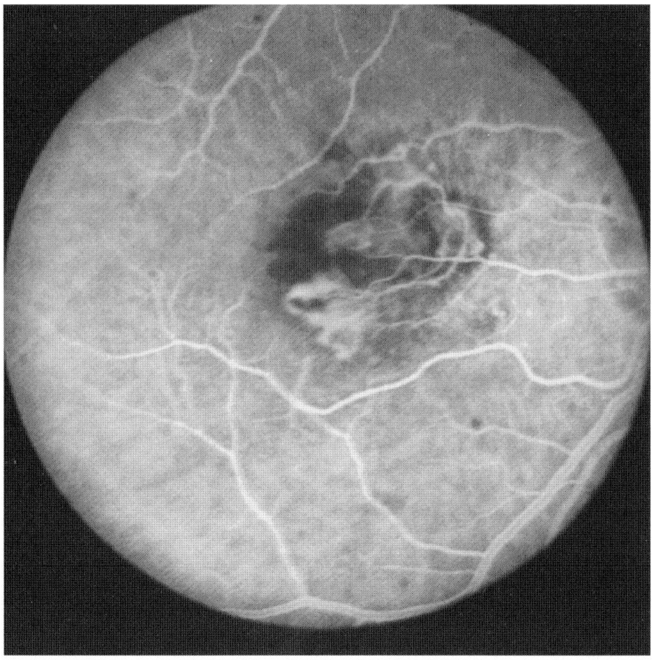
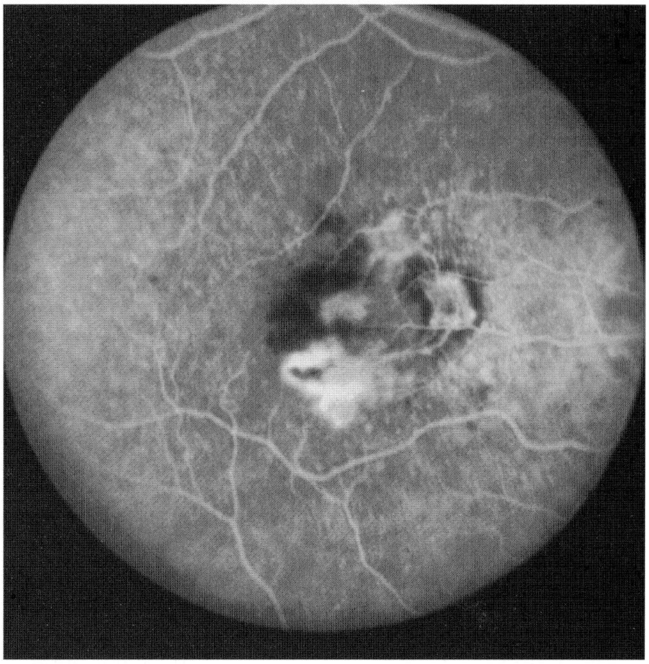
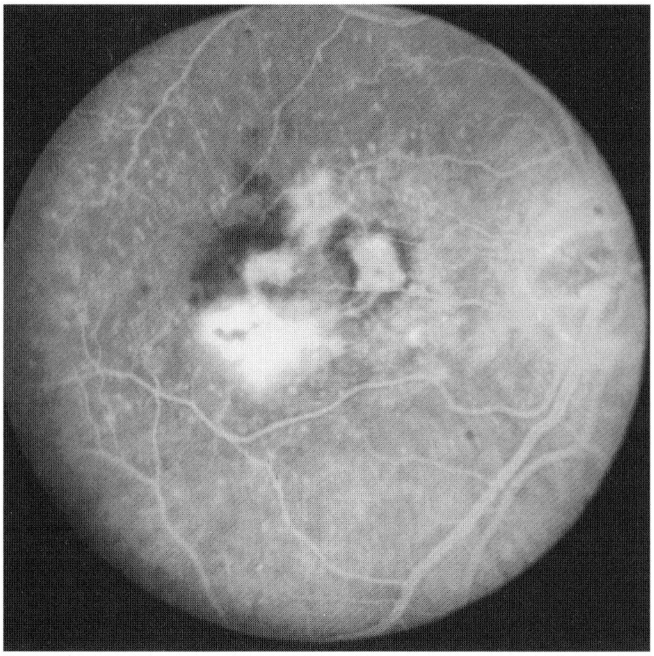
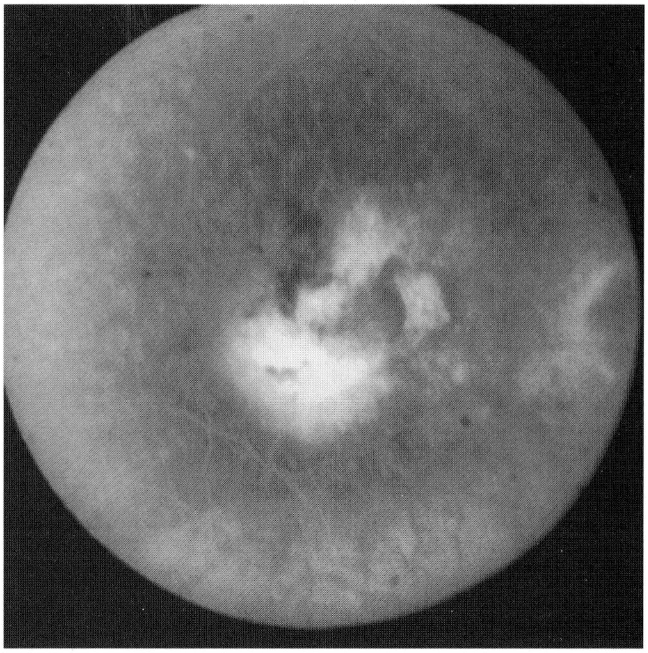

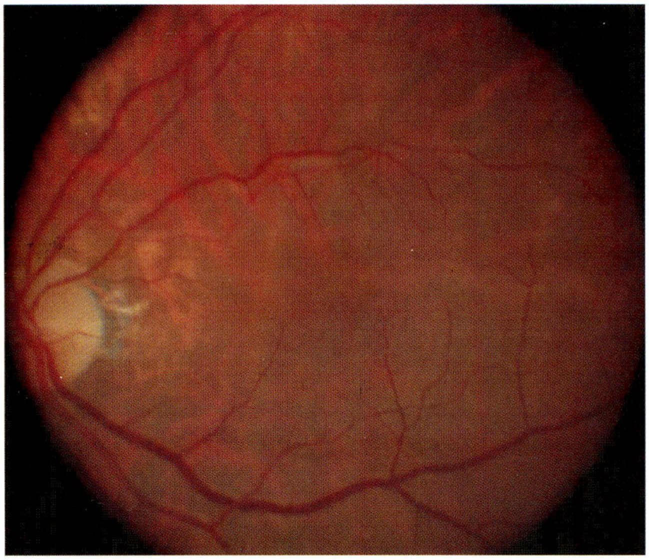

Example 10. Leakage Causing Hyperfluorescence

Diagnosis: Pseudophakic CME
Color photograph: Macular edema
Fluorescein angiogram: Early arteriovenous phase (upper left)
Arteriovenous phase (upper right)—area corresponding to edema caused by leakage of perifoveal capillaries
Arteriovenous recirculation (lower left)—increased hyperfluorescence throughout transit
Late phase (lower right)—wreath-like hyperfluorescence characteristic of CME

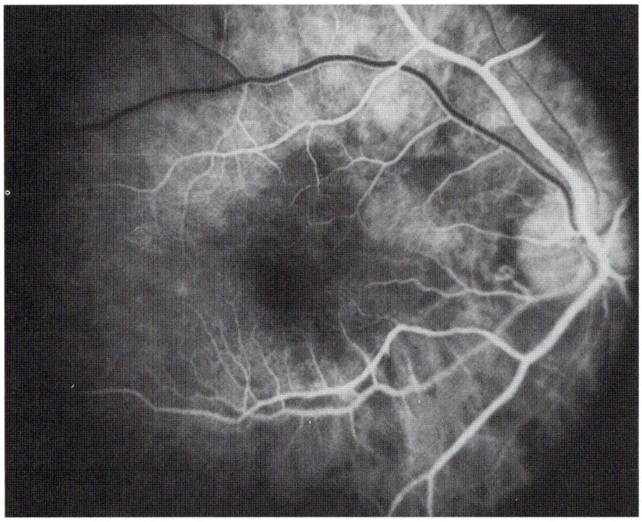

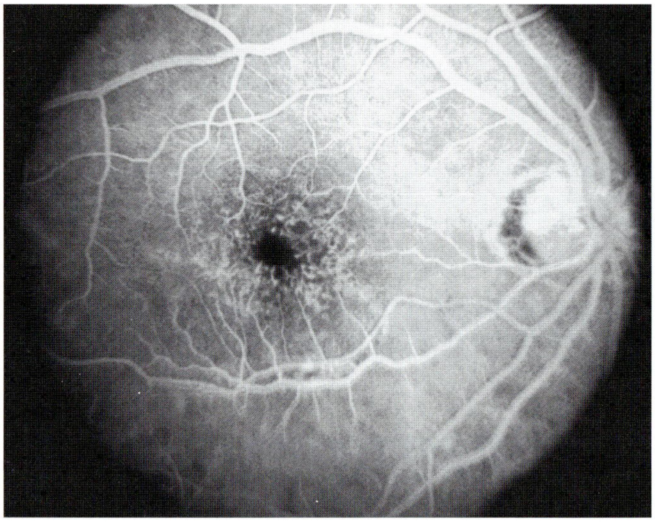

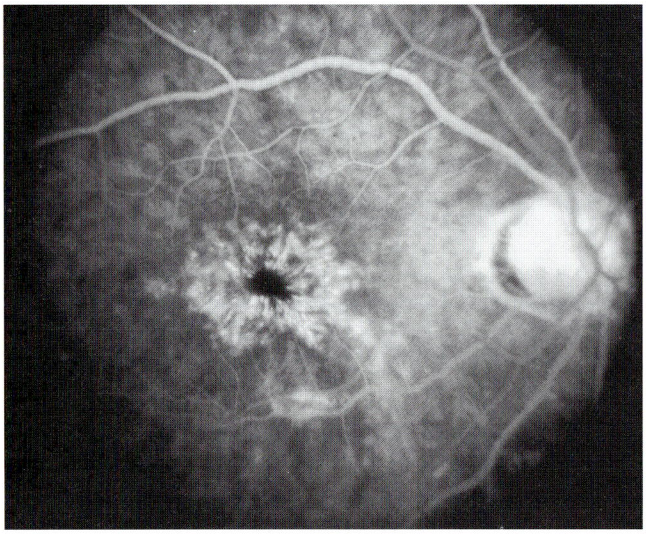

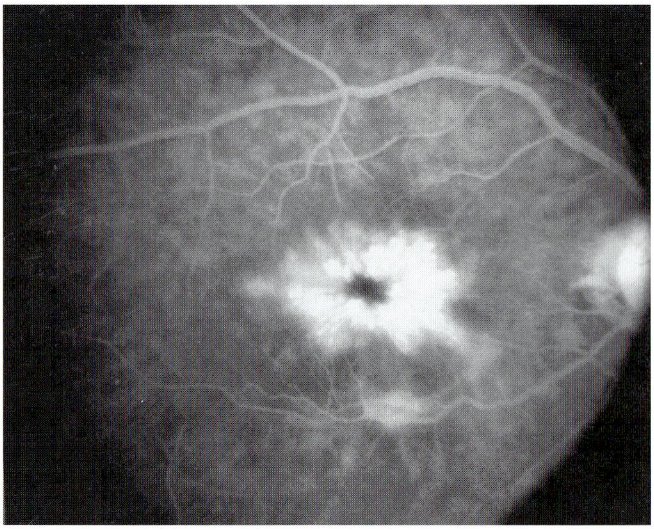

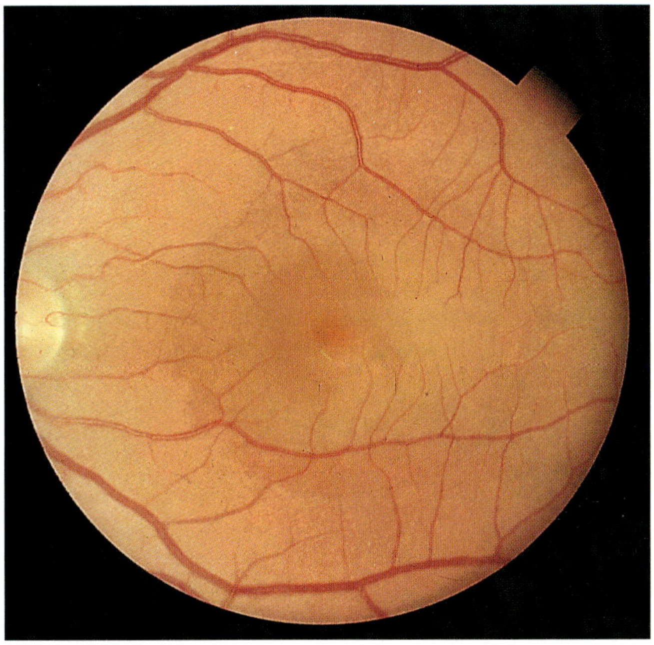

Example 11. Hyperfluorescence Caused by Leakage

Diagnosis: Idiopathic central serous choroidopathy

Color photograph: RPE disturbance
Neurosensory retinal detachment

Fluorescein angiogram: Ateriovenous phase—hyperfluorescence due to RPE disturbance and early leakage from RPE defect (upper left)
Continued progression of leakage throughout transit showing typical smokestack pattern (upper right and lower left)
Late phase—hyperfluorescence in typical "umbrella" or "mushroom cap" appearance due to slow leakage from choroid through the RPE defect (lower right)

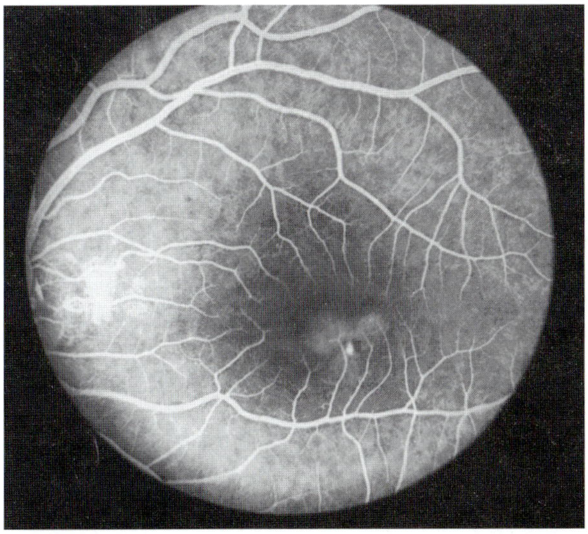

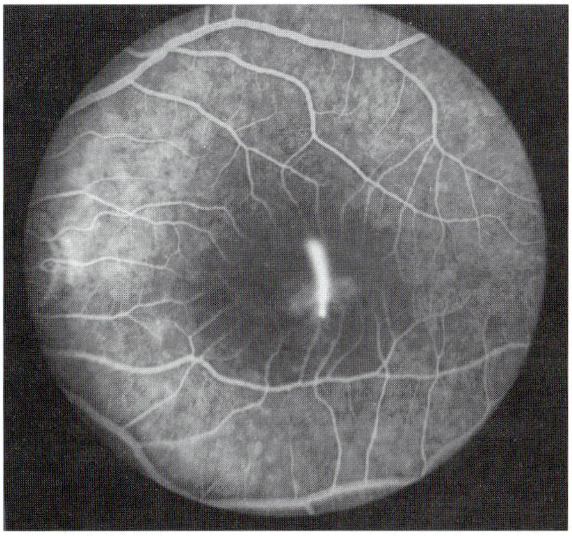

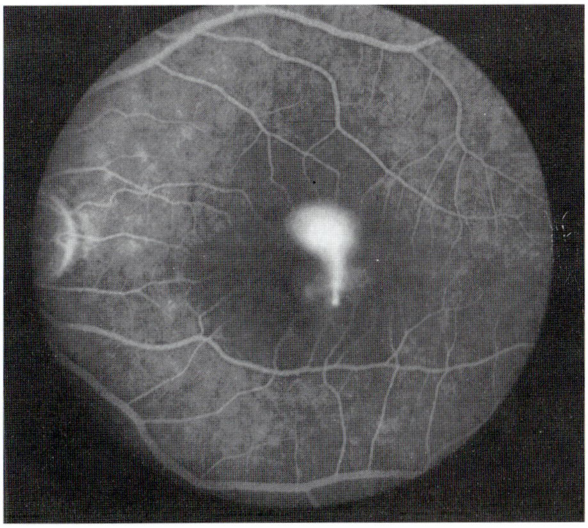

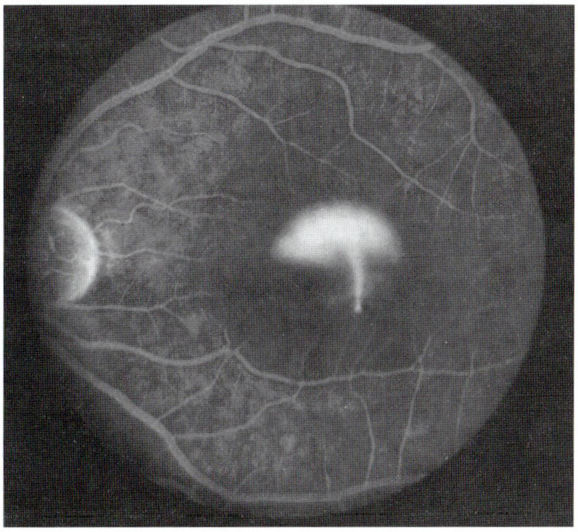

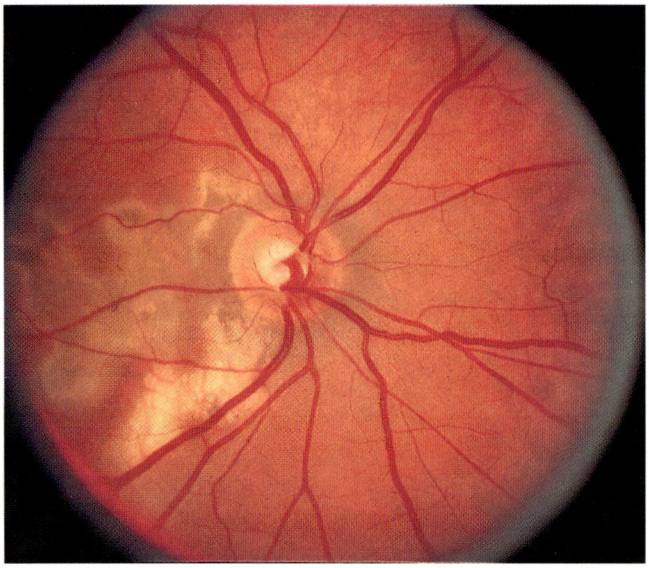

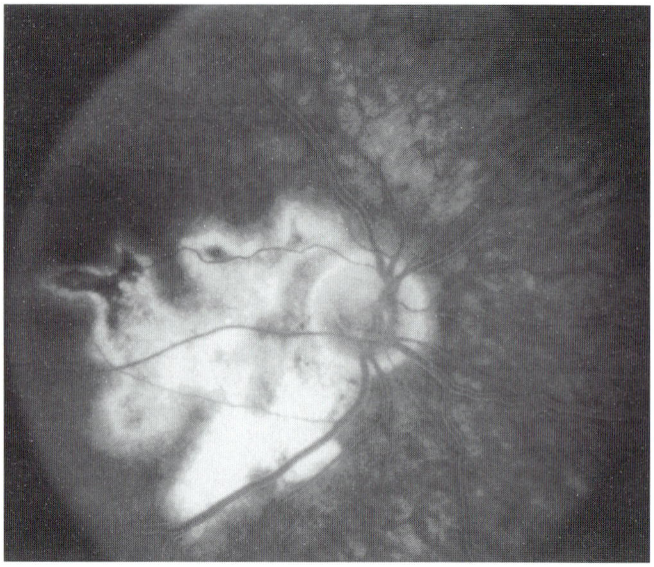

Example 12. Hyperfluorescence Caused by Staining

Diagnosis: Serpiginous choroidopathy
Color photograph: Geographic chorioretinal scarring and atrophy extending into macula and foveal avascular zone
Fluorescein angiogram: Late phase—staining in area of chorioretinal atrophy

SUGGESTED READING

Alexander K. Fluorescein Angiography. In DK Roberts, JE Terry (eds), Ocular Disease (2nd ed). Boston: Butterworth, 1996;77–91.

Bartsch D, Intaglietta M, Bille JF, et al. Confocal laser tomographic analysis of the retina in eyes with macular hole formation and other focal macular diseases. Am J Ophthalmol 1989;108:277–287.

Bursell S. A video-based fluorescein angiography system. N Engl J Optom 1987;3:12–16.

Cavallerano J. Fluorescein Angiography. In JB Eskridge, JF Amos, JD Bartlett (eds), Clinical Procedures in Optometry. Philadelphia: Lippincott, 1990;609–620.

Chopdar A. Manual of Fundus Fluorescein Angiography. London: Butterworth, 1989.

Coppinger JM. Ophthalmic Photography, Ophthalmic Technical Skills Series. Thorofare, NJ: Slack, 1990.

Destro M, Puliafito CA. Indocyanine green videoangiography of choroidal neovascularization. Ophthalmology 1989;96:846–853.

Gass JDM. Stereoscopic Atlas of Macular Disease. St. Louis: Mosby, 1987.

Guyer DR, Puliafito CA, Mones JM, et al. Digital indocyanine-green angiography in chorioretinal disorders. Ophthalmology 1992;99:287–291.

Krause FE, Burk ROW, Volcer H, et al. Reproducibility of topographic measurements of the optic nerve head with laser tomographic scanning. Ophthalmology 1989;96:1320–1324.

Nayak B. A method for fundus evaluation in children with oral fluorescein. Br J Ophthalmol 1987;71:907–909.

Porter MT. Fluorescein angiography: A clinical review. Clin Eye Vis Care 1992;4:44–54.

Porter MT, Cavallerano AA, Gutner RK. Fluorescein angiography. Part II: Interpretation of the abnormal angiogram. Clin Eye Vis Care 1993;5:131–138.

Schatz H. Essential Fluorescein Angiography. San Anselmo, CA: Pacific Medical, 1983.

Schatz H, Burton TC, Yannuzzi LA, Rabb MF. Interpretation of Fundus Fluorescein Angiography. St. Louis: Mosby, 1978.

Wolf S. Video fluorescein angiography: Method and clinical application. Arch Ophthalmol 1989;227:145–151.

Yannuzzi LA. Macular Disease. Baltimore: Williams & Wilkins, 1979.

Yannuzzi LA, Rohrer KT, Tindel LJ, et al. Fluorescein angiography complication survey. Ophthalmology 1986;15:1084–1086.

PART

II

Clinical Findings in the Diagnosis of Macular Disease

The following five chapters are designed as a guide for the clinician in developing a diagnosis and management strategy when the etiology of a macular disorder is initially unclear. Using an unconventional categorization of macular lesions based on the objective, general clinical findings, an outline for the differential diagnosis is presented. Once a diagnosis is determined, a suggested initial plan, as well as additional considerations in management of the patient, is presented for more common macular disorders.

CHAPTER

7

Lightly Colored Macular Lesions

Leonard J. Oshinskie, Anthony A. Cavallerano, and Rodney K. Gutner

The clinical category of lightly colored macular lesions includes lesions that are predominantly white, gray-white, yellow, yellow-white, or beige. To categorize these lesions further, the clinician should consider their size, depth, and accompanying pigment changes. The retinal blood vessels are an excellent reference for establishing the depth of a lesion; stereoscopic observation will greatly improve the ability to localize lesions within the layers of the retina. In many cases, deep lesions disrupt the retinal pigment epithelium (RPE) so that pathologic changes, atrophy, or clumping of the pigment may be noted near or over them. Drusen are the most common cause of lesions in this category, principally in patients 60 years and older (Figure 7.1). Small singular drusen are quite common and may be seen throughout the fundus. Numerous conditions resulting in a breakdown of the inner blood-retinal barrier produce hard exudates, and retinal ischemia produces soft exudates or cotton wool spots (CWS).

Lightly colored lesions, especially small lesions, may be refractile or bright, indicating reflectance, or they may be nonrefractile or dull. The brightness of a retinal lesion or its ability to reflect incident light (refractile nature) are both helpful characteristics in differentiating small, lightly colored macular lesions. For example, unless drusen are calcified, they do not appear to glisten, and although some drusen appear bright, most are dull in appearance. Therefore, if a small, lightly colored lesion is refractile or bright and does not appear to be a druse based on appearance, depth, or risk profile, several other conditions must be considered. As with all retinal lesions, determining the depth of these lesions is critical in making the diagnosis since certain refractile or bright lesions may also be deep or superficial.

Large lesions, as described here, often vary in size but are typically larger than 1 disc diameter (DD). Some of the same conditions described under small, lightly colored lesions may also present as larger lesions. An additional consideration is the potential for accompanying pigment changes surrounding or within larger, lightly colored macular lesions. The following lists summarize characteristics of both small and large lesions.

SMALL, DEEP MACULAR LESIONS (FREQUENTLY SMALLER THAN 1 DD)

Nonrefractile

Common
- Age-related drusen
- Punched-out lesions of presumed ocular histoplasmosis
- Laser photocoagulation scars

Less common
- Drusen in younger patients
  - Dominantly inherited drusen
  - Basal laminar drusen
- Hereditary conditions
  - Flavimaculatus
  - Vitelliform dystrophy
  - Other rare flecked retinopathies
- Active or recurrent multifocal retinochoroidopathies
  - Multiple evanescent white-dot syndrome
  - Punctate inner choroidopathy
  - Birdshot (vitiliginous) choroidopathy
  - Punctate outer retinal toxoplasmosis
- Dalen-Fuchs nodules of sympathetic ophthalmia or Vogt-Koyanagi-Harada syndrome

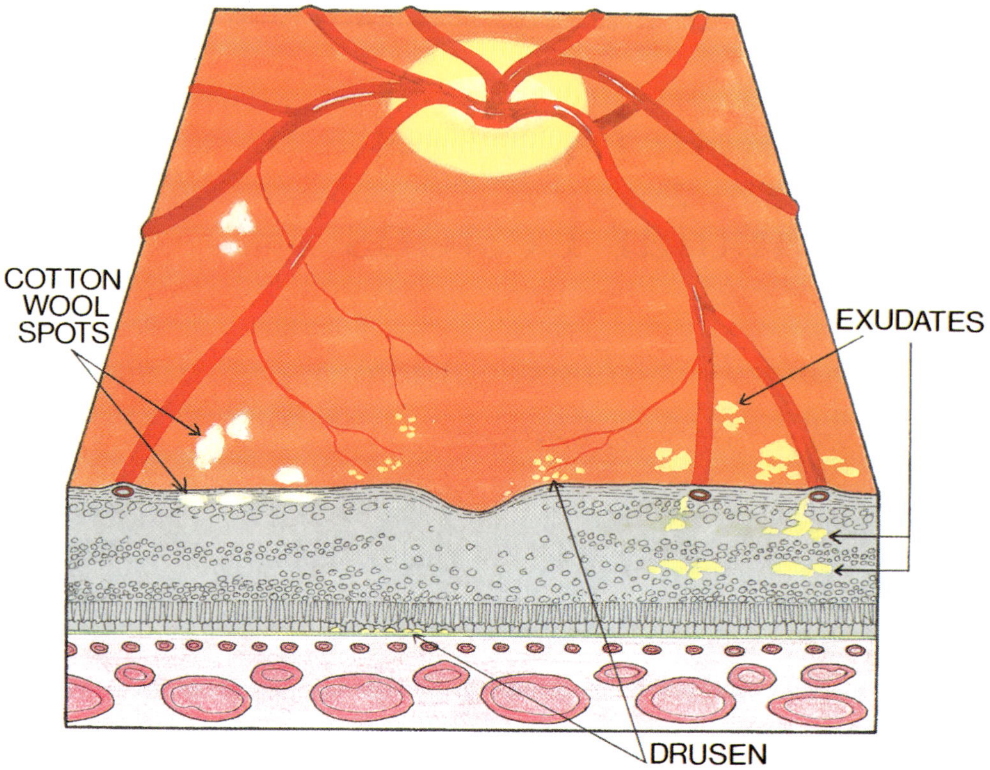

FIGURE 7.1. Illustration depicting the various examples of small, lightly colored macular lesions. The retinal vessels serve as a localizing reference for the depth of involvement within the retinal layers. Cotton wool spots lie in the superficial retinal layers and are evidence of capillary nonperfusion and retinal ischemia; hard exudates originate from the retinal vessels in the inner layers of the retina and eventually settle in the outer plexiform layer; drusen involve the outer retinal complex and lie between and within the retinal pigment epithelium and Bruch's membrane.

Refractile/Bright

Common
- Hard exudates in:
  - Diabetic retinopathy
  - Retinal vascular occlusive disease
  - Hypertensive retinopathy
  - Choroidal neovascularization
- Calcified drusen

Less common
- Hard exudates associated with uncommon retinal vascular disease
- Hard exudates associated with optic nerve head disorders (may be superficial or deep)

SMALL, SUPERFICIAL MACULAR LESIONS (FREQUENTLY SMALLER THAN 1 DD)

Nonrefractile

Common
- CWS
- Prevailing conditions causing CWS
  - Diabetic retinopathy
  - Venous occlusive disease
  - Collagen vascular disease
    - Systemic lupus erythematosus (SLE)
    - Polyarteritis nodosa
    - Giant cell arteritis
    - Scleroderma
  - Human immunodeficiency virus (HIV) or acquired immunodeficiency syndrome (AIDS) retinopathy
  - Hypertensive retinopathy
  - Embolic events

Conditions encountered less frequently
- Stasis retinopathies
- Hematologic disorders
  - Associated with malignancy
  - Associated with infection
- Active retinochoroiditis
  - Toxoplasmosis
  - Cytomegalovirus (CMV) retinitis
- Myelinated nerve fibers

Less common
- White-centered retinal hemorrhages
- Candida endophthalmitis

Refractile/Bright

Common
- Physiologic reflections from the internal limiting membrane of the retina and the vitreoretinal interface

- Epiretinal membrane or macular gliosis
- Retinal cholesterol emboli (Hollenhorst plaque)

Less common

- Tamoxifen retinopathy
- Talc retinopathy
- Bietti's crystalline tapetoretinal dystrophy and autosomal dominant crystalline dystrophy
- Oxalosis, primary and secondary
- Cystinosis
- Canthaxanthin ingestion

LARGE, MACULAR LESIONS (VARIABLE SIZE, MAY BE DEEP OR SUPERFICIAL, FREQUENTLY LARGER THAN 1 DD)

Common

- Disciform maculopathy
- Active retinochoroiditis
  - CMV retinitis (common only in immunocompromised patients)
  - Toxoplasmosis (also seen in immunocompromised patients)
- Myelinated nerve fibers

Less common

- Retinitis associated with syphilis or herpes virus (seen in immunocompromised patients)
- Active or recurrent multifocal retinochoroidopathies
  - Acute multifocal placoid pigment epitheliopathy
  - Serpiginous (geographic helicoid) choroidopathy
  - Diffuse unilateral subacute neuroretinitis
- *Pneumocystis carinii* pneumonia choroidopathy (seen in immunocompromised patients)
- Choroidal granuloma as seen in sarcoidosis
- Choroidal melanoma (amelanotic)
- Choroidal metastatic disease
- Choroidal hemangioma and osteoma
- Retinal arterial occlusive disease
- *Toxocara canis*
- Intraocular lymphoma (ocular reticulum cell sarcoma)
- Lymphoid or leukemic infiltration of the uvea
- Septic emboli
- CWS (superficial)

SMALL, DEEP, NONREFRACTILE MACULAR LESIONS

Common Conditions

Age-Related Drusen

There are different types of drusen observed in the fundus. Hard drusen are usually discrete, nonrefractile, and often occur in clusters in the macular area. Certain types of isolated drusen should be differentiated from hard exudates but otherwise have little significance. Almost all drusen are less than one-third DD in size, so any lesions larger than this probably represent another disease (Figure 7.2). Small drusen are usually numerous and bilateral; if lightly colored lesions are seen singularly or unilaterally, suspect another condition.

Risk profile

- >50 years
- White
- Family history (20% of patients)
- Lightly colored irides

Symptoms

- Visual acuity normal or reduced
- Possible dysmorphopsia

Diagnostic signs

- Common
  - Bilateral and symmetrical
  - Beige, yellow, or white
  - Nonrefractile (unless calcified)
  - Pigment changes
  - Deep to RPE
  - Indistinct borders with pigment ring
- Additional
  - Pigment atrophy and clumping
  - Peripheral reticular pigment degeneration

Other diagnostic considerations

- Rule out choroidal neovascularization (CNV) with exudates, hemorrhage, elevated macula
- CNV more likely with:
  - Soft, confluent drusen
  - Focal hyperpigmentation
  - Fellow eye involvement
- Amsler grid testing
- Patient education for dysmorphopsia or reduced visual acuity
- Fundus photography
- Monitor for CNV and age-related macular degeneration
- Under age 40 consider:
  - Dominantly inherited drusen
  - Multifocal choroidopathy
  - Fundus flavimaculatus
  - Cuticular drusen

Management

- Fluorescein angiography by retinologist if:
  - Dysmorphopsia or scotoma on Amsler grid testing
  - Sudden change in visual acuity
  - Signs of CNV
- Comanage with retinologist with contralateral exudative changes

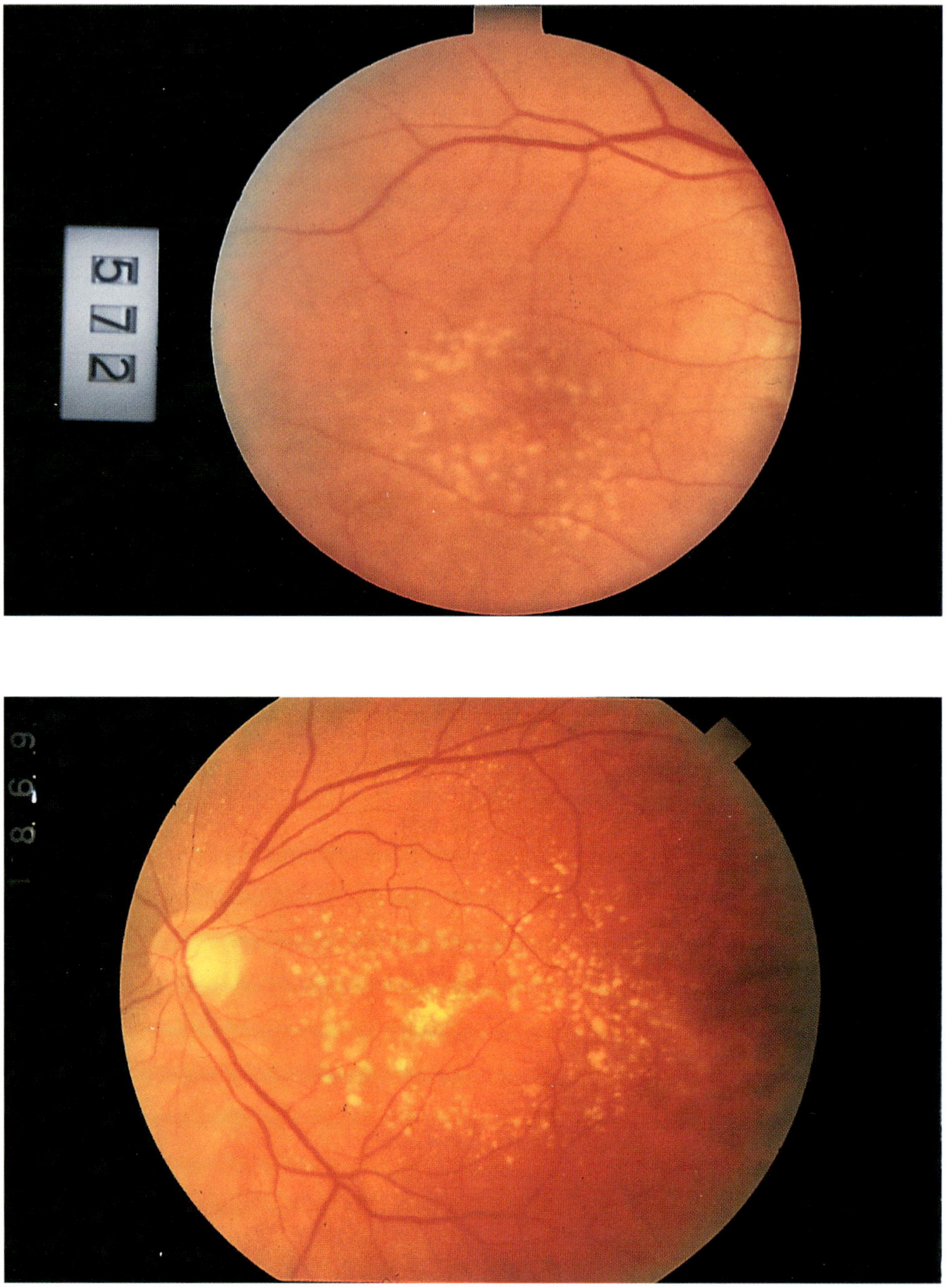

FIGURE 7.2. Two examples of hard drusen as a cause of small, lightly colored macular lesions. Drusen are often discrete and multiple, with a distribution throughout the posterior pole and elsewhere in the retina.

Punched-Out Lesions of Presumed Ocular Histoplasmosis

Lesions in presumed ocular histoplasmosis syndrome (POHS) are usually larger than drusen and are found singularly throughout the posterior pole, not grouped as in the macular drusen. The lesions sometimes take on a linear configuration (Figure 7.3) and are often surrounded by pigment. These lesions are part of a triad of clinical findings including peripapillary atrophy and CNV.

Presumed Ocular Histoplasmosis Syndrome

Risk profile
- Second to sixth decade
- Rare in blacks
- Endemic to major river valley regions, e.g., Mississippi and Ohio river valleys

Symptoms
- Only with macular involvement (blurred vision, dysmorphopsia, scotoma)

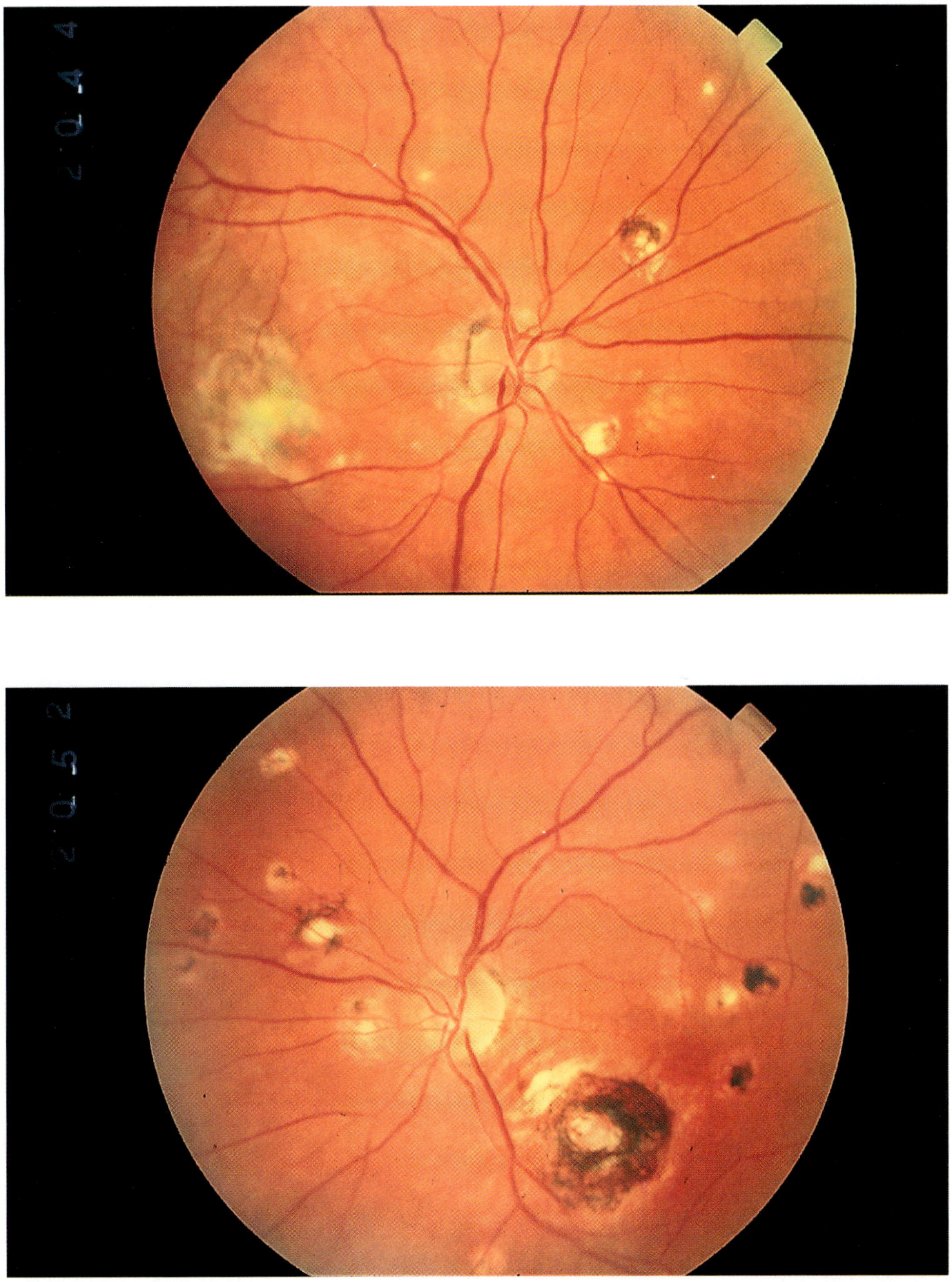

FIGURE 7.3. Examples of punched-out spots seen in presumed ocular histoplasmosis syndrome (top). Note the disciform scar in the macula caused by a hemorrhage from a choroidal neovascular membrane.

Diagnostic signs
- Common
  - Bilateral approximately 60%; asymmetrical
  - Punched-out white or yellow-white lesions with pigmented borders at level of choroid (300–1,000 μ in diameter)
  - Peripapillary atrophy approximately 85%
  - Exudative maculopathy approximately 4%
  - Absence of vitritis
- Additional
  - Vitreous hemorrhage rare
  - Disc edema (uncommon)

Other diagnostic considerations
- Rule out CNV (most common 10–20 years after punched-out macular lesions)
- Rule out other causes of choroidal neovascular membrane (CNVM)
- 75% with CNV are 30–49 years old
- Amsler grid testing
- Patient education for dysmorphopsia or reduced visual acuity
- Fundus photography
- Consider other multifocal choroidopathies

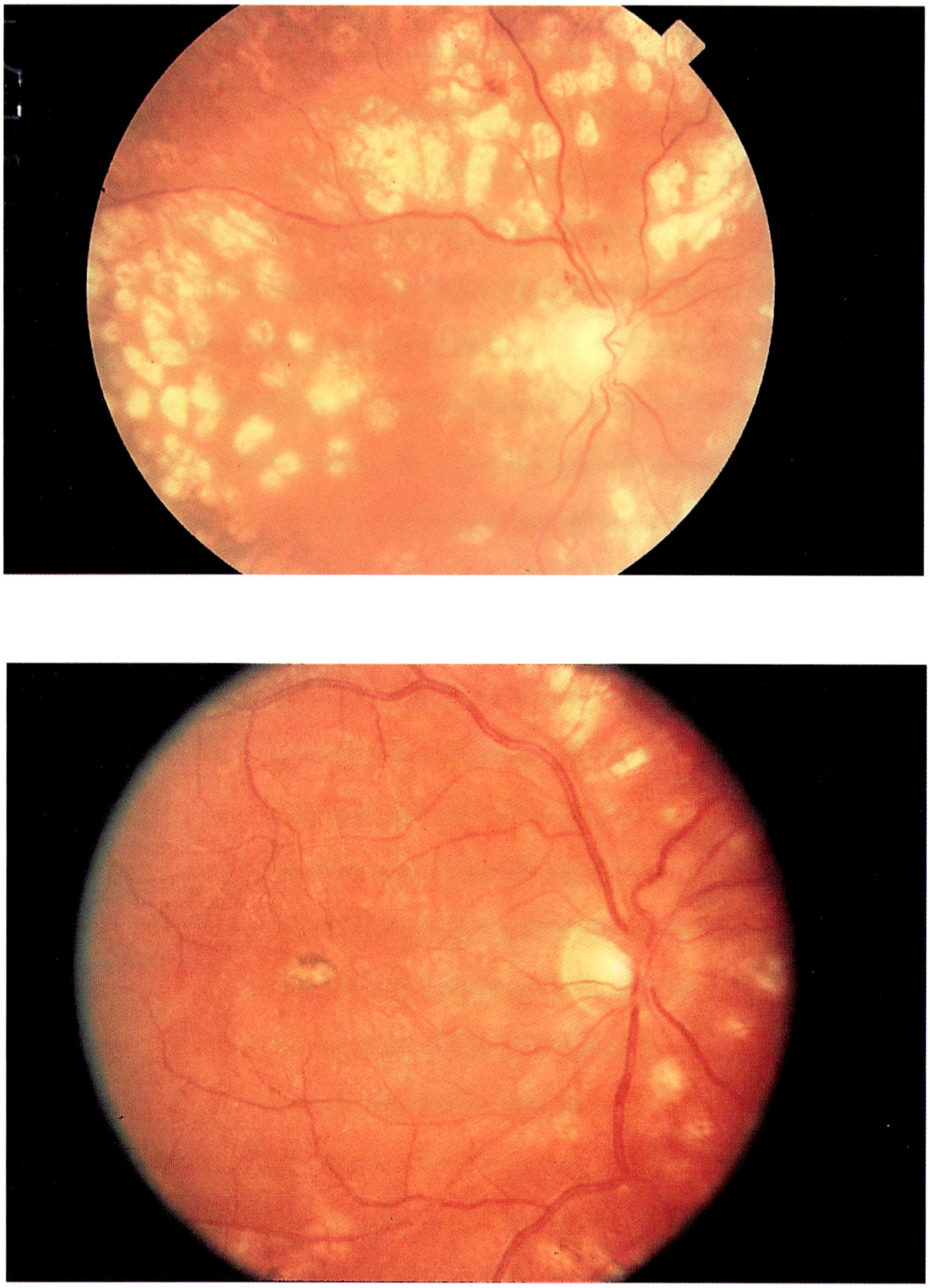

FIGURE 7.4. Examples of scars in the posterior pole from laser photocoagulation following ischemic central retinal vein occlusion.

Management

Fluorescein angiography by retinologist if:

- Dysmorphopsia or scotoma on Amsler grid
- Sudden visual acuity change
- Signs of CNV
- New or enlarging macular lesions

Laser Photocoagulation Scars

Scars from laser photocoagulation usually have accompanying pigment changes in a patient who has a corresponding history of laser therapy for edema secondary to diabetic retinopathy or branch retinal vein occlusion (Figure 7.4).

Following Laser Photocoagulation for Macular Edema

Risk profile

Laser therapy for macular edema

Symptoms

- Blurred vision
- Dysmorphopsia or scotoma
- Dyschromatopsia (typically blue-yellow defect)

Diagnostic signs
- Common
  - Obvious or faint individual yellow or white lesions
  - 200–400 μ lesions with RPE changes
- Additional
  - In diabetic patient look for:
    - Microaneurysm
    - Hemorrhage and exudate
    - Neovascularization of disc or elsewhere
  - In vascular occlusive disease look for:
    - Collateral vessels
    - Telangiectasis
    - RPE changes
    - Hemorrhage and exudate
    - Neovascularization with retinal ischemia

Other diagnostic considerations
- Look for capillary nonperfusion on fluorescein angiography in ischemic vascular occlusive disease
- Neovascularization of iris and neovascular glaucoma
- Vitreous hemorrhage possible up to 3 years following occlusive event
- Progression of nonproliferative diabetic retinopathy to proliferative diabetic retinopathy (PDR) may lead to significant loss of vision, neovascularization of iris, and glaucoma

Management
- Home Amsler grid testing
- Monitor diabetic patients with a history of macular edema every 3–6 months
- Monitor patients with vascular occlusive disease every 3 months for at least 1 year
- Fluorescein angiography by retinologist if:
  - New exudates
  - Retinal thickening
  - Dysmorphopsia/dyschromatopsia
  - Progressive blurred vision
  - Signs of neovascularization and vitreous hemorrhage

Less Common Conditions

Although age-related drusen are prevalent, many less common conditions may mimic drusen. The entities listed below should be considered when the clinical profile is not typical of age-related macular degeneration (AMD), particularly if the patient is less than age 50.

Less Common Causes of Small, Nonrefractile Lesions

Drusen in younger patients
- Dominantly inherited drusen
  - Second or third decade
  - Family history
  - Small, bright, bilateral lesions
- Basal laminar drusen
  - Bilateral
  - Fourth or fifth decade
  - Small lesions, more apparent by fluorescein angiography
- Both forms of drusen may lead to CNV; monitor for reduced visual function by home Amsler grid testing

Hereditary conditions (see Chapter 29)
- Flavimaculatus (Stargardt's disease)
  - Bilateral vision loss
  - Second or third decade
  - Usually round lesions with dark choroid on fluorescein angiography
- Vitelliform dystrophy
- Other rare flecked retinopathies
  - Fundus albipunctatus
  - Retinitis punctata albescens
  - Flecked retina of Kandori's
  - Kjellin's syndrome
  - Hallervorden-Spatz syndrome

Less common small, deep, nonrefractile lesions
- Multifocal retinochoroidopathies
  - Multiple evanescent white-dot syndrome
  - Punctate inner choroidopathy
  - Birdshot (vitiliginous) choroidopathy
- *Pneumocystis carinii* pneumonia choroidopathy
  - HIV+ patients
  - Bilateral, pale yellow, round lesions
  - 300 μ to 2 DD lesions at level of choroid
- Adult vitelliform macular dystrophy
  - Fifth to seventh decade
  - Bilateral, circular, raised yellow lesions
  - 300–750 μ in size
- Choroidal granuloma seen in sarcoidosis
  - Young adult blacks
  - Lightly colored lesions
  - Differentiate larger lesions from metastases
- Dalen-Fuchs nodules seen with
  - Vogt-Koyanagi-Harada syndrome
  - Sympathetic ophthalmia

SMALL, DEEP, REFRACTILE/BRIGHT MACULAR LESIONS

Common Conditions

A compromised retinal vasculature allows leakage of either or both lipids and protein and results in intraretinal or subretinal exudates. The three primary causes of hard exudates are retinal vascular disease, including diabetic retinopathy, CNV in AMD, and less commonly, compromised capillaries of the optic nerve head.

In diabetes, the duration of the disease is significant. In retinal venous occlusive disease, hypertension is a significant risk factor. In the case of CNV, exudates are an associated finding and may be differentiated from drusen by their brightness and the absence of RPE changes around the lesions.

Hard Exudates from Diabetic Retinopathy (see Chapter 24)

Risk profile
- Increased duration of diabetes
- Male > female subjects
- Blacks
- Longer duration of insulin-dependent diabetes
- Increased glycosylated hemoglobin
- Higher systemic blood pressure and increased proteinuria

Symptoms
- Visual acuity may be normal, blurred, or fluctuating
- Possible dysmorphopsia, dyschromatopsia (with macular edema)
- Scotoma if associated with RPE detachment

Diagnostic signs
- Common
  - Small, bright yellow lesions, frequent circinate or stellate pattern
  - Associated with macular thickening and microaneurysms
- Additional
  - Retinal hemorrhages
  - PDR
  - Intraretinal microvascular abnormalities

Other diagnostic considerations
- Rule out macular thickening indicating significant edema
- Decreased color vision or spatial contrast sensitivity testing when associated with macular edema
- Amsler grid testing

Management
- Fluorescein angiography by retinologist if:
  - Dysmorphopsia or scotoma on the Amsler grid
  - Sudden visual acuity change
  - Signs of macular edema
  - Comanagement after focal or grid laser photocoagulation treatment

Hard Exudates from Venous Occlusive Disease (see Chapter 25)

Risk profile
- Sixth and seventh decades
- Male > female subjects
- Hypertension and hyperlipidemia
- Hypercoagulation states and increased blood viscosity

Symptoms
- Visual acuity may be normal to significantly reduced depending on extent of macular involvement

Diagnostic signs
- Common
  - Unilateral exudates (limited to one quadrant of the retina in branch occlusion)
  - Hemorrhages and microaneurysms
  - CWS
  - Macular thickening
- Additional
  - Telangiectatic collateral vessels
  - Neovascularization at the disc or neovascularization elsewhere
  - Vitreous hemorrhage

Other diagnostic considerations
- Rule out macular thickening indicating edema
- Decreased color vision or spatial contrast sensitivity testing when associated with macular edema
- Amsler grid testing

Management
- Medical evaluation to rule out systemic disease
- Fluorescein angiography by retinologist if:
  - Dysmorphopsia or scotoma on Amsler grid testing
  - Sudden visual acuity change (especially if visual acuity <20/40)
  - Signs of macular edema
  - Comanagement after photocoagulation treatment

Hard Exudates from Hypertensive Retinopathy (see Chapter 25)

Risk profile
- Accelerated hypertension with diastolic pressure >110 mm Hg

Symptoms
- Visual acuity may be normal, fluctuating, or significantly reduced from macular thickening
- Diplopia (secondary to associated cranial nerve palsy)
- Mild-to-severe headache

Diagnostic signs
- Common
  - Vascular tortuosity and arteriolar narrowing
  - Stellate pattern of hard exudates and CWS

Flame-shaped hemorrhages
Disc edema, blurred margins, and hyperemia
Macular thickening
Additional
Choroidal hemorrhage with pigment changes
Other diagnostic considerations
May appear similar to venous occlusive disease but is bilateral
Exudates may remain after other signs have resolved
May be sign of chronically elevated blood pressure
Management
Immediate medical evaluation to control blood pressure
Blood pressure should be lowered gradually to avoid ischemic optic nerve changes and optic atrophy

Hard Exudates from Choroidal Neovascularization (see Chapters 12–15)

Risk profile
Patients at risk for CNV from:
AMD
POHS
Angioid streaks
Degenerative myopia/lacquer cracks
Choroidal rupture
Symptoms
Blurred vision
Dysmorphopsia, dyschromatopsia
Scotoma with RPE detachment
Diagnostic signs
Common
Unilateral presentation
Circinate or small groups of exudates
Intraretinal or subretinal hemorrhage
Serous neurosensory retinal detachment with elevation
Pigment changes and drusen
Additional
Vitreous hemorrhage
Other diagnostic considerations
Rule out other causes of hard exudates
Management
Immediate fluorescein angiography with retinologist to identify treatable CNVM
Home Amsler grid testing

Hard exudates are uniformly bright and have distinct borders. A circinate distribution emanating from a focus of vascular leakage is typical. They are usually found in the outer plexiform layer in the early stages of retinal vascular disease, but may be found subretinally in association with CNV or in the superficial sensory retina when macular edema becomes extensive.

A stellate or radial pattern may be apparent when exudates reside near the center of the macula, in the fiber layer of Henle (Figure 7.5). Hard exudates may remain visible for months after other fundus findings such as hemorrhages or disc abnormalities have resolved.

Calcified Drusen

Calcified drusen usually indicate long-standing drusen. This form of drusen may be seen in association with RPE geographic atrophy, and differentiating this form from lipid exudates may be difficult. Drusen are always deep to the RPE, whereas exudates are usually more superficial. Look for associated findings of AMD such as pigment changes and other noncalcified drusen. If viewed with high magnification, the examiner may recognize individual glistening particles within a single calcified drusen.

SMALL, SUPERFICIAL, NONREFRACTILE MACULAR LESIONS

Cotton Wool Spots

CWS are white or grayish-white and are often associated with retinal hemorrhages; drusen are usually not associated with hemorrhage unless CNV is present. CWS are a manifestation of capillary nonperfusion and retinal ischemia resulting from a retinal vascular or systemic disorder (see Chapter 26). The underlying cause of the CWS is a compromised retinal vessel endothelium or a blockage of a precapillary arteriole by abnormal blood components or emboli.

CWS may be differentiated from drusen and hard exudates based on their depth, shape, borders, color, and associated findings. Since they are found in the inner retinal layers, specifically the nerve fiber layer, CWS will often obscure a retinal blood vessel (Figure 7.6). CWS are usually elongated along one axis perpendicular to the nerve fiber layer, and the borders of CWS are feathered and blended compared with drusen and hard exudates, which have more distinct borders. Drusen often have accompanying pigment changes, whereas exudates and CWS generally do not.

The presence of one CWS requires a medical evaluation to rule out the numerous diseases that are associated with these lesions, with special emphasis placed on diabetes mellitus, hypertension, embolic disease, or collagen vascular disease. Numerous unilateral CWS with intraretinal hemorrhage in an older patient suggest retinal venous occlusive disease. Patients with risk characteristics for HIV should be carefully tested and monitored if CWS are detected. CWS associated with ischemic retinal venous occlusive disease tend to be slightly larger than in diabetes, HIV, and hypertension.

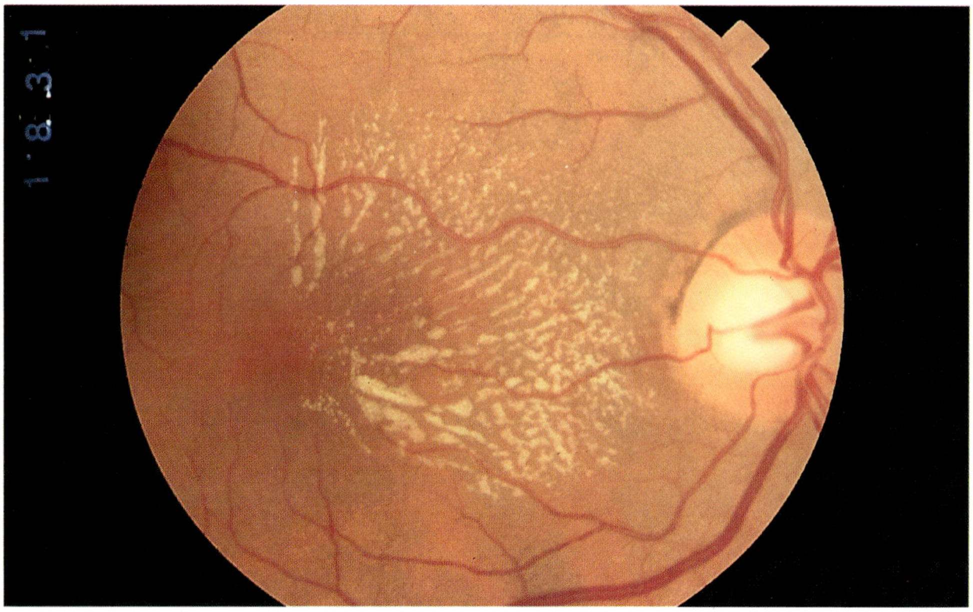

A

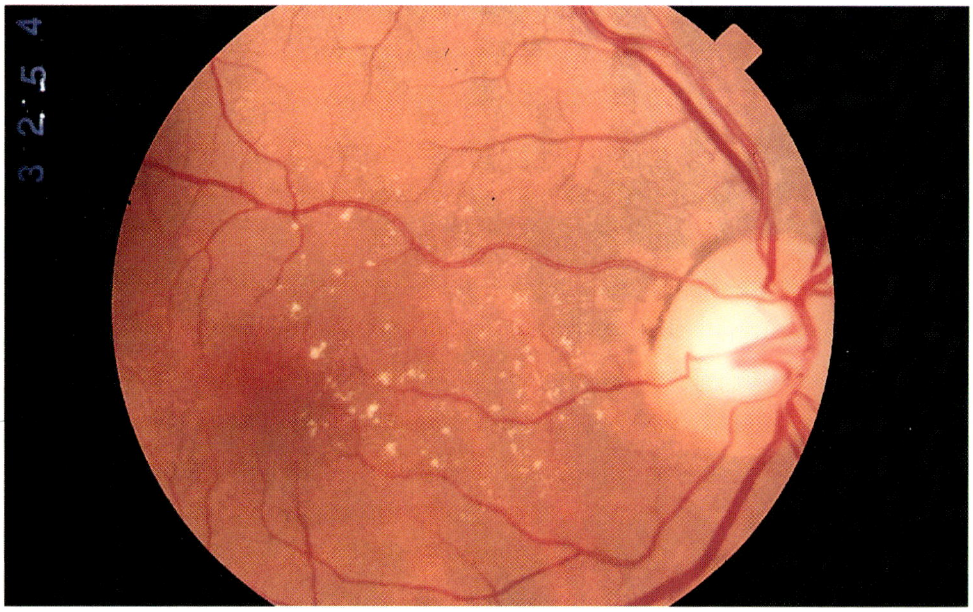

B

FIGURE 7.5. A. Hard exudates in a stellate pattern in the macula from a branch retinal vein occlusion in the right eye. B. Hard exudates in the same patient 3 months after the venous occlusion. The exudates consist of lipid material that deposits in the outer plexiform layer of the retina.

Cotton Wool Spots Associated with Diabetes Mellitus (see Chapter 24)

Risk profile
- Young or old diabetic patient
- Usually long-standing diabetes but may be the presenting clinical sign
- Poorly controlled blood glucose level

Symptoms
- Asymptomatic unless capillary nonperfusion is present
- Isolated, discrete scotoma

Diagnostic signs
- Common
  - Unilateral or bilateral
  - Usually within 3 DD of optic disc
  - Vary from 1–20 in number (average 4–5)
  - White or gray-white superficial lesions (nerve fiber layer)
  - Feathered, blended borders
  - 100–1,000 μ in size
- Additional
  - Capillary dilatation
  - Intraretinal microvascular abnormalities and venous beading

FIGURE 7.6. Cotton wool spots in a patient with AIDS with no other accompanying fundus changes (A) and along the inferior temporal arcade in a patient with a central retinal vein occlusion (B).

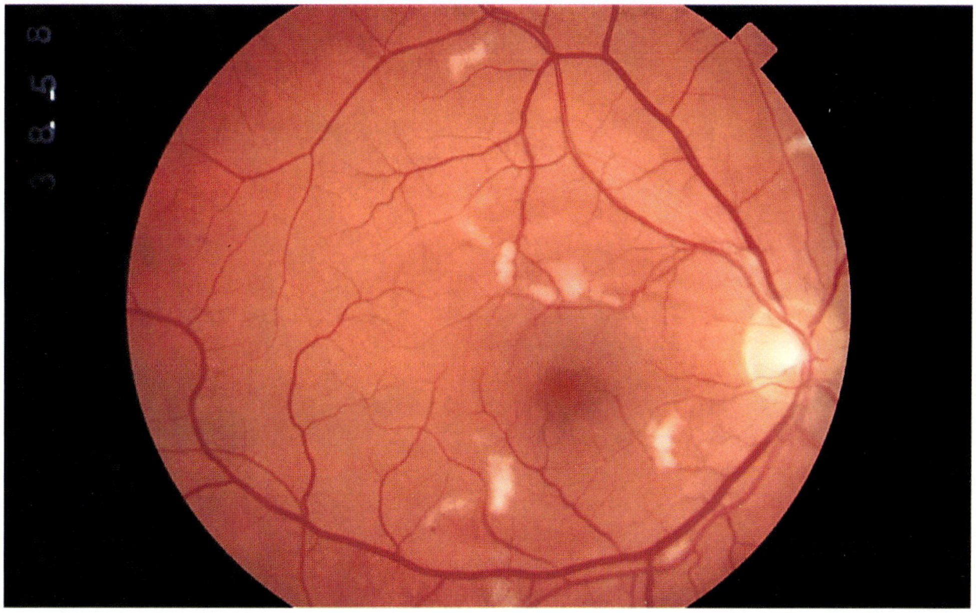

A

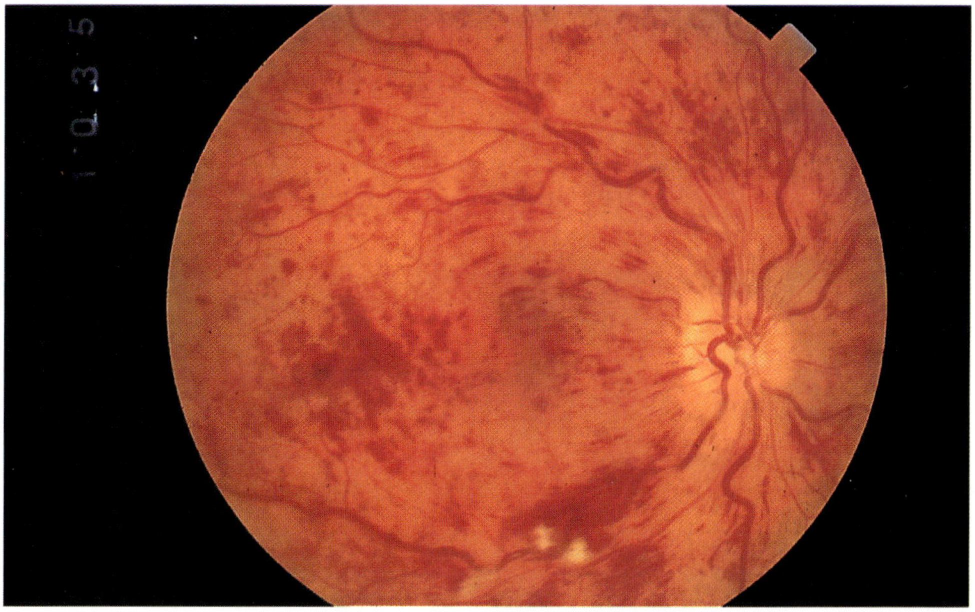

B

Other diagnostic considerations
- Indicate moderate or severe nonproliferative diabetic retinopathy
- CWS resolve slowly in diabetic patients (>8 months) compared with other causes of CWS (1–2 months)

Management
- Fluorescein angiography by retinologist if numerous CWS are present to rule out extensive capillary nonperfusion
- Rule out poorly controlled hypertension and diabetes

If unilateral in diabetic patient, rule out:
- Retinal venous occlusive component
- Carotid artery disease
- Glaucoma (to account for asymmetry of diabetic retinopathy)

Cotton Wool Spots in Hypertension

Risk profile
- Blood pressure >110 mm Hg, especially if rapid increase in blood pressure (accelerated hypertension)

Symptoms
- Usually visually asymptomatic

Diagnostic signs
- Common
  - CWS found within 2–3 DD of the disc; more commonly in temporal distribution and along arteries
  - Often bilateral

Additional ocular signs
- Flame-shaped intraretinal hemorrhage
- Attenuated arterioles
- Disc edema
- Choroidal hemorrhage and pigment changes
- Exudates in chronic hypertension

Other diagnostic considerations
- Clear in 6 weeks to 6 months depending on the severity of the hypertension; therefore, may be present after blood pressure has been elevated and then controlled. Measure blood pressure and discuss with patient's internist

Management
- Patients with hypertension and new CWS need immediate evaluation of their blood pressure (diastolic pressure is often >110 mm Hg) because of neurologic complications

Cotton Wool Spots Associated with Ischemic Venous Occlusive Disease

Risk profile
- Seventh decade
- Systemic diseases
  - Hypertension
  - Hypercoagulation and hyperviscosity states
  - Diabetes mellitus

Symptoms
- Sudden blurred vision
- Central scotoma

Diagnostic signs
- Common
  - Disc edema
  - Macular edema
  - Numerous CWS along vascular arcades
  - Dot, blot, and flame-shaped hemorrhages
- Additional
  - Neovascularization at the disc or neovascularization elsewhere
  - Neovascularization of iris with secondary glaucoma
  - Rule out primary open-angle glaucoma

Other diagnostic considerations
- Hard exudates and macular edema may also be present

Management
- Fluorescein angiography by retinologist to rule out extensive capillary nonperfusion
- Rule out hypertension
- Topical antiglaucoma agents if intraocular pressure >20 mm Hg or other signs of glaucoma are present
- Anticoagulant therapy
- Medical evaluation

Cotton Wool Spots Associated with the Human Immunodeficiency Virus and Acquired Immunodeficiency Syndrome Retinopathy

Risk profile
- High-risk characteristics for HIV and AIDS including intravenous drug abuser, homosexual men, bisexuals, heterosexual contact with an infected person, transfusion recipients

Symptoms
- No visual symptoms unless concurrent CMV retinitis is present
- May have discrete scotomas

Diagnostic signs
- Common
  - Peripapillary distribution of CWS near vascular arcades, 3–4 DD from optic disc
- Additional
  - Lesions tend to be smaller than those found in diabetes, hypertension, and venous occlusive disease
  - Usually found in the absence of retinal hemorrhages

Other diagnostic considerations
- Differentiate from CMV retinitis (vitritis)
- AIDS patients with CMS have a guarded prognosis, since CWS is associated with a low CD4 count and worsening medical condition
- CMV retinitis may advance rapidly

Management
- Medical evaluation
- Retinology consult to consider treatment with ganciclovir or foscarnet for CMV retinitis

Cotton Wool Spots in Systemic Lupus Erythematosus

Risk profile
- Female
- Less than 40 years of age
- Patients with exacerbation of systemic disease

- Symptoms
  - May have visual field loss corresponding to area of infarction
- Diagnostic signs
  - Common
    - CWS with or without intraretinal hemorrhages
- Additional ocular signs
  - Vasculitis
  - Papilledema
  - Ischemic optic neuropathy
  - Retinal artery occlusions
  - Retinal vein occlusions
  - Serous retinal detachment
- Other diagnostic considerations
  - Retinopathy often associated with exacerbation of systemic disease
  - May have concurrent hypertension
  - Systemic signs and symptoms include rashes, malaise, joint pain, arthritis, fever, weight loss, enlarged spleen, and adenopathy
  - Many patients with SLE take hydroxychloroquine or prednisone, which have side effects of retinopathy, cataracts, and glaucoma and thus require frequent monitoring
- Management
  - Consultation with an internist or rheumatologist to control systemic disease
  - Patient education regarding symptoms of retinal vascular occlusive disease and monitor every 4–6 months

CWS are also observed in collagen vascular disease and often represent one of the first manifestations of the condition. A diverse group of diseases is included in the category of collagen vascular diseases, including SLE (the most common), polyarteritis nodosa, scleroderma, dermatomyositis, and giant cell arteritis.

SLE usually begins in the third or fourth decade and affects mostly white or black women who have other systemic findings, including rash, malaise, joint pain, arthritis, fever, weight loss, enlarged spleen, and adenopathy. Retinopathy is reported to occur in about 8% of patients. CWS are the most common retinal finding and are found in approximately 50% of patients with retinopathy. Other retinal findings include retinal hemorrhages, vasculitis, papilledema, ischemic optic neuropathy, central retinal artery occlusion, central retinal vein occlusion, and serous retinal detachment. Retinopathy usually coincides with the active stage of SLE and is associated with a shorter survival time. Patients with only CWS or hemorrhages generally have good visual acuity. Hypertension and renal disease are commonly found in patients with retinopathy and active SLE. These patients are often taking hydroxychloroquine or oral corticosteroids that have well-known ocular side effects.

Polyarteritis nodosa occurs in middle-aged men and causes a necrotizing arteritis of many organ systems, particularly the renal system. Asthma, hypertension, myalgia, and neuropathy are associated conditions. CWS may be the only ocular abnormality; retinal vasculitis and ischemic optic neuropathy are other retinal abnormalities found in patients with this disease.

Scleroderma causes vascular and degenerative changes in connective tissue, including rigidity of the skin, renal disease, gastrointestinal disorders, pulmonary involvement, and heart disease. CWS are reported in this condition as well and may be related to associated hypertension.

Retinopathy in dermatomyositis is more common in children than adults. CWS are the most common retinal finding in these patients.

Giant cell arteritis, an autoimmune vasculitis, is known to be associated with anterior ischemic optic neuropathy. Disc hemorrhages and CWS may be seen in an older patient with sudden vision loss often associated with headache, scalp tenderness, jaw claudication, weight loss, and malaise. Altitudinal visual field defects are often seen with anterior ischemic optic neuropathy. If these conditions are suspected, additional diagnostic considerations include obtaining an erythrocyte sedimentation rate and immediate referral for a medical evaluation, especially if giant cell arteritis is suspected on the basis of age and symptoms.

Conditions Encountered Less Frequently

CWS may occur due to occlusion of an arteriole or due to damage to the endothelial lining of the retinal vessel. They may be a sign of carotid occlusive disease or cardiac valvular disease due to embolic disease. As with retinal cholesterol emboli, if these conditions are suspected, palpation and ascultation of the carotid artery as well as referral for a vascular evaluation is warranted.

Less Common Causes of Cotton Wool Spots

This list is adapted from GC Brown et al. Cotton-wool spots. Retina 1985;5:206–214; and JD Sapira. An internist looks at the fundus oculi. Dis Mon 1984;30:20–22.

- Embolic causes
  - Cardiac valvular disease
  - Partial central retinal arterial occlusion
  - Intravenous drug abuse, talc emboli
  - Purtscher's retinopathy
    - Posttraumatic
    - Fat or air emboli
    - Leukocyte aggregation
  - Acute pancreatitis
  - Chronic renal failure
  - Lupus anticoagulant retinopathy

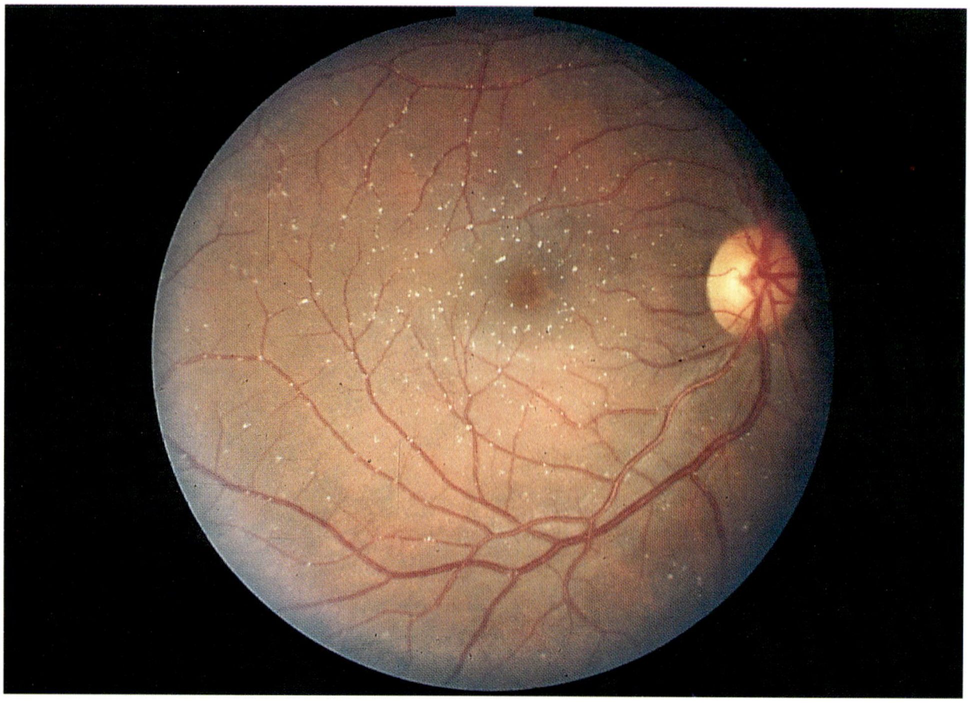

FIGURE 7.7. Lightly colored lesions distributed throughout the macula in the left eye of a patient with talc retinopathy. (Courtesy of G. Selvin.)

- Stasis retinopathies
  - Carotid occlusive disease
  - Aortic arch disease
  - Ocular ischemic syndrome
- Hematologic disorders
  - Leukemia
  - Multiple myeloma
  - Macroglobulinema
  - Sickle cell disease
  - Cryoglobulinemia
  - Aplastic or pernicious anemia
  - Dysproteinemia
  - Acute blood loss
- Malignancy related
  - Radiation retinopathy
  - Following bone marrow transplantation
  - Hodgkin's disease
  - Metastatic carcinoma
- Infectious causes
  - Rocky Mountain spotted fever
  - Leptospirosis
  - Septicemia
  - Onchocerciasis
  - Toxoplasmosis
- Other causes
  - Toxemia of pregnancy
  - Renal failure
  - High-altitude retinopathy
  - Papilledema
  - Papillitis

Other embolic diseases cause CWS by occluding small retinal vessels. Talc emboli are seen in intravenous drug abusers (Figure 7.7). Fat or air emboli as well as leukocyte aggregation have also been suggested as the cause of Purtscher's retinopathy, a condition that manifests CWS and hemorrhage following a severe Valsalva's maneuver, and in severe crushing trauma to the thorax and abdomen. A Purtscher-like retinopathy has been described in patients who suffer emboli as a result of other conditions such as acute pancreatitis, chronic renal failure, or long bone fractures.

Multiple arteriole and venous occlusions with CWS are seen in lupus anticoagulant retinopathy. This condition is seen in patients of both sexes, usually aged 30–40, who have lupus anticoagulant immunoglobulin in the serum. Abnormal platelet embolization may be responsible for the retinopathy. Many of these patients do not have clinical signs consistent with SLE and may have one of several other systemic diseases.

Severe stenosis of the carotid arteries in older patients or gradual occlusion of the aortic arch and branches (pulseless disease) in younger patients has been reported in association with CWS. Associated ischemic ocular signs may include engorged conjunctival vessels, corneal changes, including stromal edema and folds in Descemet's membrane, anterior chamber cells, retinal or iris neovascularization, and resultant complications.

CWS seen in association with leukemia or anemia are often observed with retinal hemorrhages. This retinopathy seems to occur in patients with both low platelet counts (thrombocytopenia) and severe anemia (Hgb <6.6–8.0 g/dl).

Approximately 30–40% of patients with radiation retinopathy have CWS as part of their presentation, which generally occurs 6 months to 3 years following radiation to the head or eye and is a progressive condition appear-

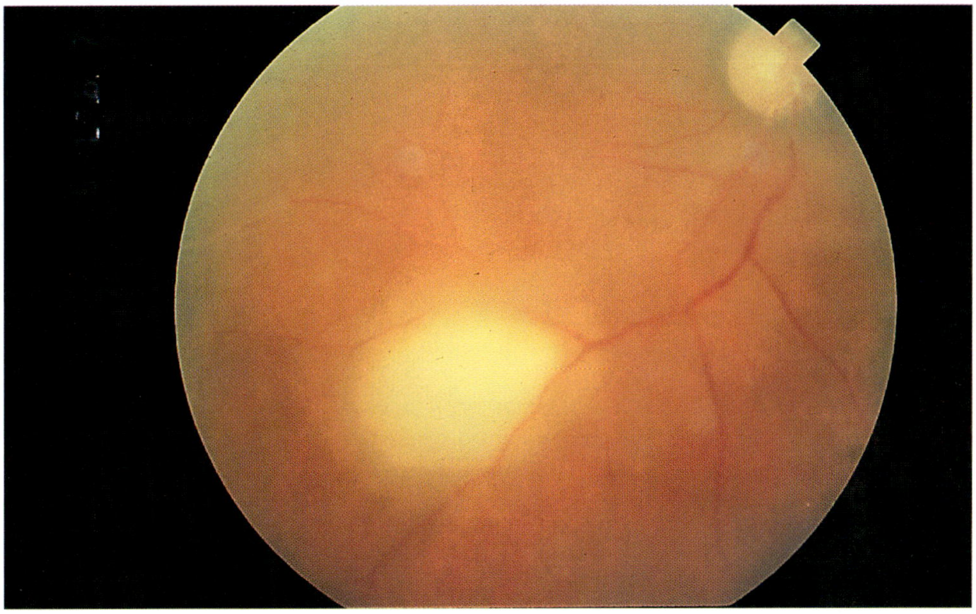

FIGURE 7.8. Reactivation of toxoplasmosis retinochoroiditis manifests with lightly colored lesions of varying sizes. Active toxoplasmosis retinochoroiditis is also a cause of large white lesions with indistinct borders. Satellite lesions are sometimes observed, and cells, including hemorrhage, and inflammatory material in the vitreous are a constant finding with toxoplasmosis.

ing similar to diabetic retinopathy. Bilateral, reversible CWS have also been reported in patients following bone marrow transplantation who also received total body irradiation and cyclosporin.

Infectious diseases such as Rocky Mountain spotted fever and leptospirosis may cause CWS along with the fever, myalgia, and malaise observed with these conditions. Other retinal changes in Rocky Mountain spotted fever include venous engorgement, retinal edema, hemorrhages, and papilledema.

Toxemia usually occurs after the sixth month of pregnancy and is associated with a diastolic pressure of greater than 100 mm Hg. High-altitude retinopathy occurs in over one-third of patients who are exposed to altitudes over 5,000 m, especially those who are not acclimatized. Associated fundus findings include tortuosity and engorgement of retinal vessels, disc hyperemia, and intraretinal hemorrhages. CWS are found in a small minority of these patients. CWS are also associated with disc swelling as in papillitis, papilledema, or central retinal vein occlusion, so any patient with CWS should have a careful examination of the disc.

Active Retinochoroiditis Caused by Toxoplasmosis

Toxoplasmosis retinochoroiditis may cause superficial nonrefractile lesions in the posterior pole and the macular area (see Chapter 20). These lesions occur with reactivation of the disease and are observed in patients with a history of exposure to the Toxoplasma gondii organism during pregnancy or in AIDS patients, where the disease is one of the most common opportunistic infections.

The lesions of toxoplasmosis may be small and superficial or they may enlarge during the acute, reactivation stage (Figure 7.8). There is an accompanying vitritis, and there may be an anterior chamber reaction. Toxoplasmosis must be differentiated from CMV retinitis and herpes simplex retinitis, two common causes of retinochoroiditis in the immunocompromised patient.

Toxoplasmosis Retinochoroiditis

- Risk profile
  - Initial attack approximately 30 years of age (range, 7 to >60 years)
  - Whites > blacks
  - Family history—mother infected with toxoplasmosis during pregnancy
  - Ingestion of uncooked meat
  - HIV+, AIDS
- Symptoms
  - Floaters
  - Blurred vision
  - Eye sometimes painful
  - Photophobia
- Diagnostic signs
  - Common
    - White or yellow-white, fluffy, elevated lesion in posterior pole
    - Active lesion usually unilateral
    - Size varies from specks to 4–5 DD
    - Old pigmented chorioretinal scar adjacent to active lesion and in fellow eye
    - Vitritis
  - Additional
    - Anterior chamber reaction
    - Hemorrhage (less common and less extensive than in CMV retinitis)

- Optic atrophy
- Other diagnostic considerations
  - Often associated with optic neuritis and encephalitis in AIDS patients
  - Elevated IgG and IgM titers
  - Consider other causes of retinochoroiditis, especially if titer results are negative
    - Toxocariasis
    - Herpes simplex retinitis
    - Acute retinal necrosis
- Management
  - Retinal consultation
  - Mydriatics or cycloplegics for anterior uveitis
  - Systemic and sub-Tenon's injection of corticosteroids
  - Trisulfapyrimidones and clindamycin
  - Vitrectomy

Cytomegalovirus Retinitis

- Risk profile
  - Male > female subjects, any age
  - HIV+, AIDS
  - Immunocompromised states resulting from:
    - Chemotherapy
    - Malignancies
    - Organ transplantation
- Symptoms
  - Floaters
  - Blurred vision
  - Dysmorphopsia or scotoma
  - Photopsia
- Diagnostic signs
  - Common
    - Large patches of white or yellow-white retina
    - Large intraretinal hemorrhage along arcardes ("brushfire hemorrhage")
    - One-third of cases are bilateral
    - Mild-to-moderate vitritis
  - Additional
    - Nongranulomatous anterior uveitis
    - Rhegmatogenous retinal detachment
- Other diagnostic considerations
  - HIV+ status usually already established
  - CWS may be present
  - Consider other causes of retinochoroiditis:
    - Syphilis
    - Toxoplasmosis
    - Herpes simplex retinitis
  - Life expectancy <1 year
- Management
  - Immediate retinal consultation
  - Therapy with ganciclovir and foscarnet

Medullated Nerve Fibers

Medullation of nerve fibers may mimic the appearance of CWS if it occurs along the retinal vascular arcades away from the macula. The absence of associated retinal hemorrhage, the singular nature of medullation, plus the striated, feathered borders, location along the nerve fiber layer distribution, and lack of progression or regression of the lesion all help establish the diagnosis.

Less Common Conditions

Superficial nonrefractile lesions may be observed in the retina as a result of rare conditions that cause CWS. Other conditions presenting as superficial nonrefractile lesions include white-centered retinal hemorrhages and candida endophthalmitis.

White-Centered Retinal Hemorrhages

A white-centered retinal hemorrhage has commonly been referred to as a Roth spot (see Chapter 27). The white center is often composed of a platelet and fibrin aggregate, although it may also be composed of leukocytes. Occasionally, an infarction of the nerve fiber layer, a CWS, lying over or near a retinal hemorrhage may mimic a white-centered retinal hemorrhage. A number of systemic conditions have been known to cause white-centered retinal hemorrhages; diabetes and leukemia are two of the more common conditions associated with them.

This list is modified from JD Sapira. An internist looks at the fundus oculi. Dis Mon 1984;30:30–34.

- Causes
  - Diabetic retinopathy
  - Leukemia
  - Subacute bacterial endocarditis
  - Septicemia
  - Multiple myeloma
  - Anemia
  - Thrombocytopenia
  - Hypertension
  - Collagen vascular disease
  - Following hemorrhaging, child battering, and anesthetic intubation
  - Oral contraceptives
  - AIDS
  - High-altitude retinopathy

A septic embolus may mimic a white-centered retinal hemorrhage. An infective endocarditis should be considered as the underlying systemic cause. Patients with infective endocarditis commonly have a history of rheumatic valve disease or other risk factors, including drug use, mitral valve prolapse, prosthetic heart valves, aortic systolic murmur, or other congenital heart conditions. Systemic symptoms include fever, fatigue, weight loss, backache, arthralgias, or abdominal pain.

Candida Endophthalmitis

Intraocular candida infection occurs in patients who are immunosuppressed by malignancy, medications, or other conditions such as HIV, alcoholism, diabetes, or dysproteinemia, as well as in hospitalized postsurgical patients or patients receiving intravenous fluids. The typical presentation is multiple white, fluffy lesions projecting into the vitreous in the posterior pole.

Associated ocular findings include anterior chamber reaction, white-centered retinal hemorrhages, and papillitis. Referral for amphotericin B or surgical treatment is indicated.

SMALL, SUPERFICIAL, REFRACTILE AND BRIGHT MACULAR LESIONS

Incidental Fundus Reflections and Epiretinal Membrane

Patients under age 40 commonly demonstrate normal retinal reflections near the vascular arcades and as a perifoveal annular reflex. As the light of the examining instrument moves across the fundus, these multiple reflections appear and disappear. This is unlike other intraretinal refractile lesions, such as hard exudates or calcified drusen, which remain visible regardless of the direction of illumination or viewing angle.

Reflections in Epiretinal Membrane

- Risk profile
  - Sixth to seventh decade in idiopathic cases
  - Whites
  - Family history (20% of patients)
  - Female > male subjects
  - History of:
    - Intraocular surgery or laser photocoagulation
    - Blunt trauma
    - Chronic inflammation
    - Branch retinal vein occlusion or hypertensive retinopathy
- Symptom
  - Blurred vision/dysmorphopsia
- Diagnostic signs
  - Common
    - Wrinkling of the internal limiting membrane
    - Macular reflections
    - Posterior vitreous detachment
    - Macular cyst or hole
  - Additional
    - Reflections are fleeting (as with incidental reflexes)
    - Associated with traction lines or folds in the retina
- Other diagnostic considerations
  - Myopia
  - Chronic uveitis
  - History of retinal vascular occlusive disease
- Management
  - Retinology consult if:
    - Visual acuity <20/60
    - Macular hole in fellow eye or vitreoretinal traction
    - Associated with cystoid macular edema

Idiopathic epiretinal membrane occurs in adults in the sixth or seventh decade. The membrane is not secondary to any specific ocular disease state and visual acuity is only minimally affected (see Chapter 18).

Not all retinal reflections are normal. Abnormal reflections are often found in association with other macular lesions such as epiretinal membranes, wrinkles or folds, pigment changes, hemorrhage, or vascular abnormalities. Refractile lesions in the sensory retina located slightly deeper than the internal limiting membrane usually represent a pathologic state. For example, a single reflection in or on an arteriole may indicate a retinal cholesterol embolus, whereas multiple refractile particles may occur in conditions such as tamoxifen or talc retinopathy.

Retinal Cholesterol Emboli (Hollenhorst's Plaque)

Retinal cholesterol emboli are observed in the more superficial level of the retina, usually at the bifurcations of retinal arterioles. There are generally no pigment changes, hemorrhages, edema, or exudates associated with these lesions, and therefore, they may be easily differentiated from other causes of bright refractile lesions. The emboli are frequently transient and may be mistaken for incidental reflections. They are flat, plate-like, highly glistening, and often appear larger than the vessel width and may sometimes be dislodged by applying pressure on the globe (Figure 7.9).

- Risk profile
  - Sixth decade or beyond
  - History of hypercholesterolemia, hyperlipidemia
  - History of vascular disease of the carotid artery, heart, or large vessels coming from the heart
- Symptoms
  - Often asymptomatic
  - Monocular, transient loss of vision
  - Shade or curtain obscuring vision

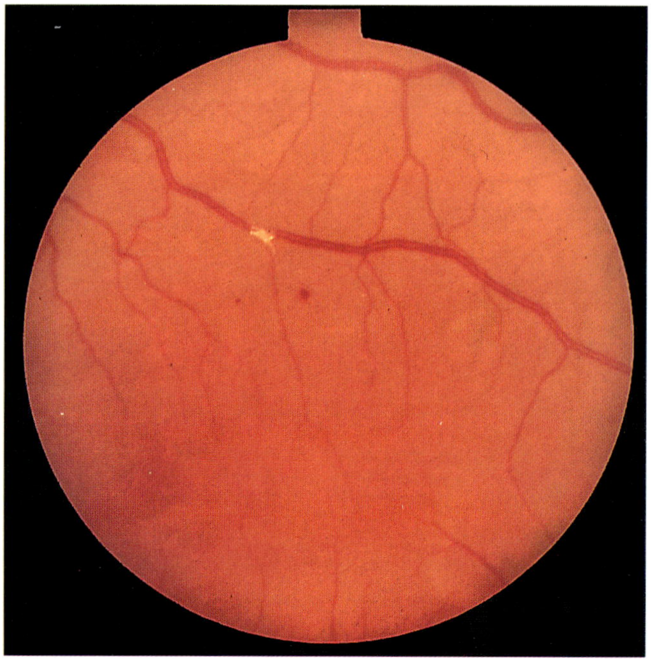

FIGURE 7.9. A cholesterol plaque in a patient with retinal arterial occlusive disease. The lesion is located in the more superficial plane of the retinal vessels.

- Hemiplegia, hemianesthesia, slurred speech
- Diagnostic signs
  - Common
    - Branch or central retinal artery occlusion
    - Attenuated and sheathed arterioles
    - Ocular ischemic syndrome
  - Additional
    - Ghost vessels
    - Cherry red spot in macula
    - Delayed arteriole filling on fluorescein angiography (arteriole may recanalize over time)
- Other diagnostic considerations
  - Auscultation and palpation of carotid arteries
  - Differentiate from fibrin or platelet, calcific, mycotic, fat, and talc emboli
  - Doppler ultrasound of carotid arteries
- Management
  - Prompt medical evaluation

Uncommon Conditions

Other retinal vascular conditions may cause hard exudates and are associated with abnormalities of the retinal vasculature, i.e., microaneurysms, telangiectasis (dilated vessels), or macroaneurysms. Exudates are often, but not always, found in proximity to abnormal vasculature. In any patient with exudate, the clinician should search for telangiectasia, microaneurysms or macroaneurysms, or saccular vessels, including the equatorial and peripheral retina.

Optic nerve conditions may also be associated with hard macular exudates. Although unusual, conditions that cause compromise of the peripapillary vasculature may give rise to hard macular exudates. Lipid and protein leak from these vessels into the outer plexiform layer between the disc and the macula, resulting in a partial or complete macular star. Optic nerve disorders, such as papilledema and optic neuritis, can be associated with hard exudates. Such findings usually indicate the chronic nature of the optic nerve disease.

Less Common Causes of Small, Refractile Lesions

- Uncommon retinal vascular disorders associated with hard exudates:
  - Radiation retinopathy
    - Patients who have received irradiation of ocular or intracranial tumors
    - Latent period of several months
    - Mimics diabetic retinopathy
  - Coats' disease
    - Unilateral; typically young men
    - Retinal telangiectasis, microaneurysms and macroaneurysms that begin in peripheral retina and extend to macula
  - Retinal macroaneurysms
    - Elderly female patient with history of hypertension and systemic vascular disease
  - Angiomatosis retinae
    - Young adults with family history
    - Bilateral 30–50%
    - Macular exudates common
  - Leber's miliary aneurysm
    - Elderly patients
    - Variation of Coats' disease with less exudation
  - Idiopathic parafoveal telangiectasis
- Optic nerve disorders associated with hard exudates
  - Leber's idiopathic stellate optic neuritis
    - Unilateral; young patients
    - Viral prodrome
    - Stellate maculopathy with vitreous cells
    - May be associated with cat scratch fever
    - Spontaneous resolution
  - Other causes of neuroretinitis
    - Lyme disease
    - Syphilis
    - Toxocara canis
    - Toxoplasmosis
    - Tuberculosis
- Less common miscellaneous causes:

Tamoxifen retinopathy
- Following mastectomy for breast cancer
- Vision loss reversible

Talc emboli
- Long-term intravenous drug use
- Small, yellow crystals in parafoveal arterioles

Bietti's dystrophies
- Rare; third decade
- Yellow-white crystals in the inner and outer layers in posterior pole with yellow crystals in peripheral cornea

Oxylosis
- Inborn error of metabolism with short life expectancy
- Black geographic lesions in macula with optic atrophy
- Calcium oxalate crystals in retina of infants

Cystinosis
- Inborn error of metabolism
- Pigmented disturbances observed in children

Canthaxanthin
- Oral synthetic suntanning agent
- Vision not affected but retinal sensitivity as measured by automated visual fields may be decreased

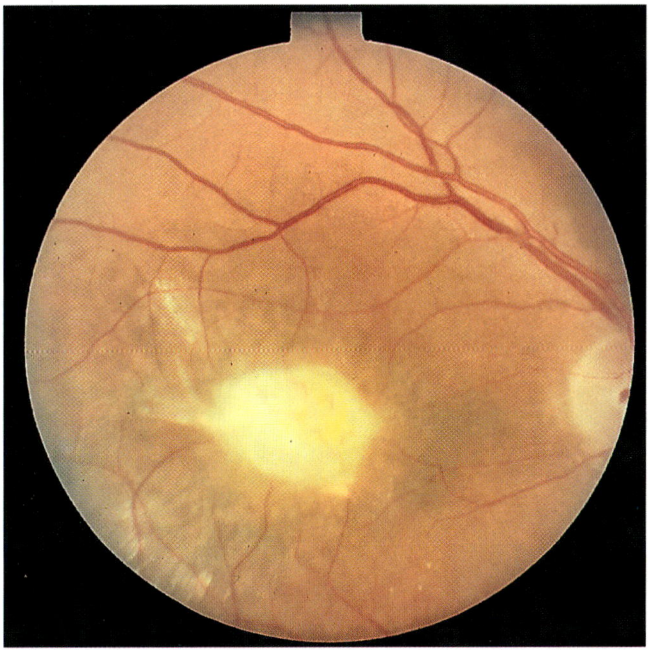

FIGURE 7.10. A disciform scar in the macula following an exudative maculopathy.

LARGE, LIGHTLY COLORED MACULAR LESIONS

Large, lightly colored macular lesions are described as typically being larger than 1 DD, uniformly white, gray-white, yellow-white, or yellow. Some of the same conditions already described under small, lightly colored lesions may present as larger lesions as well and therefore are not discussed in detail.

While pigment is often observed surrounding or within the lesions caused by toxoplasmosis or disciform maculopathy, occasionally these conditions may present as lightly colored lesions with minimal or no pigment changes and are therefore listed here as well as in the section on small, lightly colored macular lesions.

Common Conditions

Numerous conditions may cause large, lightly colored lesions, but only a few are commonly seen. Disciform maculopathy following CNV and retinochoroiditis are two of the most common entities that present in this fashion.

Retinochoroiditis may be differentiated from disciform scarring by the accompanying vitritis and occasionally other signs of ocular inflammation, including hyperemia, photophobia, pain, and anterior chamber reaction.

Disciform maculopathy may present as a large, off-white or yellow-white scar usually found in the macula (Figure 7.10). The lesion may appear elevated as a result of the fibrous tissue that infiltrates the subretinal space. Risk profile includes conditions that lead to CNVM. Associated symptoms include blurred vision and a dense scotoma since the photoreceptors are destroyed or covered over by the disciform scar. Associated ocular signs may include conditions such as drusen, or angioid streaks. Disciform scars observed in POHS tend to be smaller. Any patient with a monocular disciform scar should be monitored frequently since this condition is often bilateral (see Chapters 12–15).

Retinitis Caused by Toxoplasmosis or Cytomegalovirus

Retinitis from toxoplasmosis may manifest in a large necrotizing form with or without an associated pigmented chorioretinal scar (Figure 7.11) (see Chapters 20 and 23). These may occasionally be multifocal and bilateral. A moderate-to-severe vitritis is common, and an anterior uveitis is often present. In immunocompetent patients, toxoplasmosis is the most common form of retinochoroiditis. In AIDS patients, toxoplasmosis should be considered in the differential diagnosis of retinochorioiditis, but is much less common than CMV retinitis.

CMV retinitis, common among AIDS patients, may be extensive before the patient seeks treatment, especially since the lesions may be initially found in the peripheral fundus, where they may not produce any symptoms.

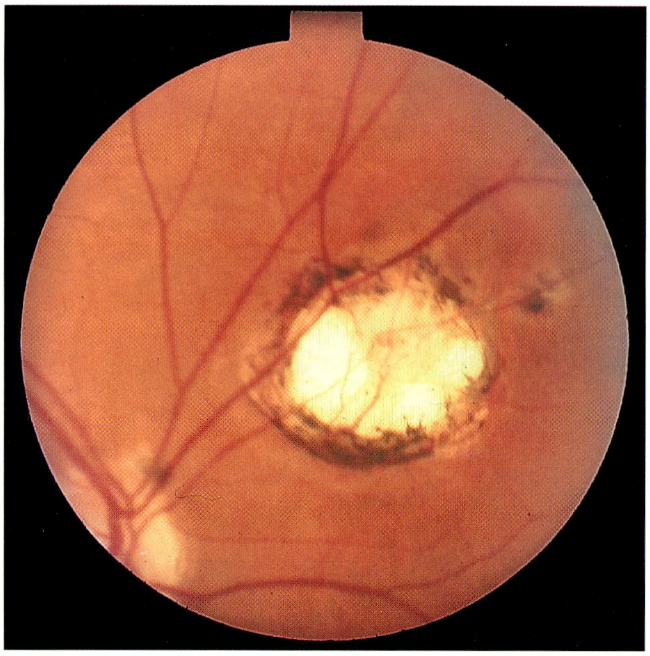

FIGURE 7.11. A large, lightly colored lesion with accompanying pigmentary degeneration surrounding the lesion in a case of inactive toxoplasmic retinochoroiditis.

Floaters due to a mild vitritis, however, are a frequent complaint in patients with CMV retinitis. With macular involvement, the patient may initially report blurred vision or dysmorphopsia. Large hemorrhages are seen in association with vascular sheathing and vitritis, which is frequently mild.

Less Common Conditions

Other Forms of Retinitis and Retinochoroiditis

Syphilis, herpes simplex virus, and varicella zoster virus are well-recognized causative organisms of retinochoroiditis. Patients are often, but not always, immunocompromised. Syphilis has many ocular manifestations, including syphilitic retinochoroiditis, which may be characterized in its active stage by areas of yellow-white necrosis, vasculitis, macular edema, vascular occlusions, or as a deep placoid lesion found in the posterior pole. Neuroretinitis (disc swelling with retinal edema) secondary to syphilis has also been described. Ocular syphilis may be associated with systemic findings of fever, malaise, lymphadenopathy, and skin rash. Several cases of concurrent ocular syphilis and HIV positivity have been reported in patients who also commonly have neurosyphilis.

The herpes viruses, herpes simplex, and varicella zoster have been implicated in causing several types of retinitis that manifest as large, lightly colored lesions. The most common is acute retinal necrosis, which presents as a peripheral necrotizing retinitis with retinal and choroidal vasculitis and vitritis that only sometimes affects the macula late in the disease process. Both the herpes simplex and varicella zoster virus have been implicated as the causative agents of acute retinal necrosis. Affected patients are either healthy or have encephalitis. It is characterized by white patches with retinal hemorrhages, sheathing of vessels, and vitritis. Patchy vasculitis with focal necrosis as well as multifocal choroiditis have been described following herpes zoster ophthalmicus.

Less Common Causes of Large, Lightly Colored Lesions

- Syphilitic retinitis
  - Symptoms include:
    - Blurred vision
    - Floaters
    - Photophobia
  - Male > female subjects, fifth decade
  - Immunocompromised state
  - Areas of yellow-white necrosis
  - Vasculitis
  - Neuroretinitis
  - Macular edema
  - Numerous ocular manifestations
    - Scleritis
    - Anterior uveitis
    - Optic nerve disease
    - Vitritis
- Herpes virus retinitis
  - Bilateral one-third of cases
  - Male > female subjects, third to sixth decade
  - Acute retinal necrosis
  - Peripheral necrotizing retinitis with retinal and choroidal vasculitis
  - Vitritis
- Choroidal metastatic disease
  - History of breast or lung malignancy
  - Yellow or beige subretinal lesion
  - Flat choroidal infiltration
  - Exudative retinal detachment
  - Anterior chamber reaction
- Additional conditions
  - Branch retinal arterial occlusion
  - Toxocara canis (see Chapter 26)
    - Unilateral, children or young adults
    - White subretinal granuloma
  - Acute multifocal placoid pigment epitheliopathy
  - Serpiginous (giant helicoid) choroidopathy
  - Intraocular lymphoma

- Seventh decade
- Vitritis and anterior chamber reaction
- Subretinal exudates

Lymphoid infiltration of the uvea

- 2:1 ratio of males to females
- Glaucoma, retinal detachment
- Extension to other ocular tissue and adnexa

Choroidal melanoma

- Exudative retinal detachment
- One-fourth are amelanotic
- Older, white adults

Acute syphilitic posterior placoid chorioretinitis
Choroidal osteoma
Choroidal hemangioma
Vogt-Koyanagi-Harada disease
Leukemic infiltration of the uvea

Multifocal Retinochoroidopathy

This class of retinal and choroidal disease may cause lesions of varying size and shape. The active stage is characterized by creamy-white lesions of various sizes found in young adult patients. Symptoms include decreased vision, scotoma, and photopsia. A viral-like prodrome has been described in association with several of these conditions, and a vitritis and anterior chamber reaction have been reported in some conditions (see Chapter 21).

SUMMARY

Lightly colored lesions are common fundus findings, especially in the macular area. The lesions may occur in any level of the retina and represent various manifestations of ocular and systemic disease. Localization, size, and distribution of the lesions provide the insight as to their nature and often provide the clinician with enough information to make an etiologic diagnosis. Retinal and systemic vascular disease, age-related fundus degeneration, and chorioretinal inflammatory disease should be considered.

SUGGESTED READING

Albert DM, Diaz-Rohena R. A historical review of sympathetic ophthalmia and its epidemiology. Surv Ophthalmol 1989;34:1–14.

Bernauer W, Gratwohl A, Hahn M, et al. Microvasculopathy in the ocular fundus after bone marrow transplantation. Ann Intern Med 1991;115:925–930.

Blacharski PA. Fundus Flavimaculatus. In DA Newsome (ed), Retinal Dystrophies and Degenerations. New York: Raven, 1988;135–159.

Bolling JP, Buettner H. Acquired retinal arteriovenous communications in occlusive disease of the carotid artery. Ophthalmology 1990;97:1148–1152.

Brezin A, Girard B, Rosenheim M, et al. Cotton wool spots in AIDS-related complex. Int Ophthalmol 1990;14:37–41.

Brown GC, Brown MM, Hiller T, et al. Cotton wool spots. Retina 1985;5:206–214.

Brown GC, Shields JA, Sanborn G, et al. Radiation retinopathy. Ophthalmology 1982;89:1494–1501.

Campo RV, Aaberg TM. Choroidal granuloma in sarcoidosis. Am J Ophthalmol 1984;97:419–427.

Culbertson WW. Infections of the retina in AIDS. Int Ophthalmol Clin 1989;29:108–118.

Dreyer RF, Hopen G, Gass JDM, et al. Leber's idiopathic stellate neuroretinitis. Arch Ophthalmol 1984;102:1140–1145.

Duker JS, Blumenkranz MS. Diagnosis and management of acute retinal necrosis syndrome. Surv Ophthalmol 1991:35:327–343.

Friedman CT, Knox DL. Variations in recurrent active toxoplasmosis retinochoroiditis. Arch Ophthalmol 1969;81:481–493.

Freeman WR, Chen A, Henderly DE, et al. Prevalence and significance of acquired immunodeficiency syndrome-related retinal microvasculopathy. Am J Ophthalmol 1989;107:229–235.

Gass JDM. A clinicopathologic study of a peculiar foveomacular dystrophy. Trans Am Ophthalmol Soc 1974;72:139–156.

Gass JDM. Diseases of the optic nerve that may simulate macular disease. Trans Am Acad Ophthalmol Otolaryngol 1977;83:763–770.

Gass JDM. Stereoscopic Atlas of Macular Diseases: Diagnosis and Treatment (3rd ed). St. Louis: Mosby, 1987.

Gass JDM, Gilbert WR, Guerry RK, Scelfo R. Diffuse unilateral subacute neuroretinitis. Ophthalmology 1978;85:521–545.

Gass JDM, Jallow S, Davis B. Adult vitelliform macular detachment occurring in patients with basal laminar drusen. Am J Ophthalmol 1985;99:445–459.

Gazes PC. Clinical Cardiology. Philadelphia: Lea & Febiger, 1990:335–345.

Graham EM. The investigation of patients with retinal vascular occlusion. Eye 1990;4:464–468.

Gutman I, Walsh JB, Knapp AB. Cotton-wool spots as a sign of leptospirosis. Ophthalmologica 1983;187:133–136.

Harnois C, Cortin P, Samson J, et al. Static perimetry in canthaxanthin maculopathy. Arch Ophthalmol 1988;106:58–60.

Hayreh SS, Servais GE, Virdi PS. Cotton wool spots (inner retinal ischemic spots) in malignant arterial hypertension. Ophthalmologica 1989;198:197–215.

Imperia PS, Lazarus HM, Lass JH. Ocular complications of systemic cancer chemotherapy. Surv Ophthalmol 1989;34:209–230.

Jalkh AE, Trempe CL. Macular edema in branch retinal vein occlusion: Types and treatment. Ophthalmic Surg 1989;20:26–32.

Jost BF. Dominantly Inherited Drusen. In DA Newsome (ed), Retinal Dystrophies and Degenerations. New York: Raven, 1988;105–113.

Kaiser-Kupfer MI, Lippman ME. Tamoxifen retinopathy. Cancer Treat Rep 1978;62:315–320.

Karesh JW, Goldman EJ, Reck K, et al. A prospective ophthalmic evaluation of patients with acute myeloid leukemia: Correlation of ocular and hematologic findings. J Clin Oncol 1989;7:1528–1532.

Kleiner RC, Najarian LV, Schattan S, et al. Vaso-occlusive retinopathy associated with anti-phospholipid antibodies (lupus anticoagulant retinopathy). Ophthalmology 1989;96:896–904.

Lam S, Tessler HH, Lam BL, et al. High incidence of sympathetic ophthalmia after contact and noncontact neodymium: YAG cyclotherapy. Ophthalmology 1992;99:1818–1822.

Lemange JM, Michiels X, Causenbroeck S, et al. Purtscher-like retinopathy after retrobulbar anesthesia. Ophthalmology 1990;97:859–861.

Lesser RL, Kornmehl EW, Pachner AR, et al. Neuro-ophthalmologic manifestations of Lyme disease. Ophthalmology 1990;97:699–706.

Levine DR, Crafts JW, Lesser GR, et al. Visual symptoms associated with the presence of a lupus anticoagulant. Ophthalmology 1988;95:686–692.

Lopez PF, Green WR. Peripapillary subretinal neovascularization. Retina 1992;12:147–171.

Mansour AM, Jampol LM, Logani S, et al. Cotton wool spots in acquired immunodeficiency syndrome compared with diabetes mellitus, systemic hypertension, and central retinal vein occlusion. Arch Ophthalmol 1988;106:1074–1077.

Margo CE, Hamed LM. Ocular syphilis. Surv Ophthalmol 1992;37:203–220.

McFadden DM, Hauston CS, Sutton JR, et al. High-altitude retinopathy. JAMA 1981;245:581–586.

McLane NJ, Carroll DM. Ocular manifestations of drug abuse. Surv Ophthalmol 1986;30:298–313.

Michealson IC. Textbook of the Fundus of the Eye. Edinburgh: Churchill Livingstone, 1980.

Morris AT, Sanders MD. Macular changes resulting from papilledema. Br J Ophthalmol 1980;64:211–216.

Ohno S, Char DH, Kimura SJ, et al. Vogt-Koyanagi-Harada syndrome. Am J Ophthalmol 1977;83:735–740.

Presley GD. Fundus changes in Rocky Mountain spotted fever. Am J Ophthalmol 1969;67:263–267.

Sapira JD. An internist looks at the fundus oculi. Dis Mon 1984;30:1–64.

Schatz H, Johnson RN, McDonald HR. Differential diagnosis of dots, spots, flecks, and specks of the fundus. Retina 1992;12:67–69.

Seibert DA, Terry JE. Atypical foveomacular vitelliform degeneration, adult type. J Am Optom Assoc 1988;10:798–801.

Shami MJ, Freeman W, Friedberg D, et al. A multicenter study of Pneumocystis choroidopathy. Am J Ophthalmol 1991;112:15–22.

CHAPTER

8 Granular Pigment Changes

Leonard J. Oshinskie, Rodney K. Gutner, and Anthony A. Cavallerano

This section addresses conditions that exhibit granular pigment changes, sometimes referred to as retinal pigment epithelium (RPE) mottling, as the predominant macular presentation. Those conditions associated with course clumping or large areas of RPE dropout are discussed in Chapter 10. Some conditions cause fine granular pigment changes initially and coarse clumping later in the disease process, or both may occur simultaneously. For example, age-related macular degeneration (AMD) may first present with granular pigment changes and then progress to an exudative form of the disease resulting in pigment clumping. Some of these conditions are discussed in Chapters 12 and 24, and the reader should determine the predominant change and use that as a guide for developing a differential diagnosis.

Fine Granular Pigmentary Changes (Retinal Pigment Epithelium Mottling)

Common
- Atrophic (dry) AMD
- RPE detachment
- Following idiopathic central serous chorioretinopathy
- Following chronic cystoid macular edema (CME) associated with:
  - Vascular occlusive disease
  - Intraocular surgery
  - Chronic inflammation
  - Diabetes mellitus
- Following focal laser photocoagulation

Less common
- Hereditary or congenital ocular conditions without systemic disease (see Chapter 29)
  - Macular pigment epithelial dystrophies (pattern dystrophies)
  - Cone dystrophy
  - Fundus flavimaculatus (Stargardt's disease)
  - Juvenile retinoschisis
  - Central areolar choroidal dystrophy
  - Best's vitelliform dystrophy
  - Retinitis pigmentosa and related systemic conditions, e.g., Usher's syndrome
- Systemic conditions associated with granular pigment changes
  - Congenital rubella or syphilis
  - Disorders of amino acid or protein metabolism, lysosomal storage diseases, and others
  - Myotonic dystrophy
- Pharmaceutically induced pigment changes, including the following agents:
  - Hydroxychloroquine
  - Chloroquine
  - Thioridazine
  - Chlorpromazine
  - Deferoxamine
  - Indomethacin
  - Tilorane
  - Cisplatinum or methotrexate
- Following central retinal artery occlusion
- Following certain multifocal choroidopathies
- Following unilateral acute idiopathic maculopathy (UAIM)
- Parafoveal telangiectasia

Fine granular pigment changes are commonly seen in patients with AMD (Figure 8.1). Older patients with drusen and an elevated, circular lesion containing granular pigment changes should be suspected of having a pigment epithelial detachment and the possibility of an underlying choroidal neovascular membrane.

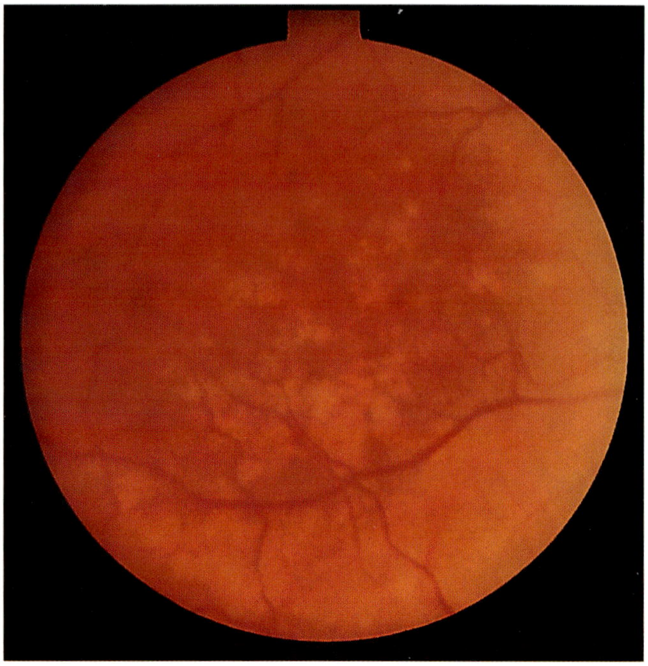

FIGURE 8.1. Fine pigment changes found in age-related macular degeneration.

Granular Pigmentary Changes in Atrophic Age-Related Macular Degeneration

Risk profile
- Seventh decade or beyond
- White
- Family history
- Lightly colored irides
- Hyperopia
- Hypertension; cardiovascular disease
- Cigarette smoking

Symptoms
- Gradual onset of blurred vision
- Dysmorphopsia
- Scotomata

Diagnostic signs
- Common
  - Bilateral drusen
    - Pigment mottling and clumping
    - Focal or large areas of RPE dropout
- Additional
  - Pigmentary atrophy and clumping
    - Disciform scar in fellow eye
    - Peripheral reticular pigmentary degeneration

Other diagnostic considerations
- If atrophic AMD converts to exudative form, look for:
  - Hemorrhage and exudates
  - Elevation caused by RPE detachment
  - RPE tear
  - Vitreous hemorrhage
- Choroidal neovascularization more likely when associated with:
  - Soft, confluent drusen
  - Focal hyperpigmentation
  - Fellow eye involvement
- Amsler grid testing
- Patient education for dysmorphopsia or reduced visual acuity
- Photodocumentation

Management
- Fluorescein angiography by retinologist if:
  - Dysmorphopsia or scotoma on Amsler grid testing
  - Sudden visual acuity change
  - Signs of choroidal neovascularization
- Comanage with unilateral exudative changes
- Antioxidant or nutrient supplement
- Ultraviolet protection

Retinal Pigment Epithelial Detachment in Age-Related Macular Degeneration

Risk profile
- Seventh decade
- AMD in fellow eye

Symptoms
- Dysmorphopsia
- Scotomata
- May be asymptomatic

Diagnostic signs
- Common
  - Elevated, circumscribed macular lesion greater than one-third DD
  - Bilateral (approximately 30%)
  - Granular pigment within lesion
- Additional
  - Often associated with soft, confluent drusen
  - Turbid exudation within lesion
  - Intraretinal or subretinal hemorrhage

Other diagnostic considerations
- Choroidal neovascularization of membrane in approximately 30% of cases

Management
- Fluorescein angiography if greater than 1 DD
- Consider laser photocoagulation if lesion meets Macular Photocoagulation Study criteria
- If outside Macular Photocoagulation Study criteria, monitor with home Amsler grid testing, periodic fluorescein angiograms, and fundus biomicroscopy

Other conditions must be considered when the patient is younger than age 60 or has a history of some of the conditions listed previously. Unilateral changes suggest a recurrent or resolved idiopathic central serous choroidopathy, chronic CME, multiple evanescent white-dot syndrome, or UAIM. Intraocular surgery and laser photocoagulation may also cause changes resulting in granular pigment distribution in the macular area.

Granular Pigmentary Changes Following Idiopathic Central Serous Choroidopathy

Risk profile
- Fourth to sixth decade
- Male > female subjects (females usually older)
- White
- High-achievement personality

Symptoms
- Episode(s) of unilateral blurring or dysmorphopsia
- Central scotoma

Diagnostic signs
- Common
  - Unilateral granular pigment changes near the macula
  - Blister-like sensory retinal elevation
- Additional
  - Blue-yellow dyschromatopsia

Other diagnostic considerations
- RPE disturbance in fellow eye indicates past episode(s)

Management
- Fluorescein angiography by retinologist if sensory detachment is suspected
- Consider laser photocoagulation if recurrent or if no vision improvement after 6 months
- Home Amsler grid testing

Granular Pigmentary Changes Following Cystoid Macular Edema

Risk profile
- Intraocular surgery
- Chronic inflammation
- Vascular occlusive disease
- Conditions associated with undiagnosed macular edema

Symptoms
- Decreased visual acuity—20/25–20/400
- Past history of sudden blurred vision long since resolved

Diagnostic signs
- Common
  - Resolving intraretinal hemorrhages
  - Granular pigment changes
  - Cystic changes in macula
- Additional
  - Collateral vessels crossing horizontal raphe or on optic disc with old vascular occlusion

Other diagnostic considerations
- Fluorescein angiography may be required to confirm diagnosis
- Check intraocular pressure in fellow eye to rule out ocular hypertension or glaucoma if old venous occlusion is suspected
- Rule out neovascularization of iris and neovascular glaucoma, which is common with ischemic central retinal vein occlusion

Management
- Fluorescein angiography by retinologist to confirm diagnosis if CME not apparent by direct fundus examination
- Monitor every 3 months for neovascularization of iris and neovascular glaucoma in vascular occlusive disease

Granular Pigmentary Changes Following Laser Photocoagulation

Risk profile
- Laser treatment for macular edema from any cause

Symptoms
- Minimal-to-moderate vision decrease depending on the extent of treatment

Diagnostic signs
- Common
  - Small punctate areas of hyperpigmentation or hypopigmentation sometimes found in a grid pattern or randomly near retinal arterioles
- Additional
  - Microaneurysms or blot hemorrhages
  - Occasional paracentral scotomata

Other diagnostic considerations
- Other signs of diabetic eye disease or complications from venous occlusive disease

Management
- Monitor for recurrence of macular edema in diabetic patient
- Home Amsler grid testing

LESS COMMON CAUSES OF GRANULAR PIGMENT CHANGES

Pigment mottling in a healthy patient under 20 years of age suggests an inherited ocular condition. These conditions should be suspected if a positive family history of vision loss is elicited; however, some patients may have no definite family history of vision loss or maculopathy. In the late stages of the disease process, several condi-

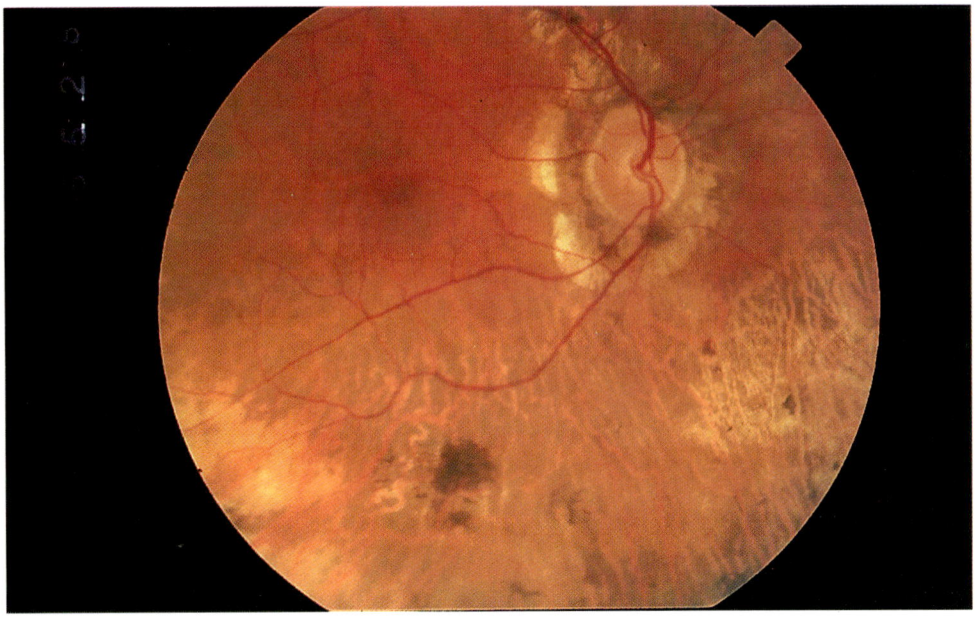

FIGURE 8.2. Macular pigment changes in a patient with retinitis pigmentosa.

tions may manifest with disciform scarring or course clumping of the RPE resembling AMD. A history of vision loss at a young age helps to rule out AMD. The following list summarizes the primary inherited causes for these pigment changes:

- Macular pigment epithelial dystrophies (pattern dystrophies)
- Cone dystrophy
- Fundus flavimaculatus (Stargardt's disease)
- Juvenile retinoschisis
- Central areolar choroidal and autosomal dominant central areolar dystrophy
- Best's vitelliform dystrophy
- Primary retinitis pigmentosa

OTHER OCULAR CONDITIONS CAUSING GRANULAR PIGMENT CHANGES

Central retinal artery occlusion may cause unilateral macular pigment changes. A history of sudden acute vision loss, attenuated retinal arterioles, and a pale optic disc associated with unilateral pigment changes are all suggestive of a previous central retinal artery occlusion.

Multifocal choroidopathies, including multiple evanescent white-dot syndrome, occur unilaterally in young patients, usually female patients, who have recently had a viral-like illness with mild vision loss. The white dots are present for only a few days or weeks and sometimes leave behind mild pigment changes.

UAIM has recently been described as a cause of an exudative macular detachment and a resulting bull's-eye appearance. The condition occurs in young patients and initially causes moderate-to-severe vision loss that resolves without treatment; vision usually improves to 20/25 or better. A flu-like prodrome has also been reported in many of these patients.

Parafoveal telangiectasis usually occurs in middle-aged or older men, but may also present in women. Microaneurysms and telangiectasis of the retinal blood vessels are the predominant fundus abnormality; unilateral or bilateral pigment changes may also be found surrounding the fovea. Exudates may also occur, with vision being slightly reduced due to macular edema.

RETINITIS PIGMENTOSA

Macular changes such as epiretinal membrane, CME, and pigment changes frequently occur in patients with retinitis pigmentosa (RP) (Figure 8.2). RP must be considered on the basis of nyctalopia, family history, or additional retinal findings, including bone spicule formation or other peripheral pigment changes. A visual field and an electroretinogram are indicated; for the differential diagnosis, dark adaptometry and an electro-oculogram may be helpful.

Macular pigment changes are found in some patients with systemic conditions. Many of these patients develop symptoms during the first decade of life and have other systemic findings such as mental disabilities, developmental delays, facial or skeletal abnormalities, or seizure disorders. Other ocular findings may include optic atrophy, attenuated retinal vessels, corneal clouding, or nystagmus. The peripheral fundus should be examined in any patient with macular pigment changes since a number of these systemic syndromes include RP or RP-like retinopathy as an accompanying finding.

SYSTEMIC CONDITIONS CAUSING GRANULAR PIGMENTARY CHANGES

Pigment macular changes arranged in a reticular or stellate pattern have been described in adults with myotonic dystrophy. These patients have associated findings of expressionless facies, baldness, and inability to release a handshake as well as other muscle weakness. Ocular findings may include polychromatic cataracts and ptosis.

Maculopathy has also been associated with rubella, syphilis, and morbilli. Characteristic granular pigment changes occur at the level of the RPE and may be present at birth. Metabolic disorders have also been known to cause mottling of the pigment in the macular area. The changes associated with these systemic disorders are summarized below.

RP-like syndromes, e.g., Usher's syndrome
- Epiretinal membrane
- CME
- Pigment changes
- Family history
- Nyctalopia

Congenital rubella
- Blotchy or granular pigment changes
- Visual acuity normal unless associated with cataract
- Clinical signs may not be present at birth

Syphilis
- Salt and pepper fundus (bilateral)

Neurologic and neuromuscular disorders
- Myotonic dystrophy
- Kearns-Sayre syndrome

Metabolic disorders
- Cystinosis
- Cobalamin C defects
- Others (see AV Drack, EI Traboulsi. Systemic associations of pigmentary retinopathy. Int Ophthalmol Clin 1991;31:35–59)

DRUG-INDUCED MACULOPATHY

The cumulative effects of retinotoxic drugs are risk factors for the development of pigmentary retinopathy. Extensive information is available regarding the retinal toxicity of chloroquine (Aralen) and hydroxychloroquine (Plaquenil), and patients taking these medications should have a comprehensive retinal examination every 6–12 months; threshold automated visual fields, color vision testing, and Amsler grid testing should be performed at appropriate intervals. Maculopathy from these pharmaceutical agents occurs more often in patients taking chloroquine than hydroxychloroquine. Patients taking chloroquine at dosages of 250 mg per day or less and patients who have taken less than 300 g in 2–3 years are less likely to develop retinopathy. Hydroxychloroquine is relatively safe at dosages of less than 6.5 mg per kg per day, 400 mg per day or less, or when the patient has taken the drug for less than 10 years. It has been reported that patients may rarely develop vision loss at lower dosages or with shorter durations. Early maculopathy manifests as granular pigment changes with RPE dropout, leading to the development of the characteristic bull's-eye maculopathy, with generalized macular atrophy observed in the later stages. Numerous other conditions may result in macular changes producing a bull's-eye pattern in the macula. Renal or liver disease may potentiate the toxic effect of hydroxychloroquine.

Conditions Associated with Bull's-Eye Maculopathy

These data are from JM Jimenez-Sierra, TE Ogden, GB Van Boemel. Inherited Retinal Diseases: A Diagnostic Guide. St. Louis: Mosby, 1989; and E Shakin. Macular Dystrophies. In WS Tasman (ed), Clinical Decisions in Medical Retinal Disease. St. Louis: Mosby, 1994;125–140.

- Chloroquine or hydroxychloroquine toxicity
- Cone dystrophy
- Stargardt's disease
- Rod-cone dystrophy
- Olivopontocerebellar degeneration
- Sjögren-Larsson syndrome
- UAIM
- Benign concentric annular bull's-eye maculopathy
- Fundus flavimaculatus
- Fenestrated sheen macular dystrophy
- AMD

Phenothiazide derivatives, including thioridazine (Mellaril) or mesoridazine (Serentil), may cause cutaneous and ocular pigment changes, including retinal pigment disturbances. Toxicity is dose dependent, so patients taking less than 800 mg per day are at lower risk. Chlorpromazine (Thorazine) has also been reported to cause retinopathy, although the association is not as strong as for thioridazine.

The following pharmaceutical agents have also been identified as potential causes of granular pigmentary maculopathy: indomethacin, deferoxamine, and the chemotherapeutic agents cisplatinum, tilorane, and methotrexate.

SUGGESTED READING

Bernstein HN. Ocular safety of hydroxychloroquine. Ann Ophthalmol 1991;23:292–296.

Carr RE, Siegel IM. Retinal function in patients treated with indomethacin. Am J Ophthalmol 1973;75:302–306.

Chew EY, Deutman AF, Cruysberg JRM. Macular Changes in Myotonic Dystrophy. In SJ Ryan (ed), Retinal Disease. Orlando: Grune & Stratton, 1985;141–148.

Drack AV, Traboulsi EI. Systemic associations of pigmentary retinopathy. Int Ophthalmol Clin 1991;31:35–59.

Elman MJ, Fine SL, Murphy RP, et al. The natural history of serous retinal pigment epithelium detachment in patients with age-related macular degeneration. Ophthalmology 1986;93:224–230.

Finbloom DS, Silver K, Newsome DA, Guakel R. Comparison of hydroxychloroquine and chloroquine use and the development of retinal toxicity. J Rheumatol 1985;12:692–694.

Fong ACO, Schatz H, McDonald HR, et al. Central retinal vein occlusion in young adults (papillophlebitis). Retina 1991;11:3–11.

Imperia PS, Lazarus HM, Lass JH. Ocular complications of systemic cancer chemotherapy. Surv Ophthalmol 1989;34:209–230.

Jimenez-Sierra JM, Ogden TE, Van Boemel GB. Inherited Retinal Diseases: A Diagnostic Guide. St. Louis: Mosby, 1989.

Lakhanpal V, Schocket SS, Jiji R. Deferoxamine (Deferal)-induced toxic retinal pigmentary degeneration and presumed optic neuropathy. Ophthalmology 1984;91:443–451.

Miller DF, Bay JW, Lederman RJ, et al. Ocular and orbital toxicity following intracarotid injection of BCNU (Carmustine) and cisplatinum for malignant gliomas. Ophthalmology 1985;92:402–406.

Newsome DA. Pigment Epithelial Dystrophies. In DA Newsome (ed), Retinal Dystrophies and Degenerations. New York: Raven, 1988;195–231.

Ruiz RS, Saatci OA. Choroquine and hydroxychloroquine. Ann Ophthalmol 1991;23:290–291.

Schatz H. Essential Fluorescein Angiography. San Anselmo, CA: Pacific, 1983.

Yannuzzi LA. Retinal Pigment Epithelial Detachment. In LA Yannuzzi (ed), Laser Photocoagulation of the Macula. Philadelphia: Lippincott, 1989;49–63.

Yannuzzi LA, Jampal LM, Raab MF, et al. Unilateral acute idiopathic maculopathy. Arch Ophthalmol 1991;109:1411–1416.

CHAPTER

9 Dark Macular Lesions

Leonard J. Oshinskie, Anthony A. Cavallerano, and Rodney K. Gutner

Macular conditions in this category are characterized by gray, gray-black, or gray-green lesions that are typically larger than 1 disc diameter (DD) and lie deep within the layers of the outer retina and choroid. Although not necessarily confined to the macular area, these lesions are usually solitary, uniform in color, homogeneous in appearance, and have relatively distinct borders. The lesions tend to be unilateral and may be flat or elevated, an important distinction when considering the differential diagnosis. Dark lesions of a pigmentary nature may result from an increased number of cells (pigment hyperplasia) or an increase in the size of the cells (hypertrophy).

Since the etiology varies, the clinician should note any change in appearance of the lesion when viewed with the red-free filter of the ophthalmoscope or slit-lamp biomicroscope. If a pigmented lesion disappears from view with the filter in place, it is subretinal. It is sometimes difficult to differentiate a pigmented lesion, containing melanocytes, from a neovascular lesion, which takes on a dark appearance due to its location within the choroid or because of accompanying retinal pigment epithelial (RPE) cells, blood, or impending hemorrhage. A subretinal hemorrhage usually indicates a choroid neovascularization membrane (CNVM) and may have accompanying elevation if there is a serosanguinous exudation raising the neurosensory retina. Careful examination using stereoscopic techniques will aid in the differential diagnosis.

DARK, SUBRETINAL, SOLID-APPEARING LESIONS

Common conditions
- Choroidal nevus
- Congenital RPE hypertrophy
- RPE hyperplasia

Less common conditions
- Subretinal hemorrhage from:
  - CNVM
  - Macroaneurysm
- Metastatic disease to the choroid
- Choroidal melanoma
- Melanocytoma
- Other choroidal tumors

Common Conditions

Choroidal Nevus

Choroidal nevi appear as solid, dark lesions occurring throughout the fundus, including the posterior pole. They tend to be unilateral and are less common in blacks and Asians. Their borders are relatively distinct depending on the amount of elevation, and the surface may take on a mottled appearance. Although most nevi are flat, there may be as much as 2 or 3 mm of elevation. Drusen may be seen overlying the lesion in long-standing cases, and in rare circumstances, choroidal neovascularization (CNV) may develop over the lesion (Figure 9.1). Stereoscopic fundus examination techniques and β-scan ultrasonography help to differentiate a choroidal nevus from a melanoma. It is rare that nevi increase in size, and only rarely has it been reported that the lesion gives rise to a melanoma. Photodocumentation and annual evaluation are indicated in patients with a choroidal nevus.

Risk profile
- Second decade and beyond
- Whites

Symptoms
- Rare unless associated with CNVM

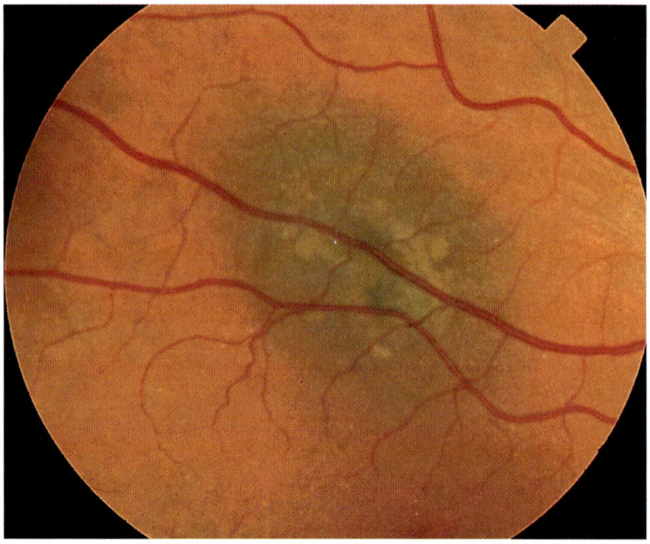

FIGURE 9.1. Choroidal nevus with well-defined borders and overlying drusen and cystic retinal changes indicating the long-standing nature of this lesion. (Courtesy of A. Bell.)

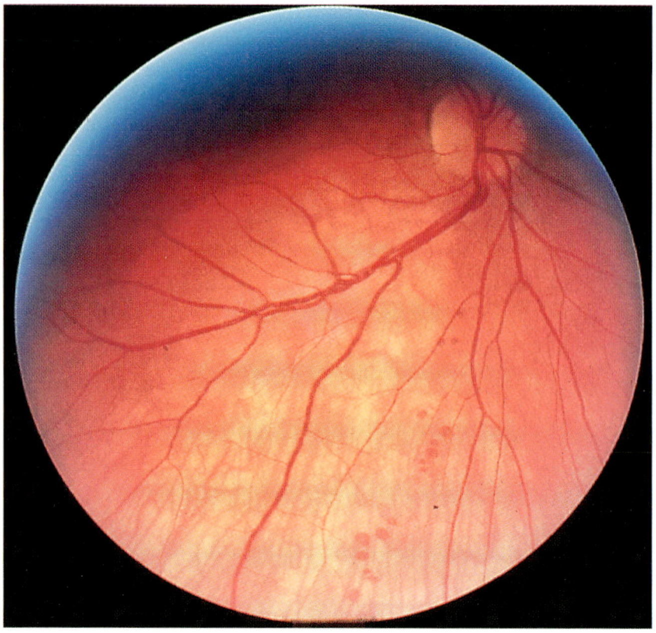

FIGURE 9.2. Congenital hypertrophic retinal pigment epithelium. The lesions are usually uniformly dark, flat, and well-defined. A lacuna of depigmented area often develops from the center of the lesion. (Courtesy of L.P. Semes, O.D.)

Diagnostic signs
- Common
  - Uniform, slate gray color
  - Feathered edges
  - Little or no elevation
  - Deep to RPE
- Additional
  - Overlying drusen possible
  - CNVM rare but possible if Bruch's membrane and choriocapillaris complex is altered

Other diagnostic considerations
- Significant elevation may indicate malignant melanoma
- Drusen is indicative of longevity

Management
- Photodocumentation
- Annual evaluation unless change is noted
- Beta-scan ultrasonography if greater than 3-mm elevation
- Fluorescein angiography when indicated
- Retinal oncology consult if elevated greater than 3 mm or increase in size is documented

Congenital Retinal Pigment Epithelium Hypertrophy

Congenital RPE hypertrophy is a benign fundus condition that manifests as a dark gray or black lesion deep in the retina. A surrounding depigmented area (halo) is often apparent, as are small areas that lack pigment (lacunae) within the lesion. Although benign, the lesions should arouse suspicion if they are multiple and bilateral, an indication that the patient may have Gardner's syndrome, a gastrointestinal disorder. This syndrome has other systemic manifestations, including soft tissue tumors that may become malignant (Figure 9.2).

Risk profile
- Present at any age
- No race or gender predilection

Symptoms
- None

Diagnostic signs
- Common
  - Gray or black flat lesion
  - Often unilateral; can be bilateral
  - Well-defined borders
  - Smooth or irregular surface
- Additional
  - Temporal fundus more common
  - Depigmented halo
  - Lacuna within lesion over time

Other diagnostic considerations
- Unchanged red-free appearance
- If multiple and bilateral, consider Gardner's syndrome (intestinal polyps, bone and teeth abnormalities, soft tissue tumors)

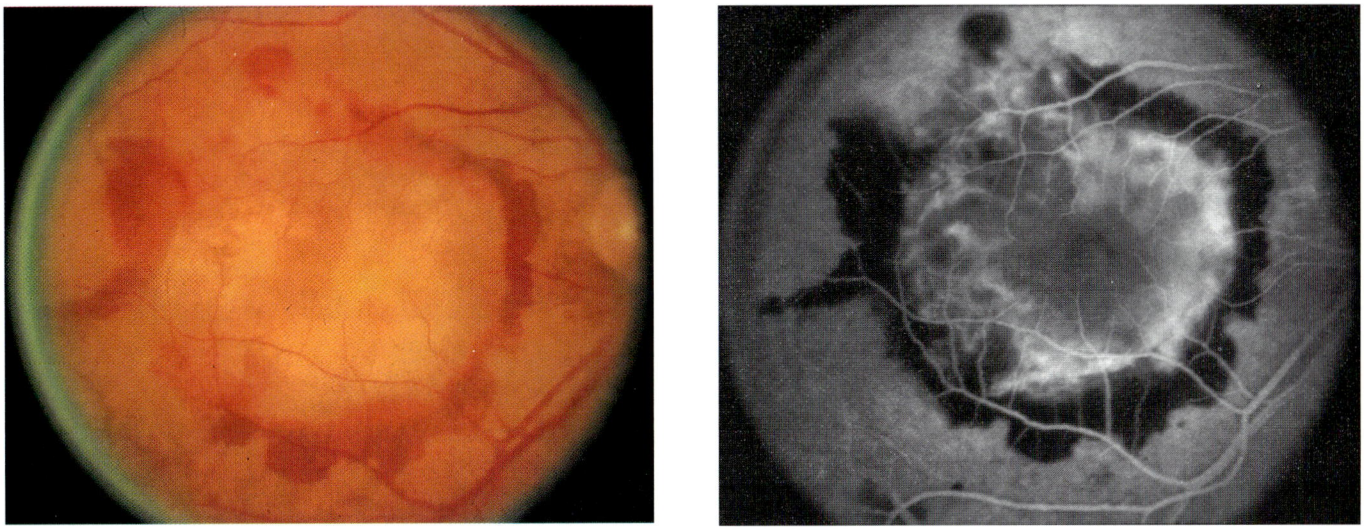

FIGURE 9.3. (Left) Large subretinal hemorrhage and neurosensory elevation in a patient with a choroidal neovascular membrane. (Right) The fluorescein angiogram of the same eye, with hyperfluorescent neovascular lesion causing the elevation and hypofluorescent surround. (Courtesy of S. Sinclair, M.D.)

Management
- Photodocumentation
- Red-free stereoscopic observation
- Gastrointestinal evaluation if multiple and bilateral

Retinal Pigment Epithelium Hyperplasia

RPE hyperplasia usually occurs secondary to trauma or chorioretinal inflammation. Regardless of the cause, the lesions are usually not uniformly pigmented but contain areas of pigment clumping interspersed with pigment dropout. The borders are often irregular, and the lesions may be found anywhere in the ocular fundus. Inactive toxoplasmosis retinochoroiditis is one of the most common causes of this pigment manifestation (see Figure 7.11), although any chorioretinal inflammation may be the cause. If thought to be due to inflammation, the clinician should educate the patient to look for signs of reactivation of the process. The patient should be evaluated periodically for signs of active inflammation.

Less Common Conditions

Subretinal Blood from Choroid Neovascularization or Retinal Macroaneurysm

When blood leaks under the RPE, a uniformly deep gray lesion may be apparent, which looks very much like a nevus (Figure 9.3). Unlike a nevus, however, there is often elevation of the retina and an associated bright red hemorrhage that breaks through the RPE. Since CNV is usually the source of subretinal blood, conditions that commonly result in or are caused by CNV must be ruled out.

Retinal macroaneuryms also may leak blood beneath the RPE, resulting in the appearance of a large dark lesion.

Metastatic Disease to the Globe

Lung and breast cancer are the most common malignancies that metastasize to the posterior uvea, producing a slightly elevated lesion that is yellow or yellow-gray in color (Figure 9.4). However, some patients may present with an elevated gray-colored lesion due to an overlying exudative, nonrhegmatogenous detachment. Patients are generally 40–60 years of age and should already carry a diagnosis of cancer. Many complain of blurred vision since metastasis to the choroid often occurs in the posterior pole, the most common site for ocular involvement.

Choroidal Melanoma

These lesions are rare and are usually found in older white patients. They have been reported in 5.5–6.0 per million of the population, and sun exposure appears to be a risk factor. Symptoms of blurred vision, decreased peripheral vision, or flashes of light may cause the patient to seek care, although many are asymptomatic. The lesions are usually solitary, elevated, and gray, often with an associated nonrhegmatogenous, usually exudative, retinal detachment (Figure 9.5). CNV may occur in some instances, and a hemorrhage is seen overlying the melanoma in such cases. Any elderly patient with a vari-

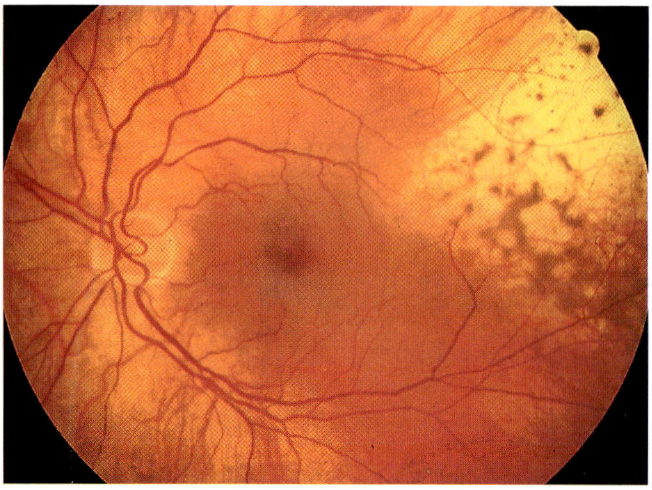

FIGURE 9.4. Metastatic lesion in the posterior pole. Note the relative absence of significant pigment but noticeable elevation of the lesion as it impinges on the temporal macular area. (Courtesy of J. Hamlin.)

ably pigmented elevated lesion should be suspected of having a choroidal melanoma, and fundus photographs should be obtained for documentation. The primary care clinician should seek consultation with a retinal specialist, preferably one whose subspecialty is oncology. If an elevated lesion is observed in the fundus, ß-scan ultrasonography and radioactive ^{32}P uptake testing along with fundus fluorescein angiography are appropriate in confirming a diagnosis of choroidal melanoma.

Melanocytoma

Melanocytoma is a tumor of the optic nerve head that may grow in the direction of the macula. The lesion is usually extremely dark, may be slightly elevated, and is often associated with a visual field defect (Figure 9.6).

Other Rare Choroidal Tumors

Although choroidal melanoma is rare, there are several other uveal tumors that may appear large and dark and are even more uncommon. An example of these is a neurilemoma. Since these tumors appear to be similar to a melanoma or may be associated with systemic disease, further evaluation by a retinal specialist is warranted.

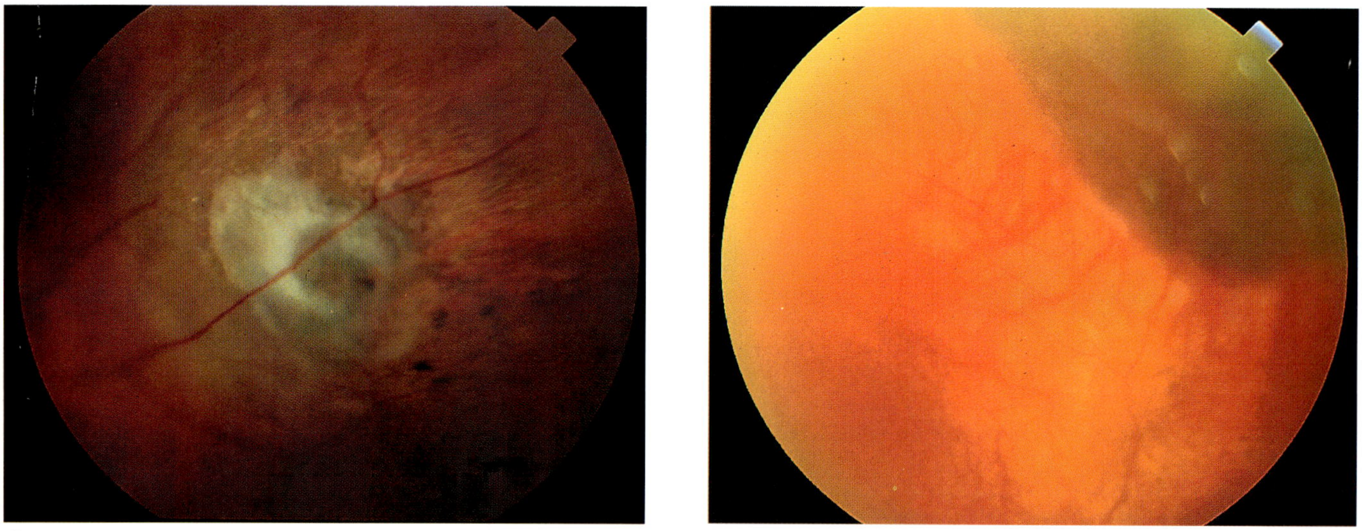

A B

FIGURE 9.5. A. A malignant melanoma in another patient, darker in appearance, following proton beam irradiation treatment. Most choroidal melanomas appear darker when viewed with indirect ophthalmoscopy compared with other methods of observation. B. An elevated, less pigmented choroidal melanoma.

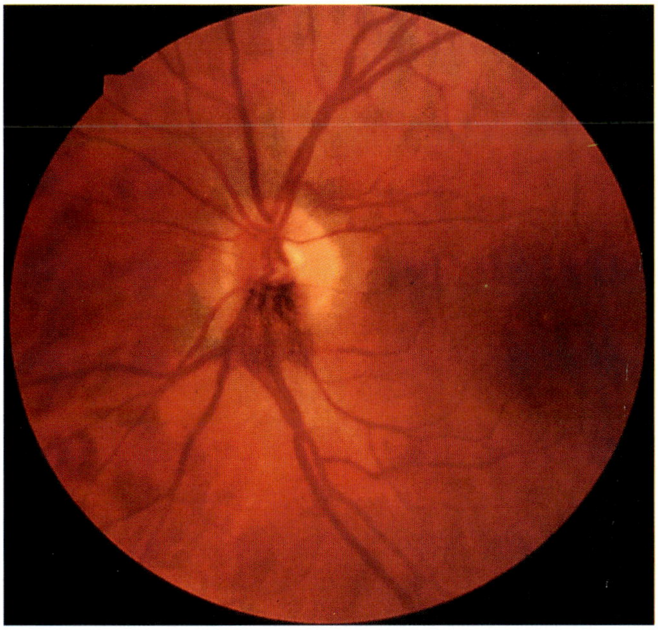

FIGURE 9.6. Example of a melanocytoma. (Courtesy of L.P. Semes, O.D.).

SUGGESTED READING

Buettner H. Congenital hypertrophy of the retinal pigment epithelium. Am J Ophthalmol 1975;79:177–189.

Freedman MI, Folk JC. Metastatic tumors to the eye and orbit. Arch Ophthalmol 1987;105:1215–1219.

Gragoudas E, Seddon J. Pigmented choroidal lesions. Clin Eye Vis Care 1988;1:8–18

Purcell JJ, Shields JA. Hypertrophy with hyperpigmentation of the retinal pigment epithelium. Arch Ophthalmol 1975;93:1122–1126.

Stein EA, Brady KD. Ophthalmologic and electro-oculographic findings in Gardner's syndrome. Am J Ophthalmol 1988;106:326–331.

CHAPTER

10

Large, Lightly Colored Macular Lesions Associated with Coarse Pigment Clumping

Leonard J. Oshinskie, Anthony A. Cavallerano, and Rodney K. Gutner

The lesions in this category are defined as those generally larger than 1 DD and are characterized by large, lightly colored fundus areas and clumping of the retinal pigment epithelium (RPE) and choroidal pigment. Establishing the diagnosis for a macular disorder that results in large, lightly colored lesions requires that the clinician determine the level of the retina involved in the process. The lightly colored appearance is generally due to a loss or migration of pigment in the RPE layer, the choroid, or from fibrous scarring, generally in the sensory retina. Additionally, infiltration into the retinal layers by degenerative, infectious, or inflammatory material may result in these pigment changes. The dark areas are due to an abnormal distribution of melanin in the RPE, choroid, or sensory retina. Typically these lesions are larger than 1 DD; however, the same conditions may also cause smaller lesions.

LARGE, LIGHTLY COLORED MACULAR LESIONS ASSOCIATED WITH COARSE PIGMENT CLUMPING

Common causes

- Disciform maculopathy
- Toxoplasmosis
- RPE geographic atrophy in age-related macular degeneration (AMD)
- Trauma
- Following laser photocoagulation

Less common causes

- Advanced Best's disease
- Other infectious or inflammatory causes of chorioretinitis such as syphilis, herpes simplex retinitis, tuberculosis, and others
- RPE window defect
- Retinitis pigmentosa
- Following acute multifocal placoid pigment epitheliopathy (APMPPE), serpiginous choroidopathy, and other multifocal choroidopathies
- Nematode infestation (diffuse unilateral subacute neuroretinitis)
- Choroidal melanoma
- Choroidal metastasis
- RPE tear (often occurs following laser photocoagulation or spontaneously with serosanguinous accumulation under RPE or neurosensory retina)
- Resolving subretinal hemorrhage

DISCIFORM MACULOPATHY

One of the most common conditions resulting in this appearance is disciform maculopathy. A choroidal neovascular membrane under the RPE can leak blood and blood elements (exudates), resulting in a disruption of the normal anatomy of RPE and sensory retina. The presence of serosanguinous fluid under the RPE eventually leads to fibrous tissue formation above the RPE layer but below the level of retinal vessels. As the scar progresses, less RPE clumping may be evident since the RPE is now covered by fibrous tissue, although pigment may be found at the borders of such a lesion. Retinal vessels are often visible overlying a disciform scar. While AMD is the most common condition associated with disciform maculopathy, angioid streaks, degenerative myopia, choroidal rupture, presumed ocular histoplasmosis, and idiopathic choroid neovascularization (CNV) are other common causes of this maculopathy.

To establish a diagnosis, the fellow eye should be examined since these conditions are often bilateral. Angioid streaks radiate out from the disc but vary in

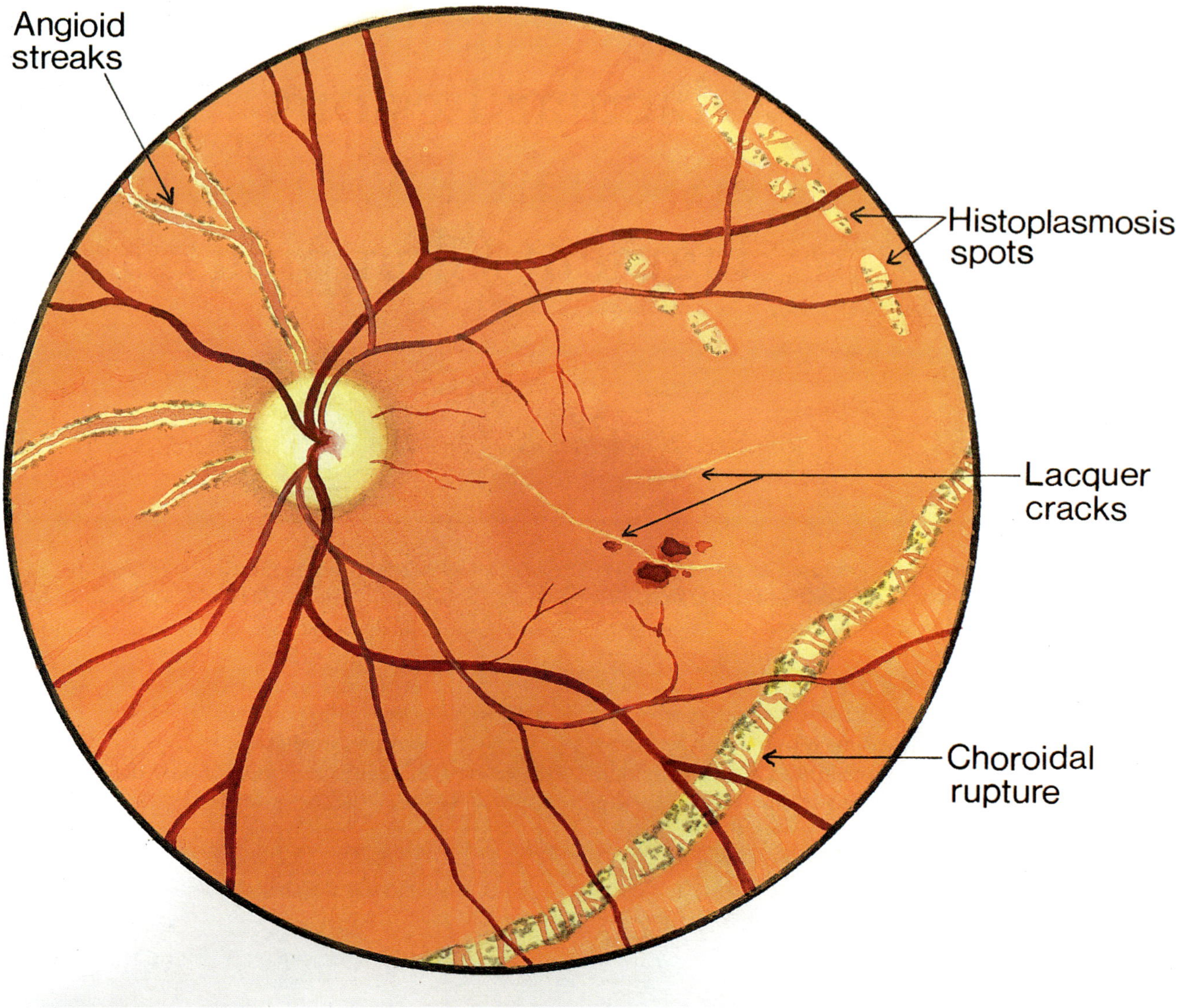

FIGURE 10.1. Illustration depicting three causes of large, lightly colored macular lesions: angioid streaks, which always appear in the posterior pole; lacquer cracks of myopic degeneration, which are finer linear lesions associated with a tesselated fundus; and traumatic choroidal rupture, often a larger lesion with more accompanying pigment changes.

length. Patients with high myopia often have abnormally shaped discs and lacquer cracks. Choroidal rupture forms a linear streak opposite from the site of injury (Figures 10.1 and 10.2). Diagnostic signs in presumed ocular histoplasmosis include the triad of fundus findings of peripapillary atrophy, punched-out lesions, and macular disciform scar that is often smaller than those seen in AMD (Figure 10.3) (see Chapter 13). Macular involvement may occur up to 40 years following discovery of other fundus lesions.

Many less common ocular diseases, which disrupt Bruch's membrane and give rise to CNV, may also result in a disciform scar. RPE geographic atrophy occurs in older patients and usually presents bilaterally with minimal clumping of pigment at the borders of the lesion. As the RPE and choroidal pigment dissipate in this degenerative process, the sclera becomes more visible, accounting for the lesion's light appearance. Large choroidal vessels are often visible through this area of RPE dropout, and drusen may be found at the periphery of this area (Figure 10.4). Fibrous tissue formation occurs in this type of AMD.

Risk profile
Conditions causing CNV
Symptoms
Central scotoma

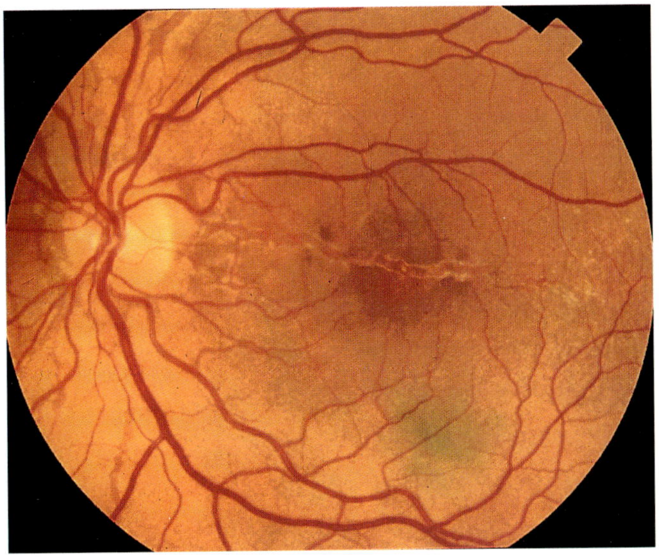

A

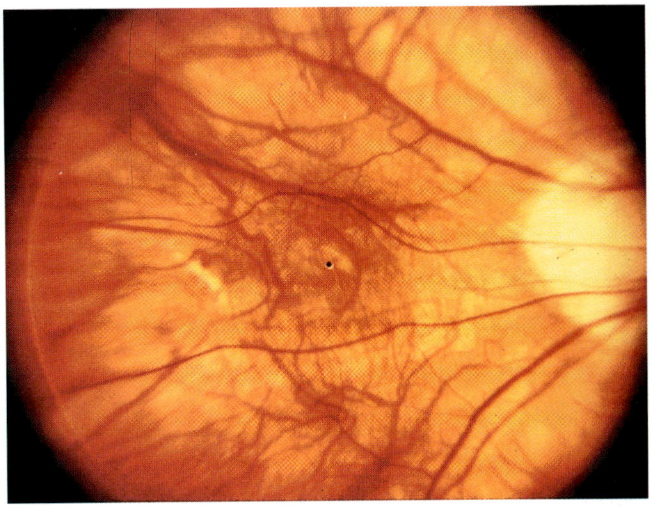

B

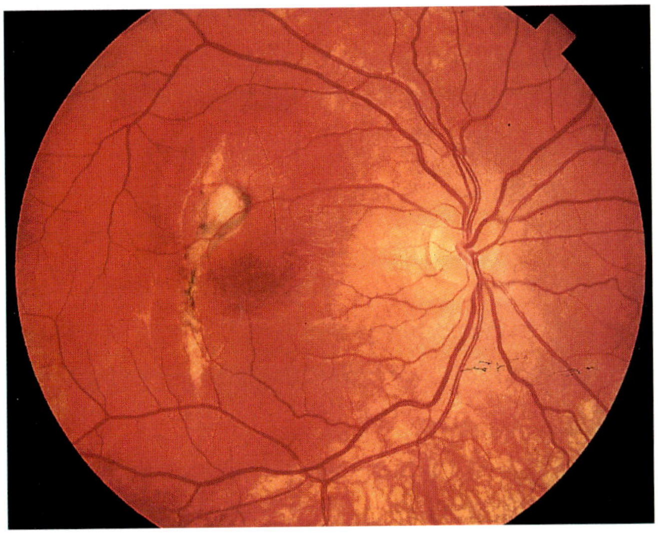

C

FIGURE 10.2. A. Angioid streaks. The linear lesion radiates from the optic disc and in this case passes directly through the center of the fovea. A choroidal nevus is apparent inferotemporal to the center of the fovea. B. Myopic lacquer cracks in a highly myopic, tesselated fundus. C. Traumatic choroidal rupture temporal to the fovea following blunt trauma to the globe. Each of these conditions can give rise to choroidal neovascular membranes.

- Legal blindness in affected eye

Diagnostic signs

- Common
  - White or lightly colored fibrous tissue
  - Retinal vessels usually remain visible
  - RPE clumping at the borders of the lesion
- Additional
  - May have retinal hemorrhage at the boundary of the lesion

Other diagnostic considerations

- Rule out all causes of CNV
- Vitreous hemorrhage possible following CNV

Management

- Monitor fellow eye every 4 months for recurrent CNV
- Home Amsler grid testing
- Photodocumentation and fluorescein angiography of fellow eye
- Polycarbonate lenses
- Ultraviolet protection
- Antioxidant therapy (advocated by some)
- Surgical excision of disciform scar (controversial)
- Low vision evaluation if bilateral

An inactive macular lesion from a previous chorioretinitis, including toxoplasmosis, may appear as RPE clumping associated with areas of pigment dropout. A key to the diagnosis of toxoplasmosis is the presence of smaller, satellite lesions at the periphery of the main lesion, which are pigmented when inactive or fluffy white when active. Symptoms of decreased vision or floaters due to vitritis may cause the patient to seek care.

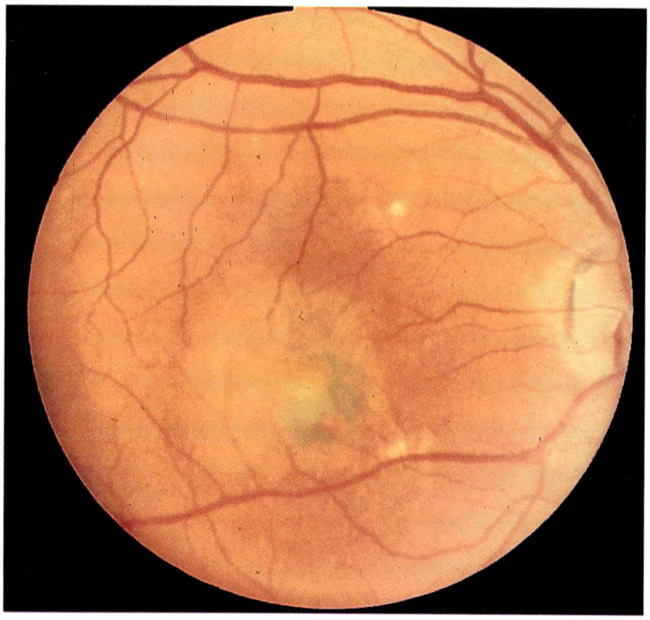

A

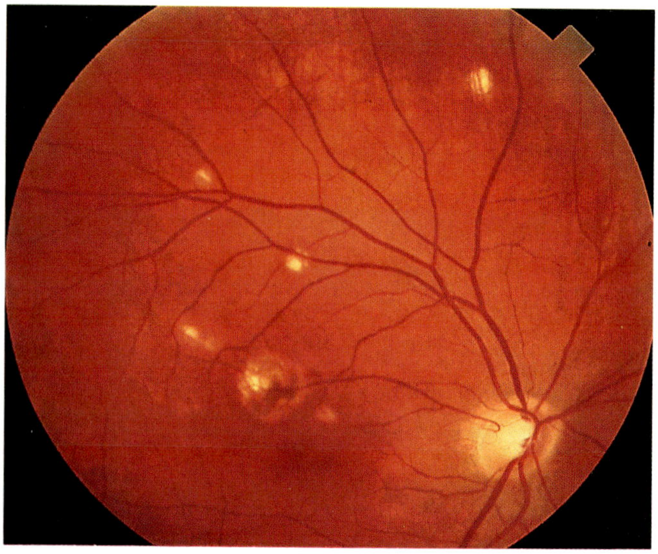

B

FIGURE 10.3. A. Ocular histoplasmosis lesions may occur as isolated punched-out spots or may take on a linear pattern that is often surrounded by dark areas. B. Histo spots may give rise to choroidal neovascular lesions, a condition that may produce a disciform scar if hemorrhage occurs.

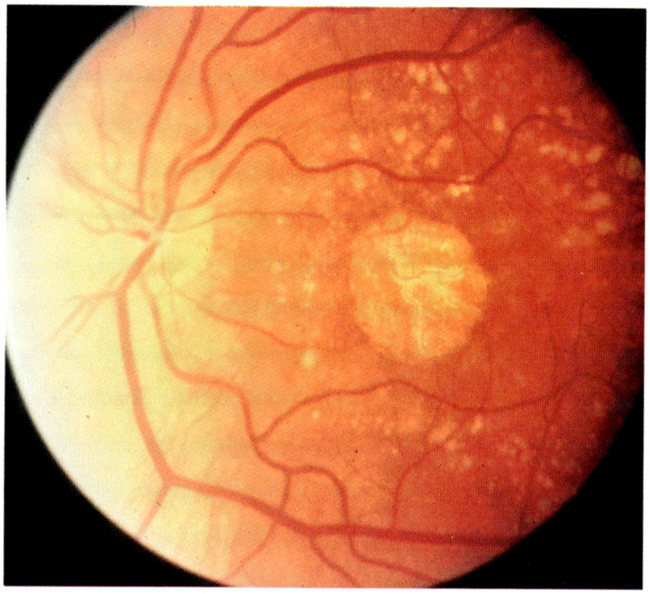

FIGURE 10.4. Extensive geographic atrophy and accompanying pigment epithelial detachment with increased visibility of the underlying choroidal structures. (Courtesy of S. Sinclair, M.D.)

Toxoplasmosis

Risk profile

Risk characteristics for toxoplasmosis (see Chapter 20)

Immunosuppressed patients

Chemotherapy

HIV+

Systemic corticosteroid therapy

Symptoms

New onset of decreased vision

Floaters

Diagnostic signs

Common

Vitritis

Cells in anterior chamber

Ocular pain and photophobia

Fluffy, white exudates with satellite lesions

Additional

Inactive stage shows RPE clumping

Other diagnostic considerations

Rule out all causes of toxoplasmosis by serologic and radiologic testing

Management

Trisulfapyrimidine therapy

Systemic and subtenon's corticosteroid therapy

Mydriatic and cycloplegic therapy

Blunt trauma can disrupt the RPE cell membranes and results in clumping and dropout in the macular area. Penetrating injuries also cause pigment clumping, often with large areas of RPE dropout.

Other Causes of Large Variegated Lesions

RPE geographic atrophy in age-related macular degeneration
- Increased age; white race
- RPE dropout
- Minimal RPE clumping and drusen at boundary of lesions
- Seldom leads to CNV
- Low vision devices helpful

Trauma
- History of contusive ocular injury
- RPE clumping with visible sclera
- Anterior segment signs of ocular injury including:
  - Hyphema
  - Angle recession
  - Iris sphincter damage
  - Lens luxation
- Monitor for late onset glaucoma and retinal detachment
- Mydriatic and cycloplegic therapy

LESS COMMON CAUSES OF LARGE, LIGHTLY COLORED LESIONS WITH RETINAL PIGMENT EPITHELIUM DISRUPTION

The RPE may be disrupted by other conditions such as inflammation, infection, hereditary dystrophies, or degenerations. Bilaterality suggests the two latter conditions, although it does not rule out the two former entities. Obtaining a family history of vision loss is helpful in the differential diagnosis since dystrophies are familial by definition. Less common causes of large, lightly colored lesions with RPE disruption include:

- Congenital/hereditary diseases
  - Best's disease
  - Fundus flavimaculatus
- Laser photocoagulation
- Multifocal choroidopathies
  - APMPPE
  - Serpiginous choroidopathy
- Nematode infestation
- Retinitis pigmentosa
- Choroidal melanoma or nevus
- Sarcoidosis

CONGENITAL AND HEREDITARY LESIONS

Although Best's disease is well known to cause a vitelliform (egg-yolk) lesion, pigment atrophy and clumping are observed in the late stages of the disease. In the late stages, Stargardt's disease may also cause an area of bilateral RPE dropout and clumping appearing similiar to RPE geographic atrophy of AMD. The early onset of vision loss and family history are keys to this diagnosis. Hereditary and congenital conditions are discussed in detail in Chapter 29.

Retinal Pigment Epithelium Window Defects

RPE window defects are usually found in the equatorial region but may be seen near the macula. These lesions are singular, with distinct borders, and have minimal RPE clumping at the edges of the lesion only; choroidal vessels are now visible through the absent RPE. Choroidal pigment is usually missing as well, but if present, the lesion appears light gray.

Laser Photocoagulation

Laser photocoagulation causes a variety of macular pigment changes depending on the fundus pigmentation, the power and spot size used, and the time since treatment. Patients with darker colored fundi produce more pigment clumping after laser therapy. Laser spots are white or yellow-white immediately following therapy, but demonstrate pigment clumping in subsequent weeks and months.

Multifocal Choroidopathies

Several forms of multifocal choroidopathy may result in light and dark patches in the macula. Serpiginous choroiditis, for example, is a bilateral but asymmetric condition occurring in patients aged 40–50. It is recurrent and is usually found starting in the peripapillary area and extending toward the macula. APMPPE initially presents as lightly colored plaques in the posterior pole of young adults, which later resolve, leaving RPE pigment changes. Vision loss is usually minimal during the pigmented stage of the disorder. Recurrent multifocal choroiditis or punctate inner choroiditis also causes clumping of the RPE in the macula (see Chapter 21).

Nematode Infestation

Previous ocular involvement by nematode infestation, particularly *Toxocara canis*, may present as unilateral RPE disruption and fibrous bands extending from the macula, usually in young men. Disc pallor is a commonly associated finding, and a nematode may occasionally be found in the vitreous. This condition is found more commonly in patients from the southeastern United States or in third world or developing countries.

Maculopathy in Retinitis Pigmentosa

Although retinitis pigmentosa is well known to cause pigment changes in the periphery, it is important to recog-

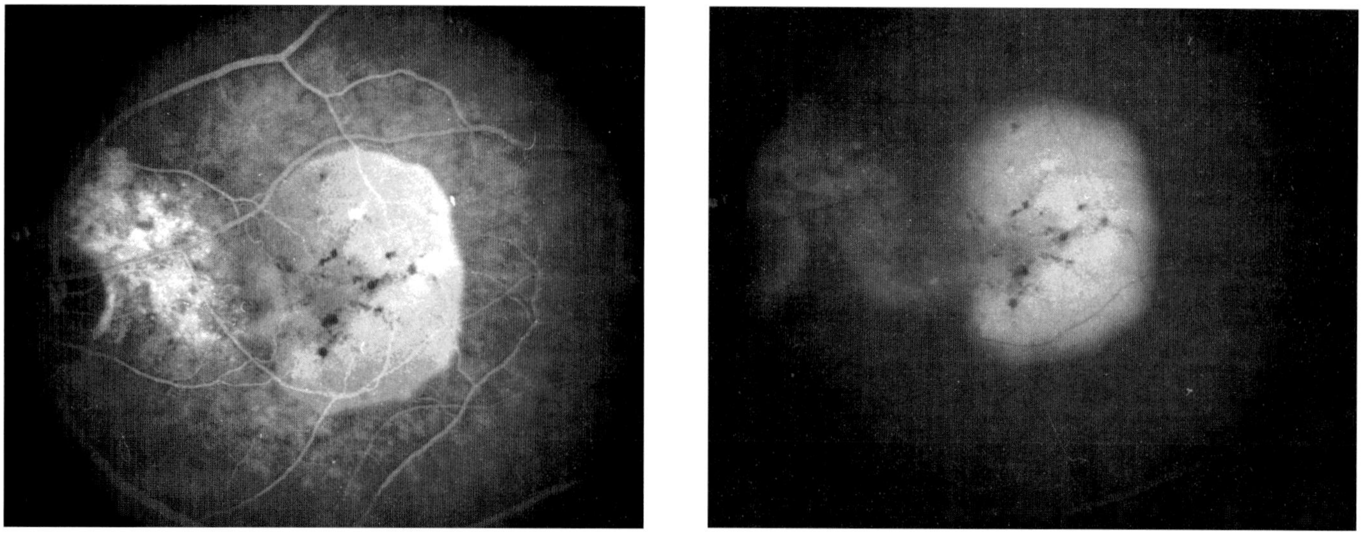

A B

FIGURE 10.5. An example of a retinal pigment epithelium tear in a patient with exudative macular degeneration. The arteriovenous phase of the angiogram demonstrates (A) hyperfluorescence with increased leakage and (B) hyperfluorescence in the late phase of the transit. (Courtesy of S. Sinclair, M.D.)

nize that a maculopathy also occurs in many patients. Severe macular involvement usually occurs relatively late in the disease process. Although macular changes such as epiretinal membranes and cystoid macular edema are more common, both RPE clumping and RPE dropout lesions have been described in retinitis pigmentosa.

Malignant Tumors of the Choroid

A rare but important cause of lesions in this category is malignancy of the choroid, namely choroidal melanoma and metastasis of systemic cancer to the choroid. Choroidal melanoma is rare, with an incidence of approximately 5.5–6.0 per million persons. Patients are usually white and elderly. The key diagnostic signs include an elevated choroidal lesion, whose dimension is greater than 5 DD, variable pigmentation, and associated, exudative retinal detachment. Any patient with a diagnosis of systemic cancer, particularly breast or lung cancer, who presents with an RPE disruption, particularly if elevated or associated with a nonrhegmatogenous retinal detachment, should be suspected of having choroidal metastasis (see Figure 9.4).

Retinal Pigment Epithelium Tears

RPE tears occur in patients with AMD following laser photocoagulation or spontaneously with exudative maculopathy. A break in the RPE at the edge of an RPE detachment followed by a retraction of this layer exposes the underlying Bruch's membrane. The fellow eye is at higher risk for vision loss secondary to RPE detachment (Figure 10.5).

LESS COMMON CAUSES OF CHORIORETINITIS

Following infection or inflammation of the choroid and retina, pigment clumping and destruction often occurs, revealing an underlying sclera that appears white or yellow-white. Infiltration of inflammatory material may also result in fibrous scarring, which will appear white with associated pigment disruption. Conditions associated with chorioretinitis include:

- Toxoplasmosis
- Syphilis
- Cytomegalovirus
- Herpes simplex
- Herpes zoster
- *Toxocara canis*
- Collagen vascular disease, systemic lupus erythematosus, sarcoidosis
- Others causes include:
  - Bacterial
  - Rickettsial
  - Viral
  - Mycotic
  - Parasitic organisms
  - Hypersensitivity
  - Toxic or irritative
  - Skin disease

SUGGESTED READING

Decker WL, Sanborn GE, Ridley M, et al. Retinal pigment epithelial tears. Ophthalmology 1983;90:507–512.

Schoeppner G, Chuang EL, Bird AC. The risk of fellow eye visual loss with unilateral retinal pigment epithelial tears. Am J Ophthalmol 1989;108:683–685.

van Knapen F. Toxoplasmosis, old story and new facts. Int Ophthalmol Clin 1989;13:371–375.

van Loon AM. Laboratory diagnosis of toxoplasmosis. Int Ophthalmol Clin 1989;13:377–381.

Weiss MJ, Velasquez N, Hofeldt AJ. Serologic tests in diagnosis of presumed toxoplasmic retinochoroiditis. Am J Ophthalmol 1990;109:407–411.

Williams DF, Mieler WF, Williams GA. Posterior segment manifestations of ocular trauma. Retina 1990;10:S35–S44.

CHAPTER

11

Red or Roseate Lesions

Leonard J. Oshinskie, Rodney K. Gutner, and Anthony A. Cavallerano

Retinal hemorrhages are frequently encountered in clinical practice and usually indicate an underlying systemic or ocular disease that may have serious implications. Although retinal hemorrhages are the most common cause of lesions in this category, it is important to recognize that other conditions, such as macular holes, macroaneurysms, or microaneurysms, may have a similar appearance to retinal hemorrhages.

As with the previous categories, lesions in this category may be separated into those that are typically small (<1 DD) or those that are large (>1 DD). Since they are typically less than 1 DD, intraretinal hemorrhages, including dot, blot, and flame-shaped hemorrhages, are discussed under small red lesions. Other retinal hemorrhages that are generally larger, including preretinal and subretinal hemorrhages, are discussed under large red lesions. Subretinal pigment epithelium (sub-RPE) hemorrhages are presented under the section on dark, solid lesions since they do not appear red, but rather gray or gray-green.

SMALL RED OR ROSEATE LESIONS

Common
- Superficial and intraretinal hemorrhages
- Microaneurysms
- Macular holes or cysts
- Cystoid macular edema

Less common
- Macroaneurysms
- Solar maculopathy
- Central retinal artery occlusion (cherry-red spot)
- High myopia
- Capillary hemangioma
- Choroidal hemorrhage

RETINAL HEMORRHAGES

Retinal hemorrhages occur secondary to vascular incompetence that results in extravasation of blood into one or several layers of the retina. This compromise may be caused by a disease limited to the eye, for example, central retinal vein occlusion or choroidal neovascularization membrane (CNVM), but is often associated with a systemic illness that results in overall vascular damage involving the retinal vessels. As with the lightly colored lesions, it is important to determine the anatomic depth of a hemorrhage, since the cause of a subretinal hemorrhage is frequently different from the cause of an intraretinal or a superficial flame-shaped hemorrhage.

Anatomic variations in the macula, including a more complicated vascular system and the propensity for choroidal neovascularization (CNV) to occur in the macula, make this area susceptible to hemorrhage. The types of hemorrhage found in the macula are preretinal, superficial (often flame-shaped), intraretinal, subretinal, sub-RPE, and choroidal. Hemorrhages at or near the optic nerve head represent a subset of retinal hemorrhages and are also presented here. White-centered retinal hemorrhages and sub-RPE hemorrhages are not discussed here since they do not strictly appear as red, pink, or orange lesions and are discussed elsewhere.

Preretinal hemorrhages are usually large and may have a boat-shaped appearance due to gravitational effects. These hemorrhages are located between the internal limiting membrane and the retinal nerve fiber layer.

Intraretinal hemorrhages may be superficial (flame-shaped) or deep (dot and blot) depending on whether the superficial or deep retinal capillaries are compromised (Figure 11.1). Flame-shaped hemorrhages are elongated lesions with feathered borders that lie along the superficial nerve fiber layer in the posterior

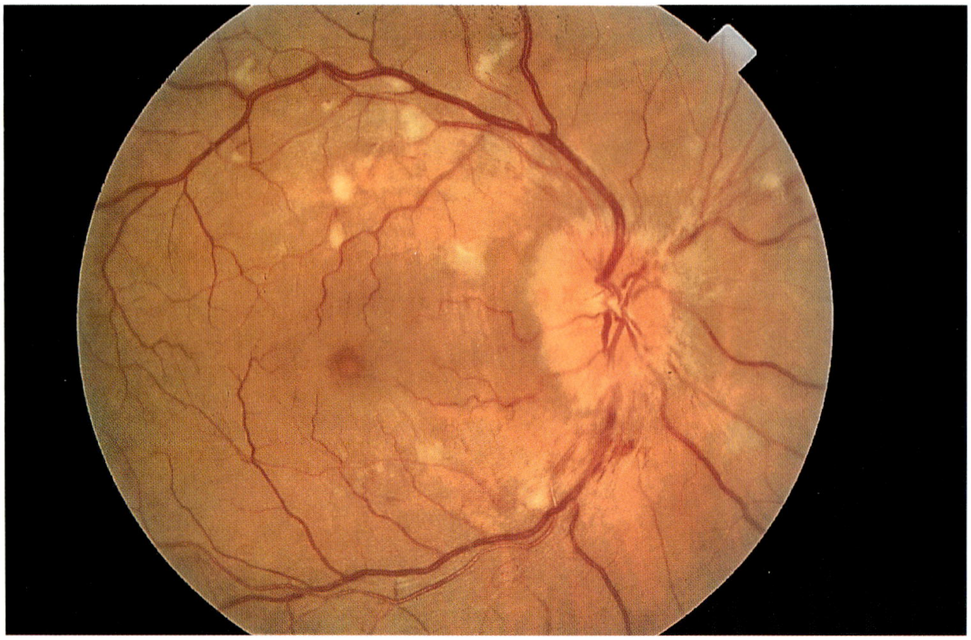

FIGURE 11.1. Hypertensive retinopathy with flame-shaped, dot and blot hemorrhages with cotton wool spots and papilledema in a patient with malignant hypertension.

pole. When located at the disc, a separate group of conditions should be considered in the differential diagnosis. A single, isolated superficial hemorrhage at or around the optic nerve head may occur in glaucoma (Drance hemorrhage) or be observed in venous occlusive disease and anterior ischemic optic neuropathy. Other conditions that are associated with disc hemorrhages include papilledema, papillitis, posterior vitreous detachment, anterior ischemic optic neuropathy, and venous occlusive disease.

Flame-Shaped Hemorrhages

- Central retinal vein occlusion
- Branch retinal vein occlusion
- Diabetic retinopathy
- Human immunodeficiency virus (HIV) retinopathy

Dot and blot hemorrhages lie in the inner nuclear and outer plexiform layers. Ophthalmoscopically, these hemorrhages are difficult to differentiate from microaneurysms; however, by fluorescein angiography (FA), microaneurysms hyperfluoresce while dot hemorrhages block choroidal fluorescence and appear dark. Blot hemorrhages lie within multiple layers of the sensory retina and indicate venous abnormalities.

Subretinal hemorrhages are located above the RPE and below the level of the photoreceptors. Their presence often indicates CNV, trauma, or severe retinal vascular disease. Choroidal hemorrhages are darker than intraretinal hemorrhages.

Intraretinal Hemorrhage

Venous occlusive disease is a common condition causing unilateral dots or blots radiating from the disc or an arteriovenous crossing. Flame-shaped, superficial hemorrhages radiating from the disc are also seen.

Numerous hemorrhages and cotton wool spots (CWS) indicate the ischemic form of the disease, a condition that frequently leads to iris neovascularization and neovascular glaucoma in central retinal vein occlusion and retinal neovascularization in a major branch occlusion. Patients are typically men older than 60. If only a few dot and blot hemorrhages are found in the absence of or with few CWS, then the nonischemic variety is suspected. This type occasionally evolves into the ischemic variety in older individuals. Patients should have a medical evaluation for hypertension, diabetes mellitus, atherosclerotic disease, and serum lipid abnormalities. Appropriate hematologic testing includes a complete blood count, lipid profile, serum protein electrophoresis, erythrocyte sedimentation rate, and prothrombin time and partial thromboplastin time. Younger male patients with a fundus picture similar to central retinal vein occlusion are categorized as having papillophlebitis, which is thought to be inflammatory in nature. Vision usually returns to normal in these patients. Hemorrhages in hypertensive retinopathy are usually flame-shaped, although dot and blot shapes may be found. CWS and sometimes vessel caliber changes accompany retinal hemorrhages in patients with a recent acute increase of diastolic blood pressure greater than 110 mm Hg. Hemorrhages remain for several weeks after the blood pressure is controlled.

Flame-Shaped Hemorrhage in Central Retinal Vein Occlusion

Risk profile
- Sixth decade or beyond
- History of:
  - Diabetes
  - Hypertension
  - Hyperviscosity syndrome
  - Hyperlipidemia
- Oral contraceptive use
- History of ocular hypertension or glaucoma

Symptoms
- Sudden, painless vision loss (20/40 to light perception)
- Unilateral
- Nonischemic type may have good vision

Diagnostic signs
- Common
  - Flame-shaped hemorrhages
  - CWS
  - Microaneurysms
  - Blot hemorrhages
  - Dilated, tortuous retinal veins
  - Disc edema
  - Macular edema
- Additional
  - Positive afferent pupillary defect (APD) in ischemic variety

Other diagnostic considerations
  - Rule out glaucoma in fellow eye
  - FA to determine ischemic versus nonischemic type
  - Rule out neovascularization of the iris and neovascular glaucoma

Management
- Treatment indicated for ischemic retinopathy or neovascularization of the iris
- Medical evaluation to rule out:
  - Diabetes
  - Hypertension
- Additional tests
  - Electrocardiogram
  - Complete blood count
  - Serum protein electrophoresis
  - Prothrombin time
  - Erythrocyte sedimentation rate
  - Serum lipid profile

Flame-Shaped Hemorrhage in Branch Retinal Vein Occlusion

Risk profile
- Sixth decade or beyond
- Hypertensive male subjects
- Hyperlipidemia
- Pre-existing ocular hypertension or glaucoma

Symptoms
- Minimal-to-moderate reduction in vision
- Dysmorphopsia with macular edema

Diagnostic signs
- Common
  - Flame-shaped and blot hemorrhages in a wedge pattern
  - Macular edema if superior temporal quadrant affected
- Additional
  - Collateral vessels crossing horizontal raphe
  - Dilated, tortuous veins

Other diagnostic considerations
- Neovascular glacoma and neovascularization of iris uncommon
- Rule out ocular hypertension and primary open-angle glaucoma

Management
- FA to rule out retinal ischemia, neovascularization of the retina, and macular edema
- Medical evaluation to rule out systemic disease

Flame-Shaped Hemorrhage in Malignant Hypertension

Risk profile
- Black males
- Noncompliance in a known hypertensive
- Family history
- Pregnancy

Symptoms
- Headache
- Decreased vision
- Dizziness and palpitations

Diagnostic signs
- Common
  - Bilateral flame-shaped hemorrhages
  - CWS
  - Hard exudates
  - Disc edema
- Additional
  - Attenuated arterioles

Other diagnostic considerations
- Elevated blood pressure
- Systolic generally >190 mm Hg
- Diastolic generally >110 mm Hg

Management
- Immediate referral for medical evaluation
- Blood pressure must be lowered gradually to avoid optic nerve and end-organ ischemia

Diabetic retinopathy is a common systemic condition associated with bilateral dot or blot hemorrhages, and if a patient is not a known diabetic, then a medical evaluation for a number of systemic conditions is indicated based on the patient's age and symptoms. Type I diabetic patients generally do not develop retinopathy for at least the first 3 years following diagnosis, whereas type II diabetic patients may have dots and blots at the time that diagnosis is established. Patients with dot and blot hemorrhages found in greater number than standard photo 2A in the Airly-House system require more frequent follow-up since proliferative retinopathy is more likely. Venous occlusive disease is sometimes superimposed on diabetic retinopathy and should be suspected in a diabetic patient with asymmetric retinal hemorrhages.

Flame-Shaped Hemorrhage in Diabetic Retinopathy

- Risk profile
  - Increases with duration of diabetes
- Symptoms
  - Minimal-to-moderate reduction in vision secondary to associated nonperfusion or macular edema
  - Dysmorphopsia with macular edema
- Diagnostic signs
  - Common
    - Flame-shaped, dot and blot hemorrhages
    - Microaneurysms
      - Bilateral, confined to posterior pole
  - Additional
    - Proliferative diabetic changes with capillary nonperfusion
- Other diagnostic considerations
  - Rule out other manifestations of diabetic eye disease
- Management
  - FA to rule out retinal ischemia and macular edema
  - Comanage with endocrinologist

Preretinal, intraretinal, subretinal, or sub-RPE hemorrhages in a patient with drusen or other signs of age-related macular degeneration strongly suggest a leaking CNVM. These patients require immediate referral for FA and consideration for laser photocoagulation. Many human immunodeficiency virus–positive (HIV+) and acquired immunodeficiency syndrome (AIDS) patients develop noninfectious microvascular retinopathy. The most common manifestation in HIV+ patients is CWS, but these patients also have retinal hemorrhages in association with CWS or retinal hemorrhages in isolation (Figure 11.2).

Patients with only HIV retinopathy are often asymptomatic. Large blot and flame-shaped hemorrhages with patches of white or yellow-white retinal necrosis and perivascular sheathing in an HIV+ patient strongly suggest an infectious process, usually CMV retinitis, although other illnesses such as syphilis and acute retinal necrosis may present in a similar fashion. An associated vitritis is often found, with patients complaining of floaters. Collagen vascular diseases, such as systemic lupus erythematosus, are also associated with dot and blot hemorrhages and CWS. These hemorrhages are secondary to necrosis of retinal vessels and usually occur in patients with exacerbation of their systemic condition.

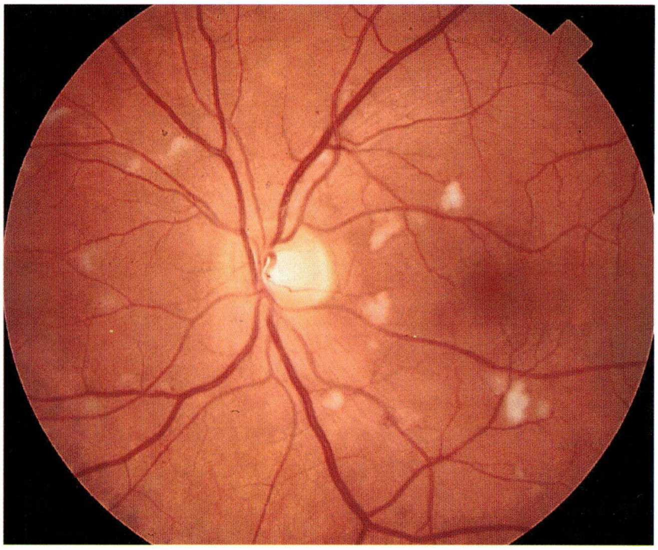

FIGURE 11.2. Acquired immunodeficiency syndrome patient with multiple cotton wool spots with occasional hemorrhage.

Severe blunt trauma to the globe may cause retinal hemorrhage, as may a crushing injury to the thorax (Purtscher's retinopathy) or long bones. Shaken child syndrome has also been reported to cause retinal hemorrhages. Retinal hemorrhages rarely occur in anemia unless the condition is severe. Hemoglobin values less than one-half the norm (8 g per 100 ml) are generally required before retinal hemorrhages occur. Retinal hemorrhages associated with anemia are usually flame shaped, but may also be of the dot and blot variety. If thrombocytopenia (low platelet count) is concurrent, hemorrhages are more likely.

Macular hemorrhage in sarcoidosis is rare but has been reported in association with other fundus lesions, including CWS. Patients with leukemia, especially the acute type, commonly have retinal involvement including round, flame-shaped, or white-centered hemorrhages and dilated and tortuous veins.

Dot and blot hemorrhages are a common finding in radiation retinopathy and are commonly associated with microaneurysms and hard exudates with a clinical appearance similiar to diabetic retinopathy. Most of these patients have had radiation therapy of greater than

Venous stasis retinopathy secondary to carotid occlusive disease usually causes blot hemorrhages outside the macula in the midperiphery, but in severe stages, hemorrhages may be found in both the midperiphery and macula (Figure 11.3).

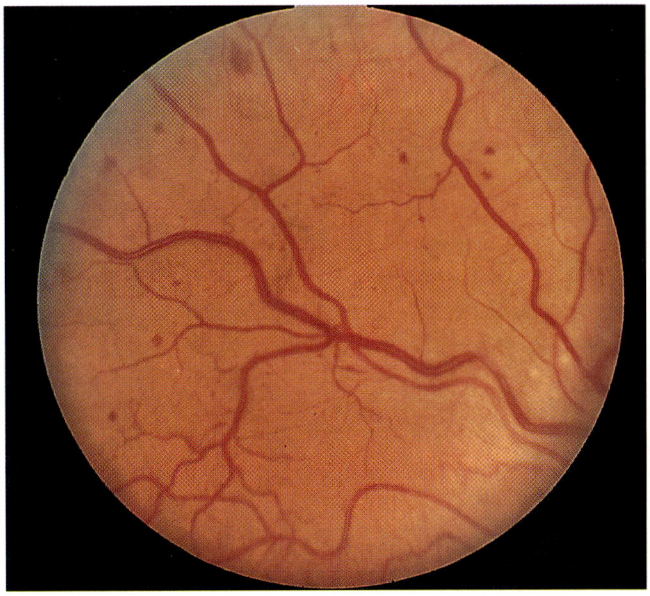

FIGURE 11.3. Venous stasis retinopathy with multiple blot hemorrhages.

Intraretinal Hemorrhage (Dot and Blot)

Risk profile
- Systemic disease
- Medications

Symptoms
- Significant decrease in visual function with subfoveal hemorrhage
- Macular edema reduces vision

Diagnostic signs
- Common
  - Dot, blot, or flame-shaped hemorrhages
  - Superficial, indicating nerve fiber hemorrhages
  - Flame-shaped hemorrhages usually found around the vascular arcades
- Additional
  - CWS
  - Microaneurysms
  - Hard exudates

Other diagnostic considerations
- Determine if treatable ocular lesions:
  - Macular edema
  - Proliferative retinopathy
  - CNVM
- Rule out ocular or systemic conditions associated with intraretinal hemorrhage

Management
- Treatment indicated for macular edema, venous occlusive disease, suspected CNVM
- Medical evaluation to rule out:
  - Diabetes
  - Hypertension
- Venous occlusive disease; additional tests include:
  - Electrocardiogram
  - Complete blood count
  - Serum protein electrophoresis
  - Prothrombin time
  - Erythrocyte sedimentation rate
  - Serum lipid profile

Conditions Associated with Intraretinal Hemorrhages

Common
- Diabetes
  - Almost always bilateral
- Venous occlusive disease
  - Sometimes in association with diabetes
  - Unilateral
  - Radiates from disc
  - Observe for macular edema, neovascularization elsewhere, and neovascularization of iris
- Poorly controlled hypertension
  - Flame-shaped hemorrhage with CWS
  - Vessel caliber changes
  - History of recent increase in blood pressure (diastolic >110 mm Hg)
- CNVM (in any patient with drusen and intraretinal hemorrhage)
- CMV retinitis (vitritis usually present)

Less common
- Collagen vascular disease (often seen with exacerbation of disease)
- Radiation retinopathy
  - 6 months to 3 years following radiation treatment to the eye or head
  - Microaneurysms, exudates, CWS
- HIV retinopathy
  - Hemorrhages and CWS
- Blood dyscrasias
- Hyperviscosity states
  - Multiple myeloma
  - Waldenberg's microglobulinemia
  - Polycythemia vera
  - Anemias and thrombocytopenia (usually flame shaped)
  - Leukemia (hemorrhage more common in acute type; round, flame-shaped, or white-centered retinal hemorrhage with dilated, tortuous veins)

- Sickle cell disease (usually peripheral retinal involvement)
- Retinal vascular disease
  - Eale's disease
  - Coats' disease
    - Massive exudation
  - Idiopathic juxtafoveal telangiectasia
    - Look for tortuous vessels temporal to macula
  - Angiomatosis retinae
  - Retinal macroaneurysms
    - Hemorrhages may be multilevel
- Following trauma
  - Child abuse
  - Purtscher's retinopathy
  - Blunt ocular trauma
  - Intracranial hemorrhage (Terson's syndrome)
- Hypoxic states
  - Carotid occlusive disease
    - Hemorrhages are usually midperipheral
    - Pulseless disease
    - High-altitude retinopathy
- Infectious disease
  - Subacute bacterial endocarditis
  - Retinitis
    - CMV
    - Toxoplasmosis
    - Herpes simplex
  - Rocky Mountain spotted fever
- Inflammatory conditions
  - Sarcoidosis
    - Hemorrhage rare; look for CWS
  - Behçet's syndrome
- Other causes
  - Optic nerve head hemorrhage
  - Hormone therapy (oral contraceptive)
  - Lymphoma (Hodgkin's disease)
  - Drugs with anticoagulant properties
  - Congenital conditions
  - Intravenous drug abuse (CWS)
  - Blood loss
  - Papillophlebitis (younger patients—clinical picture similar to venous occlusive disease)

MICROANEURYSMS

Histologically, a microaneurysm (MA) is an outpouching of a retinal vessel, usually a capillary, on the venous side of the retinal circulation. Clinically they appear as small, red dots clustered near smaller retinal vessels. It is sometimes difficult to differentiate MAs from a dot hemorrhage by direct clinical examination (Figure 11.4).

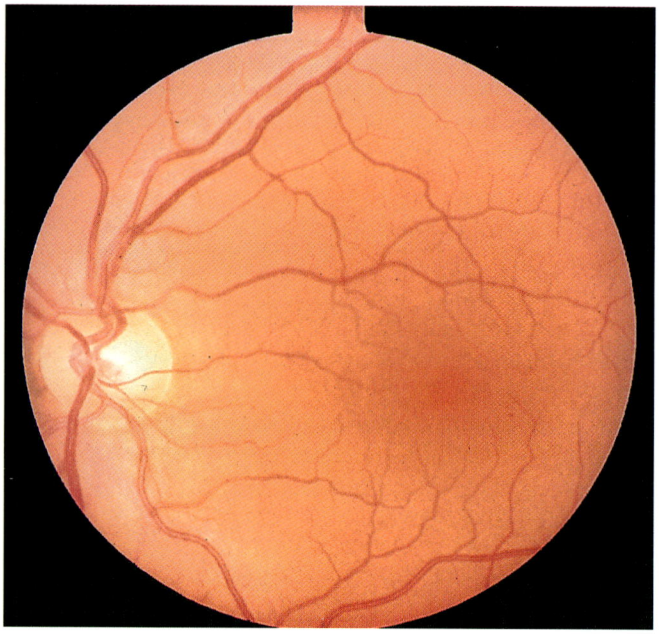

FIGURE 11.4. Paramacular microaneurysms.

FA will show hyperfluorescence corresponding to the area of MAs, whereas dot hemorrhages block fluorescence. MAs occur in several retinal vascular diseases and are often associated with hard exudates, macular edema, and intraretinal hemorrhage. Shunt vessels and neovascularization, indicative of capillary nonperfusion and retinal ischemia, may also occur in association with MAs. Common conditions associated with MAs include diabetic retinopathy, hypertensive retinopathy, and retinal vein occlusion, but many other conditions should be considered when MAs are noted.

Risk profile

- Systemic disease
  - Common
    - Diabetes
    - Hypertension
    - Venous occlusive disease
    - HIV retinopathy
  - Less common
    - Blood dyscrasias
    - Leukemia
    - Sickle cell hemoglobinopathy
    - Macroglobulinemia
    - Dysproteinemias
- Systemic lupus erythematosus
  - Coats' disease
- Eale's disease
- Posterior uveitis
- Subacute bacterial endocarditis
- Carotid insufficiency
- Radiation retinopathy
- Retinopathy of prematurity
- Idiopathic

Symptoms
- Blurred vision if associated with macular edema

Diagnostic signs
- Common
  - Small (<50 μ) red dots
  - Distinct borders
  - Sensory retina
  - Often bilateral
- Additional
  - Clustered around retinal vessels in posterior pole
  - Hard exudates
  - Dot and blot hemorrhages
  - Macular edema
  - Shunt vessels
  - Neovascularization if retinal ischemia present
  - Hyperfluoresce early on FA (dot hemorrhages block fluorescence)

Other diagnostic considerations
- May be earliest sign in undiagnosed diabetes
- If unilateral or limited to one quadrant, rule out venous occlusive disease

Management
- Evaluate for diabetes mellitus
- FA by retinologist
- Laser photocoagulation for macular edema from retinal ischemia

MACULAR HOLES

Isolated, well-circumscribed red lesions in the central macula often represent structural changes to the retinal tissue, especially in the absence of systemic vascular disease. Visual acuity may be severely impaired with full-thickness macular holes, and the clinician must determine the status of the vitreous in the fellow eye to predict the potential for hole formation. Other causes of these discrete lesions include pseudoholes, lamellar holes, which must be differentiated from full-thickness holes, and solar retinopathy (Figure 11.5) (see Chapter 19).

Risk profile
- Sixth decade and beyond
- Female > male subjects

Symptoms
- Blurred vision
- Dysmorphopsia
- Positive central or paracentral scotoma
- Entoptic symptoms

Diagnostic signs
- Common
  - Operculum attached to posterior vitreous
  - Singular red lesion
  - Centered in macula
  - 300–500 μ

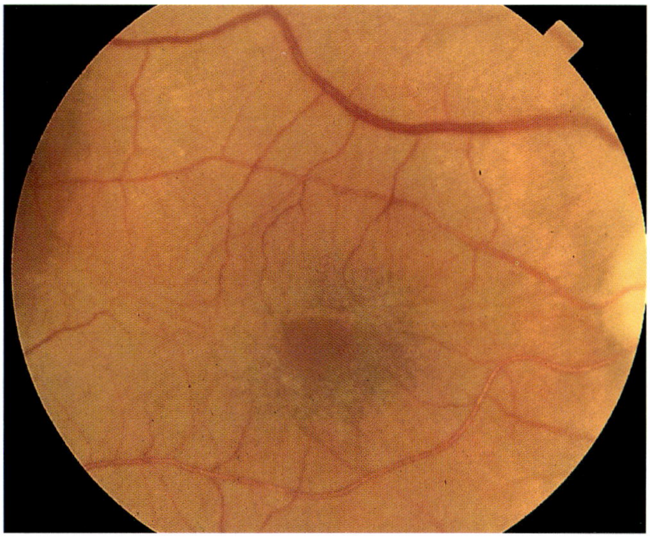

FIGURE 11.5. Well-circumscribed full-thickness macular hole.

  - Distinct borders
- Additional
  - Posterior vitreous detachment (PVD)
  - Epiretinal membrane

Other diagnostic considerations
- Check for positive Watzke's sign
- Evaluate fellow eye for impending PVD

Management
- Retinology consult to consider:
  - Vitrectomy with membrane peel
  - Tissue growth factor beta

CYSTOID MACULAR EDEMA

Cystoid changes in the macular area may produce the appearance of small red or roseate lesions (see Chapter 16). Leakage of the perifoveal vessels produces the typical appearance of cystic spaces in the foveal area. Intraocular surgery, chronic ocular inflammation, and venous occlusive disease are common causes for this clinical finding. Long-standing cystoid macular edema may result in epiretinal membrane and macular hole formation. FA will confirm the vascular leakage and the presence of the edema.

Risk profile
- Diabetic retinopathy
- After intraocular surgery
- Medications (topical epinephrine)
- Retinal vascular occlusive disease
- Trauma
- Systemic diseases
  - Leukemia
  - Behçet's syndrome

Symptoms
- Blurred vision

- Dysmorphopsia

Diagnostic signs
- Common
  - Cluster of red vacuoles in macula
  - Petalloid appearance
- Additional
  - Intraretinal hemorrhage
  - Granular pigment changes

Other diagnostic considerations
- Rule out:
  - Venous occlusive disease
  - Chronic inflammatory disease
  - Retinitis pigmentosa

Management
- Topical or retrobulbar steroids
- Topical or systemic nonsteroidal anti-inflammatory drugs
- Carbonic anhydrase inhibitors

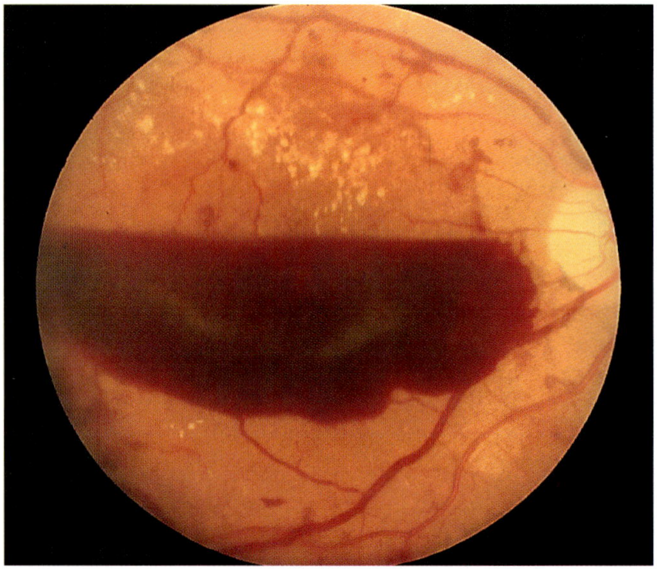

FIGURE 11.6. Large boat-shaped preretinal hemorrhage in a patient with proliferative diabetic retinopathy.

LARGE RED OR ROSEATE LESIONS

Large red lesions result from preretinal or subsensory retinal hemorrhage and occur secondary to disorders of the blood or blood-forming organs. Diabetes and hypertension are common causes of preretinal hemorrhages and patients with severe nonproliferative diabetic retinopathy and proliferative diabetic retinopathy are at high risk for severe vision loss (Figure 11.6). Other causes include sickle cell hemoglobinopathy and blood dyscrasias.

Preretinal Hemorrhage

Risk profile
- Systemic diseases
  - Diabetes
  - Hypertension
  - Leukemia
  - Anemia
  - Sickle cell hemoglobinopathy
  - Blood dyscrasias
- Head trauma (intracranial hemorrhage—Terson's syndrome)

Symptoms
- Scotoma
- Reduced vision
- Floaters with vitreous hemorrhage

Diagnostic signs
- Common
  - Superficial light to dark red lesions in posterior pole
  - Boat- or crescent-shaped hemorrhage
  - Singular or multiple hemorrhages
  - Greater than 1 DD
- Additional
  - "Thumbprint" hemorrhage
  - Color change with absorption

Other diagnostic considerations
- Vitreous hemorrhage
- PVD
- Retinal neovascularization
- Intraretinal hemorrhages
- Retinal macroaneuryms

Management
- Rule out retinal neovascularization
- Rule out subdural hemorrhage from trauma or other cause (cerebrovascular accident)
- Medical evaluation to rule out systemic diseases or trauma

Subretinal Hemorrhage

Subretinal hemorrhage results from CNVM and appears red when fresh. However, the appearance changes to a duller or dirty appearance, either gray-green or dirty brown.

Risk profile
- Ocular conditions predisposing to CNVM
- Trauma
- Anticoagulant therapy

Symptoms
- Dysmorphopsia
- Significantly reduced vision
- Scotoma

Diagnostic signs
- Common
  - Large dull to bright red macular hemorrhage
  - Singular, round or oval elevated lesion
  - Indistinct borders

Additional
- "Thumbprint" hemorrhage
- Color change with absorption

Other diagnostic considerations
- Vitreous hemorrhage
- PVD
- Retinal neovascularization
- Intraretinal hemorrhages
- Retinal macroaneuryms

Management
- Rule out:
  - Retinal neovascularization
  - CNV
  - Subdural hemorrhage from trauma or other cause (Terson's syndrome, cerebrovascular accident)
- Medical evaluation to rule out systemic diseases or trauma

Choroidal Hemangioma

Choroidal hemangioma is another cause of preretinal hemorrhage. Exudative retinal detachment often occurs and, because of their appearance, the lesions must be differentiated from choroidal metastases or amelanotic melanoma.

Risk profile
- Young to middle-aged adults
- No sex predilection
- Rare in blacks

Symptoms
- No or reduced vision
- Scotoma and other visual field defects

Diagnostic signs
- Common
  - Unilateral, round or oval elevated roseate lesion
  - Indistinct borders
  - Pigment irregularities
- Additional
  - Exudative retinal detachment
  - Conjunctival and episcleral telangiectasia

Other diagnostic considerations
- Often found temporal to the macula
- Benign lesions but can cause vision loss through retinal detachment
- Rule out choroidal metastases or amelanotic melanoma
- Rule out phakomatoses

Management
- Retinal consultation for laser photocoagulation

LESS COMMON CAUSES OF SMALL RED OR ROSEATE LESIONS

Macroaneurysms
- Seventh decade
- Male > female subjects
- Associated with hypertension or sarcoidosis

Solar retinopathy
- History of sungazing
- Central scotoma

Central retinal artery occlusion ("cherry red spot")
- Seventh decade
- Other sclerotic disease
- Carotid, cardiac, or valvular disease

Choroidal hemorrhage

Capillary hemangioma

High myopia

SUGGESTED READING

Brown GC, Shields JA, Sanborn G, et al. Radiation retinopathy. Ophthalmology 1982;89:1494–1501.

Freeman WR, Chen A, Henderly DE, et al. Prevalence and significance of acquired immunodeficiency syndrome–related retinal microvasculopathy. Arch Ophthalmol 1989;107:229–235.

Kaur B, Taylor D. Fundus hemorrhages in infancy. Surv Ophthalmol 1992;37:1–17.

Kincaid MC, Green R. Ocular and orbital involvement in leukemia. Surv Ophthalmol 1983;27:211–232.

Michealson IC. Textbook of the Fundus of the Eye (3rd ed). Edinburgh: Churchill Livingstone, 1980.

Sapira JD. An internist looks at the fundus oculi. Dis Mon 1984;30:18–38.

Witchel H, Font RL. Hemangioma of the choroid: A clinicopathologic study of 71 cases and a review of the literature. Surv Ophthalmol 1976;20:415–431.

Yanoff M, Fine BS. Ocular Pathology (3rd ed). Philadelphia: Lippincott, 1989.

PART

III

Conditions Associated with Choroidal Neovascular Membrane

CHAPTER

12

Age-Related Macular Degeneration

Anthony A. Cavallerano

Age-related macular degeneration (AMD) is a major cause of vision loss in the adult population. It was first reported over 100 years ago and historically has also been referred to in the literature as senile macular degeneration, senile macular choroidal degeneration, Kuhnt-Junius disciform detachment, and dominantly inherited drusen. The epidemiologic features have been explored, but hard data are difficult to obtain due to a poorly understood definition and the etiology of the disease.

For purposes of clinical description and definition, AMD expresses itself as changes in the outer retinal complex demonstrated by various types of drusen, alteration of Bruch's membrane, atrophy, retinal pigment epithelium (RPE) changes, and retinal changes associated with choroidal neovascularization (CNV) and exudation. When these changes result in an exudative process, the disease is referred to as the wet form of AMD; the atrophic type is designated as the dry form. AMD is generally encountered in the sixth decade and beyond, and various risk factors have been proposed to account for the disorder's etiopathogenesis.

Estimates of the prevalence of AMD range up to 9% and increase significantly with advancing age. The Framingham and Beaver Dam studies have reported a prevalence approaching a range of 30–40% in persons over age 75. The exudative form occurs in only 10% of persons with AMD; however, 90% of severe vision loss with AMD is associated with the wet or exudative form of the disease. AMD accounts for approximately 20% of all legal blindness in the United States. In spite of significant advances in laser therapy during the past two decades, relatively few patients are suitable candidates for treatment.

RISK FACTORS FOR AGE-RELATED MACULAR DEGENERATION

- Age
- Sex
- Race (rare in blacks)
- Personal factors
  - First-degree family history of AMD
  - Genetic factors
- Systemic factors
  - Hypertension
  - Cardiovascular disease
  - Cigarette smoking
- Ocular factors
  - Hyperopia >0.75 D
  - Light ocular pigmentation
  - Soft confluent drusen
  - RPE hyperpigmentation
- Environmental factors
  - Cumulative light toxicity

Risk factors for AMD include age, sex, race, family history, cigarette smoking, cardiovascular disease, hyperopia, and light-colored irides. Ultraviolet (UV) light has been implicated as a contributing factor in the pathogenesis of AMD, and studies investigating the cumulative effects of radiation are ongoing. Two hundred thousand hours of cumulative exposure to UV light is thought to be a risk factor for AMD.

An important risk factor for both types of AMD is age, with an increasing association of the exudative type occurring in older individuals. There is no clear distinction between the sexes, although random studies have demonstrated slightly higher rates among women. However, this may be due to greater longevity enjoyed by women. The exudative type seems to be more prevalent among whites compared with blacks and Asians. The hypothesis is that darker pigmentation may serve as a protective barrier for the retina, especially in the case of UV radiation, thus postponing the RPE changes that herald the onset of the disease. It is also possible that RPE cells with more pigmented populations may have an innate antioxidant effect. In addition to ocular pigmentation, hyperopia greater than 0.75 D is considered a risk characteristic for AMD.

Additional risk factors include cardiovascular disease; as it relates to AMD, it is defined as hypertension, stroke, high serum cholesterol, arterial sclerosis, left ventricular hypertrophy, circulatory problems, heart attack, or angina. Cigarette smoking appears to be a significant risk factor for neovascular AMD. It has been proposed that sclerotic changes of the choriocapillaris could be the relative factor in cardiovascular disease and AMD.

Heredity may play a role in the development of AMD. Ten to 20% of patients with AMD have at least one first-degree family member with vision loss from the disease. Family history should be explored if fundus abnormalities or other risk factors suggest a predisposition.

Other personal characteristics related to AMD include nutritional factors, intake of vitamins A, C, and E, and trace elements of zinc and selenium. Skin characteristics have also been identified as contributory factors.

Environmental factors such as cumulative sunlight exposure have been positively associated with AMD, suggesting that UV light may be related to AMD. The relationship between light absorption and cataracts has led some investigators to relate AMD to cataract.

Specifically, the Case-Control Study Group investigated the risk factors and epidemiology of AMD and concluded that there is a decreased risk of neovascular AMD with higher levels of carotenoid, with a higher horizontal cup-to-disc ratio, and in postmenopausal women taking exogenous estrogen therapy. There seems to be an increased risk associated with cigarette smoking and elevated serum cholesterol. In this particular study no change in risk was noted in sunlight exposure, serum zinc levels, and iris color.

NATURAL HISTORY OF AGE-RELATED MACULAR DEGENERATION

The natural history of AMD is poorly understood. However, the natural stages of the disorder may be divided into the atrophic or dry form and the exudative, neovascular, or wet form. Drusen is a finding common to both forms of AMD, and the progression of the disease to the exudative form is related to the nature, type, and extent of drusen.

Evolution of Age-Related Macular Degeneration

To understand the pathogenesis of AMD, it is necessary to recognize the anatomic relationships in the retina and choroid. Bruch's membrane, the choriocapillaris, and the photoreceptor–RPE complex function as a unit. Over time, the photoreceptors shed outer segments, which then become less degradable; loss of photoreceptor nuclei is an age-related phenomenon and is not specific for AMD. With continued shedding of outer receptor segments, lipofuscin accumulates, and the RPE cells lose melanin in favor of alcohol-soluble lipids. Aging changes cause a thickening and disorganization of Bruch's membrane, with a resultant alteration in the metabolism of the membrane. It becomes less permeable with age and hampers the passage of nutrients into the retina and removal of waste into the choriocapillaris. Collagen is deposited on the inner surface of Bruch's membrane, which has been referred to as "basal laminar deposits" and probably corresponds to drusen.

Since pigment epithelial cells are nonmutating, they digest their own waste products, a process that may also lead to the accumulation of lipofuscin. As cells enlarge, they may burst since there is no autoregulation. It is generally agreed that deterioration of the RPE gives rise to macular degeneration. The highly metabolic nature of the RPE, combined with the fact that these cells do not divide, results in deterioration through self-consumption. Since each pigment epithelial cell is attached to approximately 25 rods and the photoreceptors shed footplates, the RPE cells must engulf, phagocytize, and remove waste products. Undigested remnants of this process result in the accumulation of lipofuscin. The accumulation of lipofuscin affects cell metabolism. The pigment epithelial cells must also remove other waste products from metabolically active cells, a hardship that increases with further degeneration of tissue.

Drusen

Drusen have been identified as one of the earliest ophthalmoscopically detectable features of AMD. Originally referred to as colloid bodies, these crystalline-like deposits of varying size and shape consist of extracellular material that accumulates between the RPE and the inner zone layer of Bruch's membrane. The word *drusen* comes from the German *druse*, meaning nodule or bump. Certain forms of drusen are considered innocuous and are associated with advancing age; by themselves they do not cause visual loss. There are generally considered to be two types of drusen: hard and soft (Table 12.1). Both are probably derived from the breakdown of RPE cells.

Hard drusen, or hyaline, represent focal photoreceptor outer segment by-products. As seen with the

TABLE 12.1. Drusen

Type	*Histologic characteristics*	*Ophthalmoscopic features*	*Angiographic features*	*Associated risk factors*
Hard drusen	Hyaline material; inner and outer collagenous zones of Bruch's membrane; RPE changes (clumping, hypopigmentation, hypertrophy); may become calcified	Bilateral, relatively symmetric; small, well-defined; elevated; multiple; round; dense; white-yellow; RPE alteration	Transmission defects in early transit; more drusen observed angiographically than ophthalmoscopically	Age-related; low risk for vision loss from CNV; may convert to soft, serous drusen
Soft drusen (soft drusen, confluent drusen)	Amorphous material between thickened Bruch's membrane and RPE; weakened Bruch's membrane may split; serous detachment of RPE; larger area of involvement; RPE changes including hypertrophy, attenuation, or absence; may become calcified	Bilateral, relatively symmetric; ill-defined boundaries; confluent; plaque-like elevation; more obvious RPE alteration	Dye accumulation beneath Bruch's membrane; no leakage beyond margin of lesion; late pooling	Significant risk for CNV exudative changes and vision loss
Semisolid drusen (transitional drusen, combination drusen, mixed drusen)	Thickened basement membrane of RPE; RPE proliferation (less than soft); shallow separation of RPE from Bruch's membrane; fragmented hyaline material; may represent transformed hard or degenerated soft drusen	Flatter than soft drusen; semidistinct borders	Late staining but not as bright as soft drusen; more readily seen angiographically compared with ophthalmoscopically	Risk for CNV and sequellae if transforms to soft drusen

ophthalmoscope, they are small, dense, round, circumscribed, white-yellow bodies found at the level of the RPE and the remainder of Bruch's membrane. Often clustered, these lesions are usually small and are often abundant in the temporal parafoveal zone (Figure 12.1). When generalized, they may be observed along vascular arcades in the nasal region and may extend in a honeycomb pattern into the equatorial retina.

Soft drusen consist of confluent lesions of variegated size and shape with less sharply defined borders (Figure 12.2). These semisolid deposits probably represent focal layers of debris that build up on the outermost layer of the basement membrane. Soft drusen may represent a transformation from hard drusen, a change often observed with the onset of AMD (Figure 12.3).

Regardless of type, drusen can change in size, shape, and appearance over time. When there is a breakdown of the overlying RPE, the photoreceptors disappear, and the drusen tend to regress. Should this occur, there is a brighter appearance to the lesions, and they may become calcified. Atrophic changes of the overlying tissue are a typical finding, and if CNV occurs following these changes, it tends to be focal.

CLINICAL DIAGNOSIS AND CLASSIFICATION

AMD is related to retinal pigment changes, a finding that may indicate progression of the disease. In fact, there is a better correlation for visual acuity loss with pigment

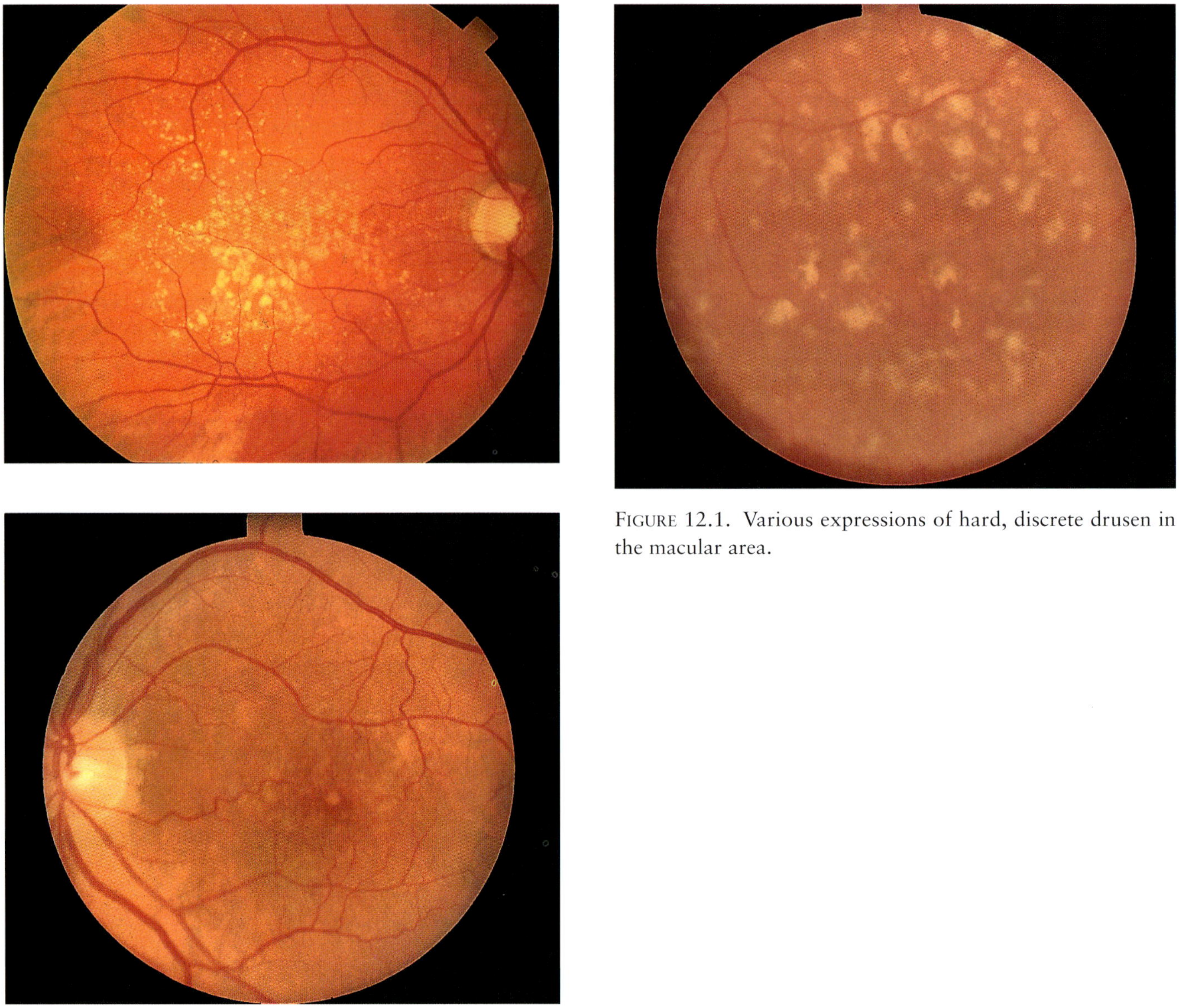

Figure 12.1. Various expressions of hard, discrete drusen in the macular area.

changes than with drusen since both forms of AMD may occur in the absence of drusen.

Atrophic Macular Degeneration

It is often difficult to separate age-related variations in the macula from the pathologic changes associated with AMD. However, atrophic changes in the macula often presage the onset of vision loss. Atrophic areas of the macula may be characterized by an incomplete annular area of hyperpigmentation around the fovea. Fixation is often spared, and drusen may or may not be present at this stage. Pigment changes often follow the distribution of drusen and may become more apparent after the drusen fade. Atrophy is also observed following the collapse of elevated RPE, which detaches secondary to the increase of confluent drusen (Figure 12.4).

Atrophic AMD is more prevalent after the sixth decade. The clinical presentation of atrophic or dry AMD is distinctive but nonspecific. Visual acuity may be minimally impaired, and subjective visual complaints are common. Although Amsler grid testing is essentially normal, focal defects may be reported. A diminished or lost foveal reflex is often the first clinically observable sign. Documentation of the status of the foveal reflex is essential for early detection of macular changes before other clinically evident findings are apparent, including loss of visual function. Mottling of the RPE is often an early clinical sign, and areas of hyperpigmentation may surround areas of pigment loss. Hyaline drusen are often present and can range from a few scattered lesions to extensive distribution. These lesions are observed deep to the retina and are easily distinguished from other lesions by fundus biomicroscopy. Pigment changes often

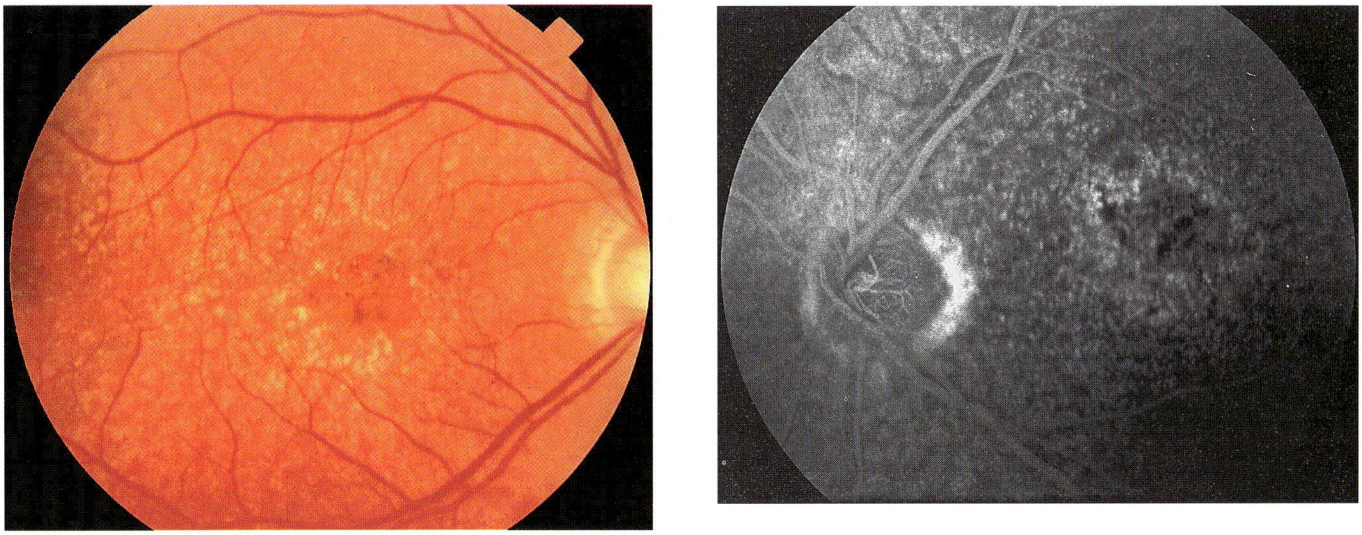

FIGURE 12.2. Drusen in conjunction with retinal pigment degeneration. Arteriovenous recirculation phase of the fluorescein angiogram reveals areas of hyperfluorescence corresponding to an absence of retinal pigment epithelium, while hypofluorescent areas represent migration and clumping of pigment.

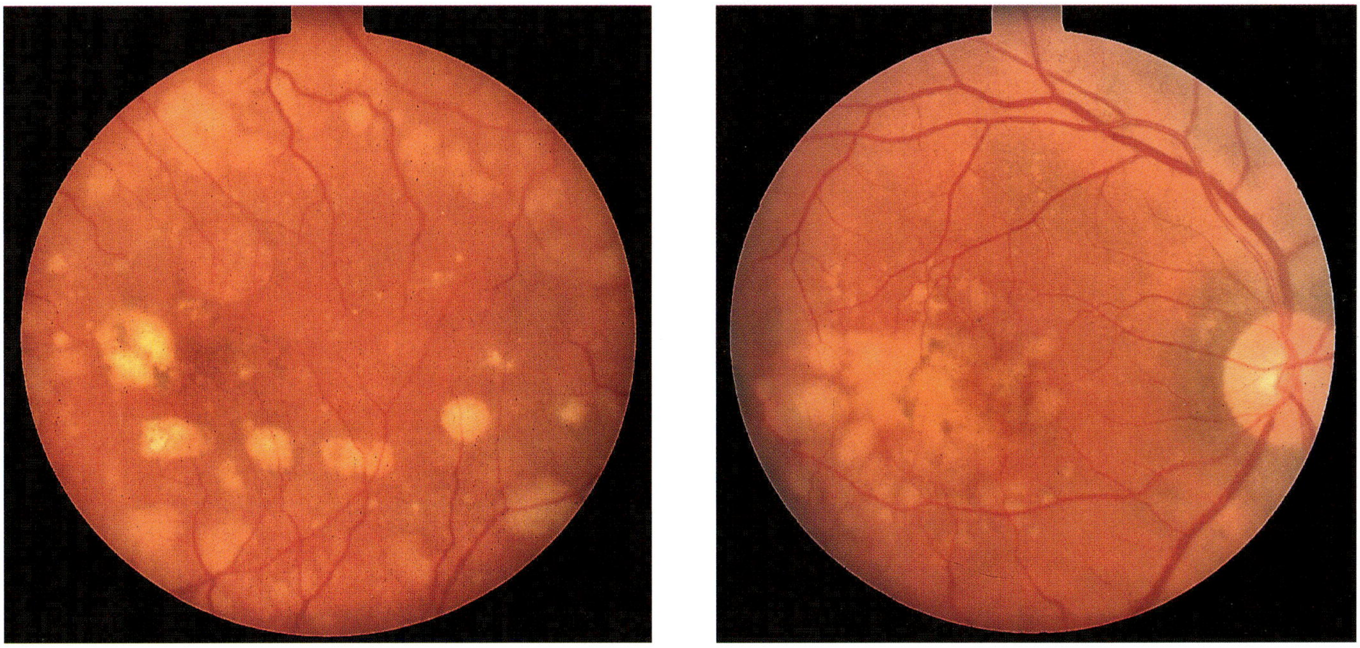

A B

FIGURE 12.3. Examples of soft drusen (A) and confluent drusen in association with pigment degeneration (B) in a patient with age-related macular degeneration.

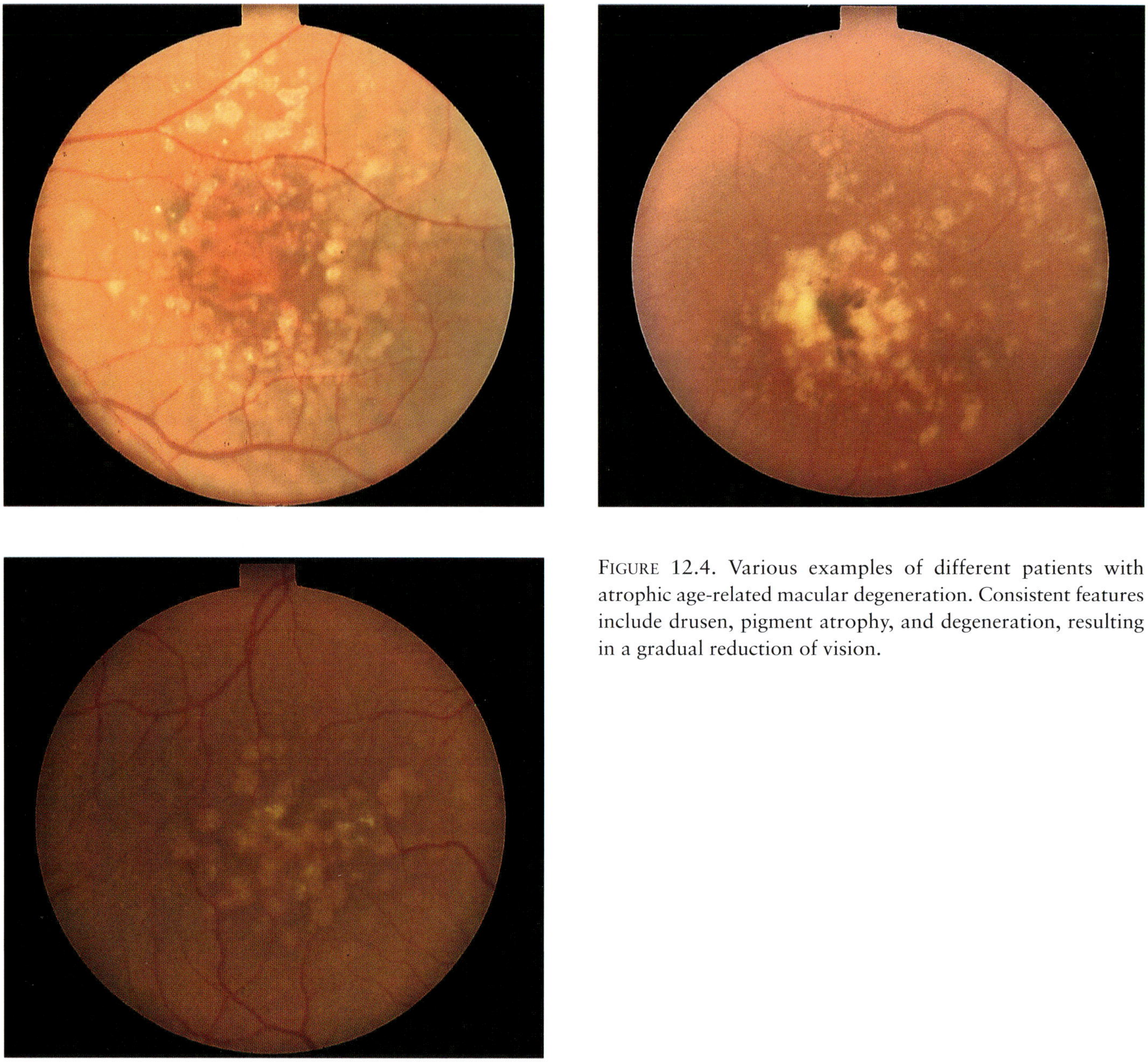

FIGURE 12.4. Various examples of different patients with atrophic age-related macular degeneration. Consistent features include drusen, pigment atrophy, and degeneration, resulting in a gradual reduction of vision.

overlie drusen and may become more apparent with the fading of the lesions. Pigment changes are demonstrated more readily by fluorescein angiography (FA) than by ophthalmoscopy.

Progression of these changes can lead to geographic atrophy, which is more extensive and involves the entire photoreceptor-RPE-choriocapillaris complex. Geographic atrophy is characterized by generalized loss of RPE associated with drusen in the perifoveal area. There is loss of photoreceptors due to blighted RPE cells and choriocapillaris atrophy. Larger choroidal vessels are observed through these areas of atrophy. Although atrophic AMD may be unilateral, it frequently presents bilaterally and symmetrically, especially in the geographic stage.

Atrophic AMD may be self-limited or may be a precursor to exudative maculopathy. For this reason, patients should be educated to look for changes in visual function and distortion on the Amsler grid. It is recommended that the patient monitor the status of his or her vision regularly, particularly for metamorphopsia. The patient should be evaluated annually, including stereoscopic macular examination using fundus biomicroscopy, as long as visual function remains stable. It should be stressed to the patient that he or she should notify the clinician immediately if any change is detected (Table 12.2).

TABLE 12.2. Clinical Considerations in Age-Related Macular Degeneration

Stage	*Visual acuity range*	*Clinical presentation*	*Clinical diagnosis and detection*	*Management guidelines*
Atrophic (dry, non-exudative)	20/20–20/70 in early stages	Minimal RPE changes—hyperpigmentation in perifoveal area; RPE dropout or atrophy; hard drusen	Amsler grid—often normal or subtle focal dysmorphopsia; FA rarely indicated; normal underlying choroidal pattern; hyperfluorescence due to transmission defects without leakage; RPE changes more apparent than ophthalmoscopic appearance. Potential for severe vision loss may occur only over a long period.	Annual examination with stable vision Patient education Home Amsler grid testing weekly; reevaluate routinely for change in vision or Amsler grid; vitamin/antioxidant therapy
Exudative	20/25–20/400 or worse	Acute onset of blurred vision and dysmorphopsia	Serous neurosensory detachment; pigment epithelial detachments; gray-green or dirty gray lesion corresponding to CNV; FA—early hyperfluorescence of CNV (lacy, nodular appearance), late hyperfluorescence, sometimes surrounded by area of hypofluorescence, visible choriocapillaris, scleral staining; ICGA—abnormal choroidal vessels hyperfluoresce, even within hemorrhage and exudate	Early treatment of well-defined CNV (FA within 48 hours of treatment); home Amsler grid; repeat FA 2 weeks after treatment; patient education for high recurrence rate and bilaterality; frequent surveillance

RPE = retinal pigment epithelium; CNV = choroidal neovascularization; FA = fluorescein angiography; ICGA = indocyanine green angiography.

Exudative Age-Related Macular Degeneration

The exudative form of AMD may represent a continuation or progression of the atrophic stage of the degenerative process. It is characterized by CNV, often in the presence of soft confluent drusen, with subsequent exudation and leakage through a compromised Bruch's membrane and RPE layer. The leakage emanating from the new choroidal vessels results in a serous detachment of the sensory retina with ensuing metamorphopsia.

Exudative or wet AMD occurs with increasing frequency after the sixth decade and is a leading cause of legal blindness in the United States and other developed countries. The onset of exudative AMD is often acute, and patients notice dysmorphopsia and sometimes blurred vision, especially at near vision. The disorder is bilateral approximately one-third of the time, and the patient is more likely to notice subtle visual changes and metamorphopsia earlier in the second eye.

Exudative macular degeneration can have a profound effect on vision, but in certain instances, this devastating result can be prevented. The clinician should carefully evaluate the macula looking for the characteristic signs of wet AMD, including choroidal neovascular membrane (CNVM), subretinal or intraretinal hemorrhage, serous detachment of the neurosensory retina, pigment epithelial detachment, drusen, hard exudate, and cystoid macular edema.

The end stage of the exudative process results in a disciform macular scar that is characterized by fibrous and pigment degeneration and destruction of the photoreceptors. RPE tears may also occur spontaneously and have also been observed following laser photocoagulation for well-defined CNV (Figures 12.5 and 12.6).

Choroidal Neovascular Membranes

Serous or hemorrhagic pigment epithelial and neurosensory retinal detachments are important findings in exudative AMD. The cause of the exudation are CNVMs originating from the choriocapillaris that protrude through breaks in Bruch's membrane, leak fluid consisting of protein and lipid, and produce a separation of the RPE or the neurosensory retina (see Figure 12.5). These new vessels are fragile, and their endothelial cells do not function as a barrier, thus allowing fluid to leak into the potential spaces of the RPE and retina. Because of their fragility, these vessels are also more disposed to hemorrhage. Blood may percolate through all the layers of the

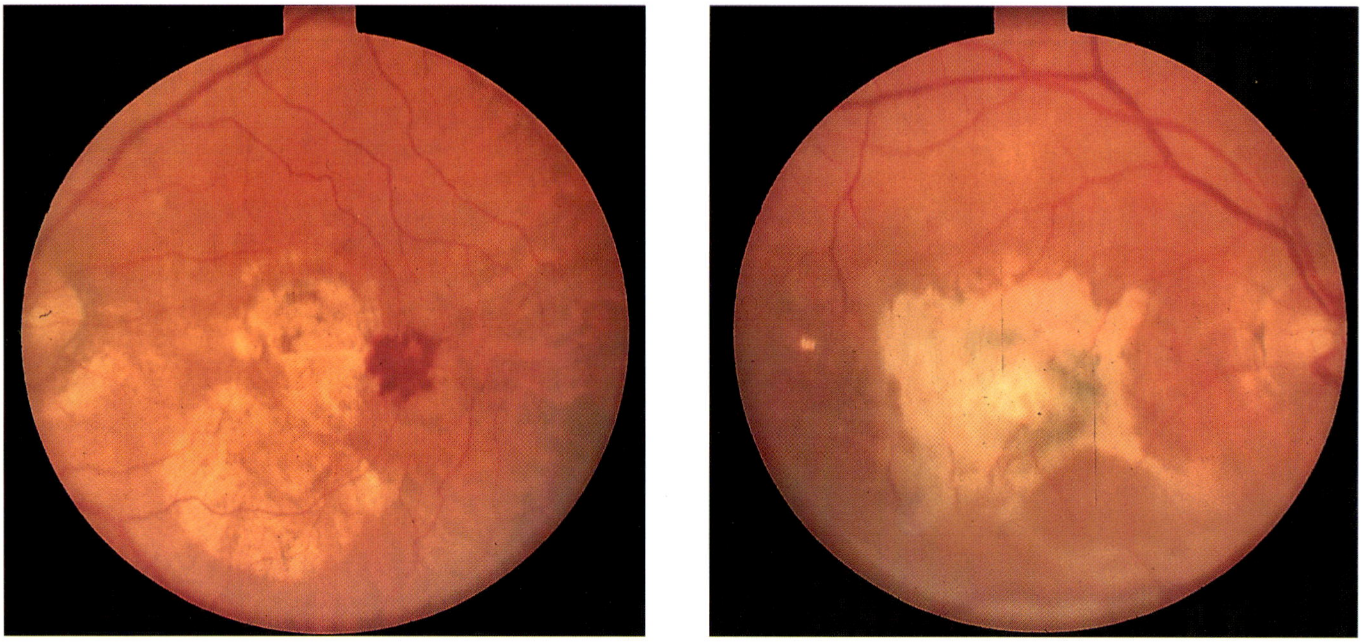

FIGURE 12.5. Various expressions of disciform macular degeneration in end-stage exudative age-related macular degeneration.

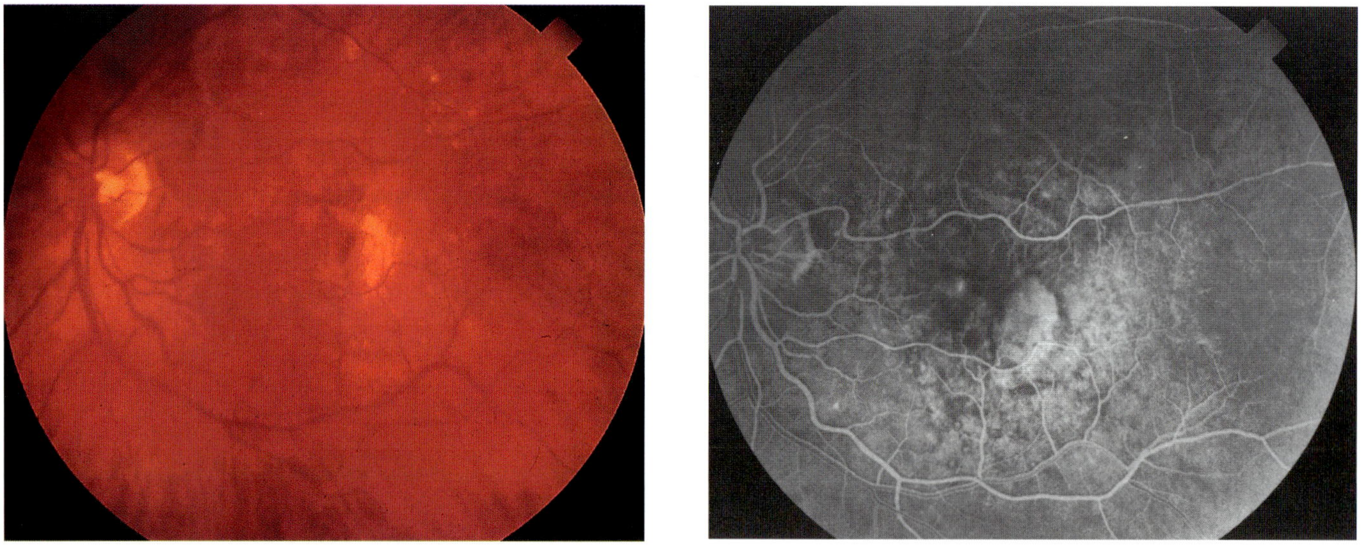

FIGURE 12.6. Retinal pigment epithelial tear in exudative age-related macular degeneration with accompanying A-V phase of the fluorescein angiogram.

retina and may find its way into the vitreous cavity. The end result of this process is a disciform scar resulting from fibrosis of the subretinal membrane and the consolidation of intraretinal and subretinal blood leads to fibrovascular scar tissue.

CNVMs are best observed with fundus biomicroscopy and appear as a gray-green lesion or "dirty" brown lesion deep to the retina. This countenance is attributed to the obscured view of the neovascular membrane through the umbra of the RPE. Serous detachment of the RPE or neurosensory retina should alert the clinician to the presence of CNV, especially when observed in the presence of other RPE changes, drusen, and hard exudates in patients over 55 years of age. The lesion is often surrounded by a pigment ring, and blood often surrounds the subretinal membrane (Figure 12.7). The presence of blood should alert the clinician to the likelihood of choroidal neovascularization; when present, the membrane may be fast-growing. The neovascular lesion may be located anywhere in the posterior pole, including the subfoveal region. Membranes located in the peripapillary area or well outside the foveal avascular zone (FAZ) may not represent a significant threat to vision. If the membranes are located between 1 and 199 μ of the FAZ center, they are termed *juxtafoveal*; those located beyond 200 μ are called *extrafoveal.* Subfoveal membranes often begin outside the fovea and progress to the subfoveal area. However, three-fourths of untreated CNVMs extend into the FAZ center.

CNVMs are observed with numerous other fundus conditions, including presumed ocular histoplasmosis syndrome (POHS), degenerative myopia, angioid streaks, and rupture of Bruch's membrane by any cause. Compared with these fundus conditions, neovascular membranes in AMD have more proclivity for the FAZ center, and the threat to vision is much greater if they exist within 2,500 μ of the FAZ center.

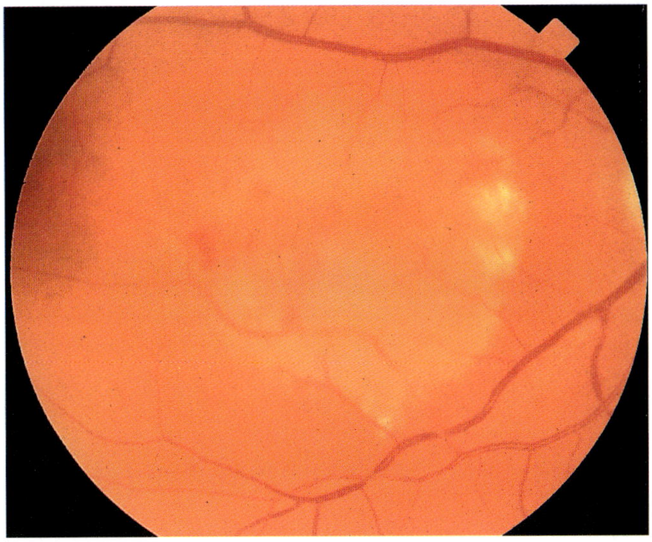

FIGURE 12.7. Example of exudative maculopathy with serosanguinous elevation of the neurosensory macula.

Ocular Conditions with Choroidal Neovascular Membrane

- AMD
- POHS
- Following laser photocoagulation
- Idiopathic CNV
- Angioid streaks
- Myopic degeneration (lacquer cracks)
- Choroidal tumors
- Chronic uveitis or chorioretinitis
- Traumatic choroidal rupture

CNVM may be well defined or poorly defined as determined by FA. The FA exhibits a classic lacy appearance to the CNV in the early stages of choroidal and arterial filling. The nodular area of hyperfluorescence is often surrounded by an area of hypofluorescence corresponding to hyperpigmentation following RPE changes. Hyperfluorescence progresses throughout the transit as the dye leaks and accumulates under the neurosensory detachment. The borders of the lesion continue to be obvious throughout the transit and into the late stages of the angiogram. There is sufficient resolution with FA to delineate the fine capillaries of neovascularization connected to larger vessels or those located at the leading edge of the neovascular membrane. Late staining of the sclera may also be evident (Figure 12.8).

Ill-defined neovascular membranes, sometimes referred to as occult or oozing CNVM, are not as readily identifiable by conventional FA. Serous or hemorrhagic neurosensory detachment, pigment epithelial detachments (PED), and other retinal changes result in patient symptoms, but delineation of the neovascular lesion is sometimes difficult. Turbid or viscous subretinal fluid and diffuse oozing of fluorescein obscure the borders of the ill-defined membrane. The membrane may be located at the borders of the nonperfused area of the choroidal capillaries (Figures 12.9 through 12.11).

Indocyanine green angiography (ICGA) is being evaluated to determine its efficacy in helping to identify and treat occult and recurrent neovascular membranes. It is useful because numerous macular disorders can cause hyperfluorescence with fluorescein. The dye does not leak into the neurosensory detachment and therefore it subtracts the leakage from beneath the RPE with only the CNV being apparent. The new vessels hyperfluoresce, but the serous elevation of the retina does not. With conventional fluorescein, both the neovascular membrane and the serous detachment hyperfluoresce in the late stages of the angiogram.

The highly recurrent nature of CNV makes effective and lasting treatment difficult or impossible to achieve. Almost two-thirds of CNV lesions recur, most of those within the first year following treatment. There are many factors surrounding the highly recurrent nature of the lesions. It is likely that incomplete identification and lineament of the lesions using conventional FA makes complete obliteration difficult. Another factor is the tendency for recurrence at the foveal border of the laser scar. Improved techniques with ICGA and videoangiography may improve these results.

TREATMENT AND MANAGEMENT OF AGE-RELATED MACULAR DEGENERATION

Currently there is no evidence to support the efficacy of treating atrophic AMD, even in the presence of signifi-

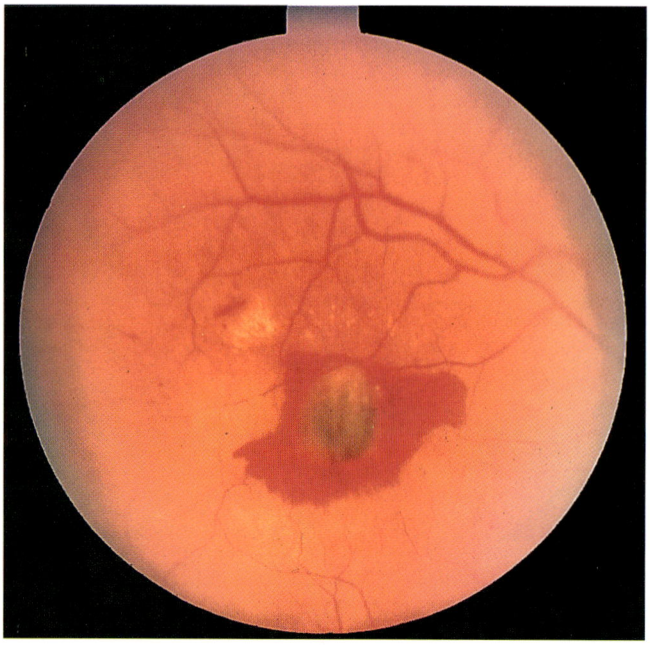

A

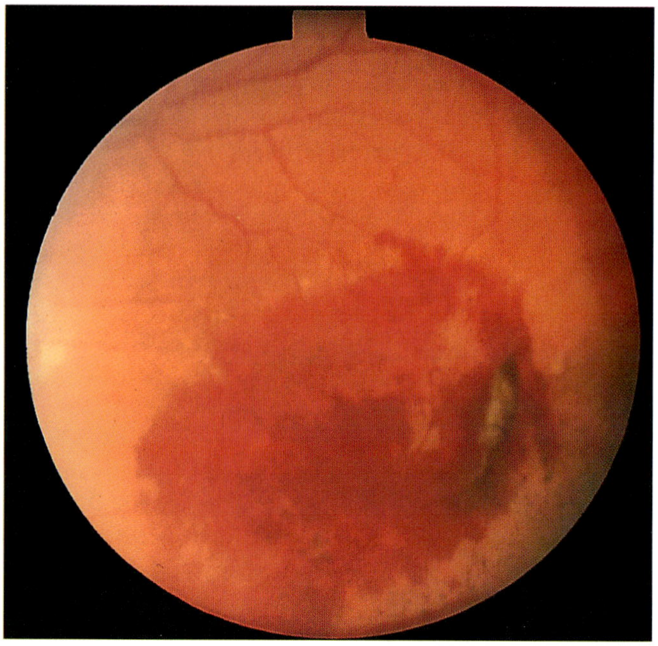

B

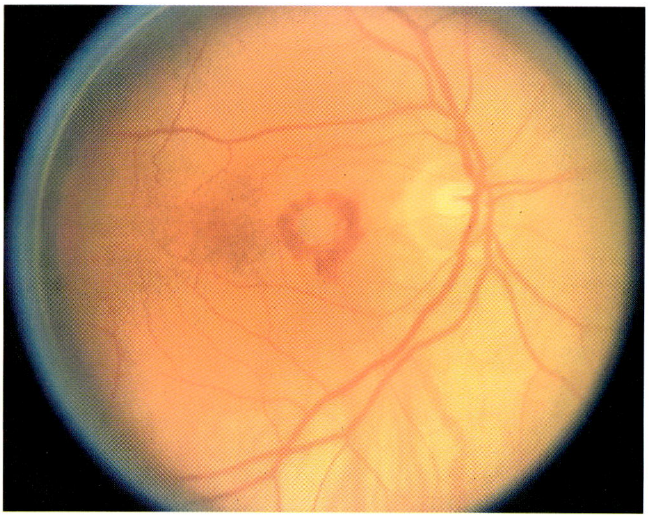

C

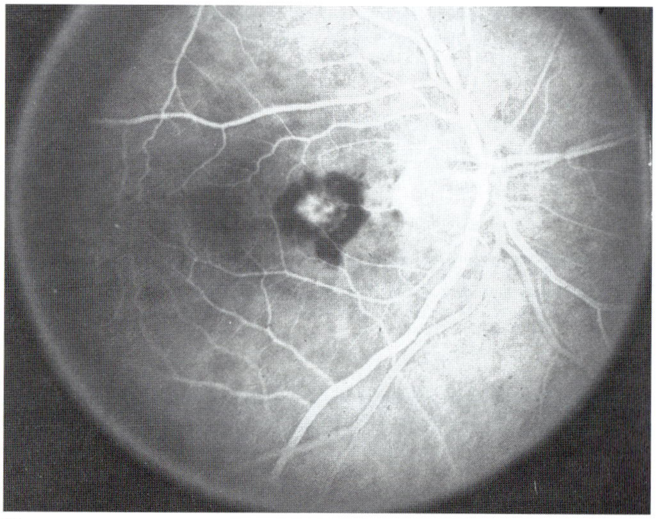

D

FIGURE 12.8. A and B. Examples of choroidal neovascularization with hemorrhage. Color photograph (C) and fluorescein angiographic patterns (D) reveal early hyperfluorescence, with continued leakage in the later phase of the transit (E).

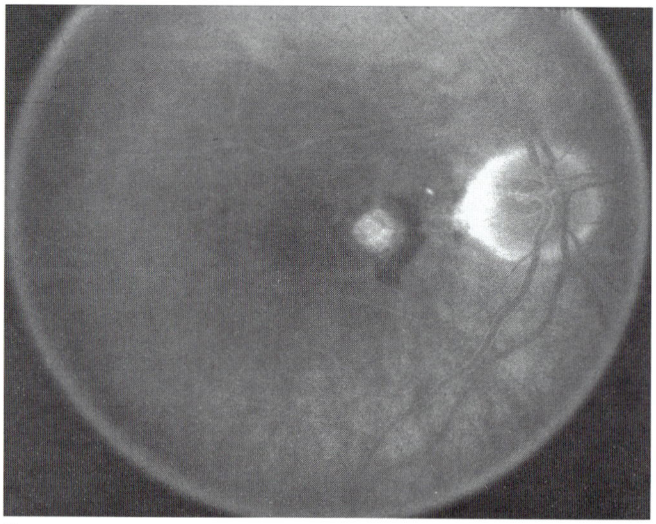

E

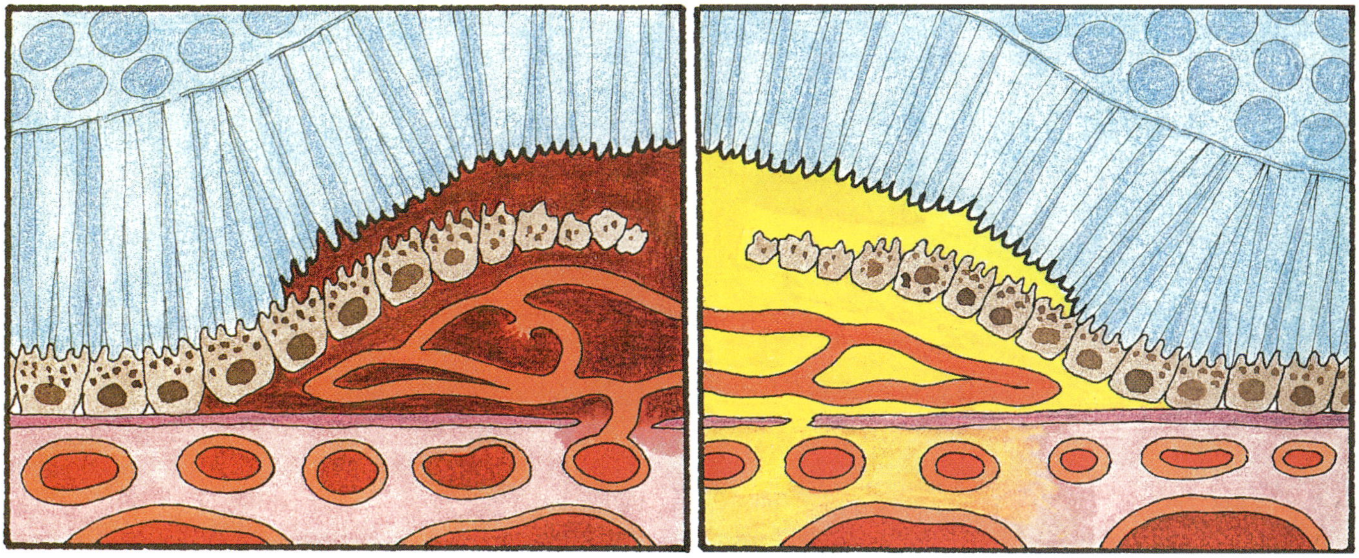

FIGURE 12.9. Illustration depicting the mechanism for serous (right) and hemorrhagic (left) leakage from a choroidal neovascularization producing a neurosensory retinal detachment in the macula.

cant pigment and drusen changes. The clinician should, however, rule out the presence of CNV in these cases because the degenerative changes in the macula may represent a transitional state. In cases of nonexudative AMD, antioxidants and other vitamin supplements may be sufficient. These medications may be taken once or twice each day, and the patient may appreciate the opportunity to feel that he or she is doing something constructive for the condition. The patient should be urged to eat green, leafy vegetables since they are high in vitamin A and beta carotene. Other important measures include UV protection and routine surveillance using the home Amsler grid test. The patient should be advised to evaluate the vision from each eye independently each day and to note subjectively any changes in vision. Additional clues may be gathered from looking at door or window frames and tile patterns in bathrooms, looking for dysmorphopsia.

Asymptomatic patients with minimal pigment changes or drusen should be evaluated annually. Those with geographic atrophy or other clinical signs of atrophic macular degeneration should be examined semiannually, with careful attention paid to subjective symptoms during the interim. New onset of dysmorphopsia should alert the patient and the clinician to the possibility of progression, and the patient should return for examination within 24 hours. Immediate referral to a retinologist for FA is indicated to rule out CNV.

Patients at risk for severe vision loss from exudative AMD have CNV and symptoms that include new onset of dysmorphopsia and scotoma, sometimes associated with blurred near vision. Leakage from the CNV results in a neurosensory, RPE serous, or hemorrhagic

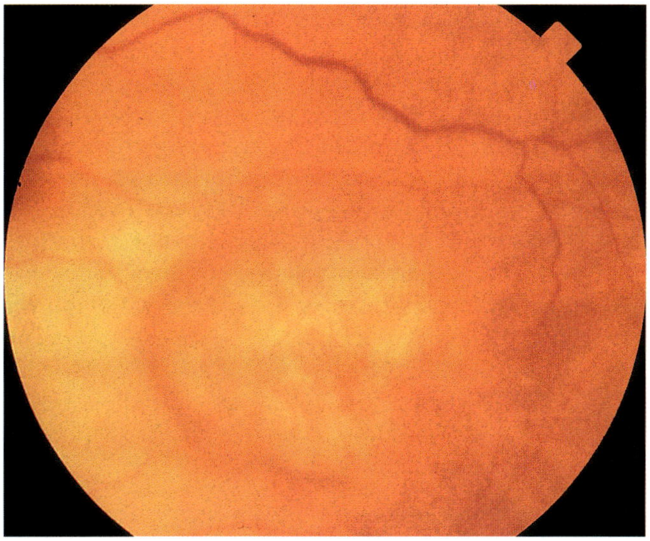

FIGURE 12.10. Exudative macular degeneration with a ring of pigment and blood surrounding the choroidal neovascular lesion.

detachment. Location of the CNV is critical since lesions whose borders are located beneath the center of the FAZ portend the worst prognosis. Seventy percent of patients with subfoveal CNV have visual acuity worse than 20/200 two years after observation. An immediate consultation or referral to a retina specialist should be obtained if clinical signs and symptoms of CNV are present. Fundus FA should be performed to determine the patient's eligibility for laser treatment of extrafoveal or

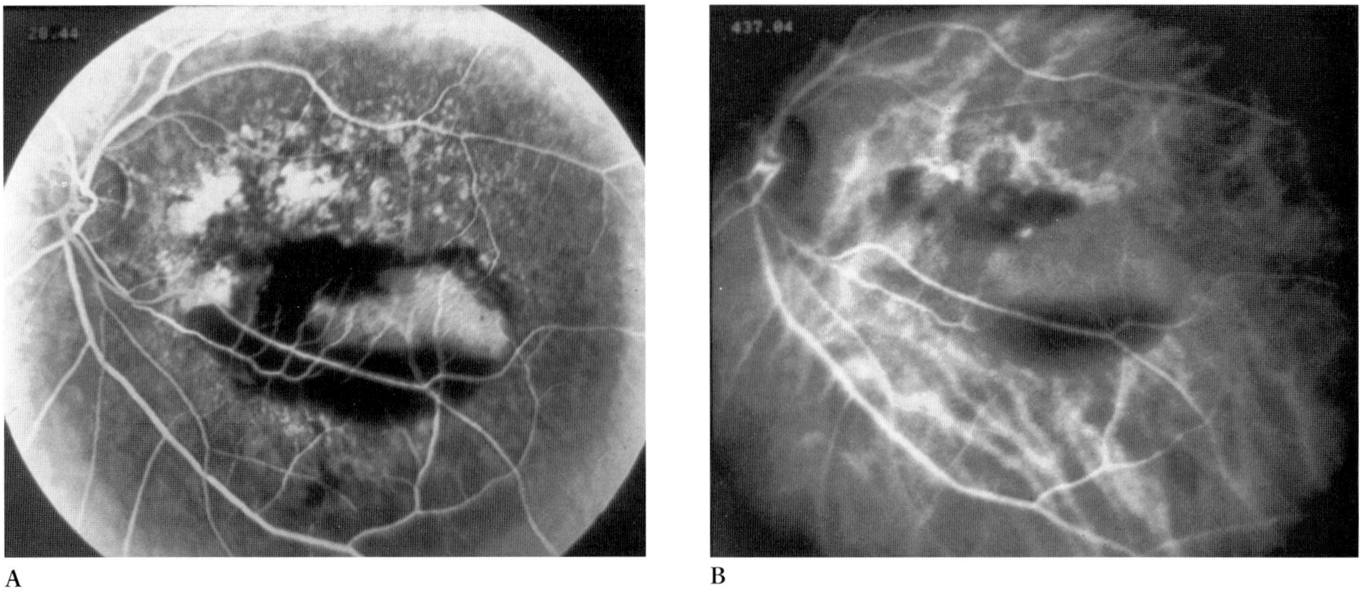

FIGURE 12.11. Ill-defined choroidal neovascularization as observed with fluorescein angiography (A) and indocyanine green angiography (B). (Courtesy of A. Dreicker.)

subfoveal CNV. Timely intervention may reduce the risk of significant vision loss from recurrence of CNV. The FA should be obtained within 72 hours prior to treatment due to the rapid growth of CNVM. The patient should be examined 2 weeks posttreatment and a repeat FA obtained to determine the efficacy of treatment, to determine if the entire CNV was obliterated, and to rule out recurrence. If no further leakage is detected, the patient should be examined again in 6 weeks, every 3 months for 1 year, and every 4–6 months thereafter. This is necessary to assess the risk for recurrence and to predict the likelihood of CNVM formation in the fellow eye based on risk characteristics of soft confluent drusen and retinal pigment abnormalities. Signs of recurrence include:

- Decrease in visual acuity
- New scotomas or dysmorphopsia
- New areas of focal hypopigmentation at the edge of an area of laser treatment
- Persistent subretinal or sub-RPE fluid
- New specks of subretinal blood

Patients who have cardiovascular disease or hypertension or are current cigarette smokers should be monitored more closely due to the higher frequency of CNV recurrence in this population. Antioxidant nutrient supplements and UV and blue light protection should be recommended to the patient because these measures will serve to provide additional protection to the RPE while allowing the patient to participate in the care process.

Fewer than 20% of patients with CNV are suitable for laser photocoagulation based on the criteria set forth by the Macular Photocoagulation Study Group. The highly recurrent nature of the lesion combined with the necessity for exact identification and delineation of the membrane make treatment a formidable challenge. For the most part, well-defined membranes are more suited to laser treatment, and even then, the lesion must lie outside of the 200 μ zone from the center of the fovea (Figure 12.12).

The Macular Photocoagulation Study Group was convened in 1982 to evaluate the long-term and short-term effectiveness of argon laser photocoagulation for extrafoveal neovascular membranes resulting from AMD, POHS, and idiopathic membranes. The Senile Macular Degeneration Study was one component of this multicenter, randomized, controlled clinical trial. The study concluded that for eyes meeting the criteria for treatment, argon green or blue-green laser photocoagulation is effective for extrafoveal membranes located 200–2,500 μ from the center of the fovea. Eligibility criteria included no previous laser treatment, well-defined extrafoveal CNV with the posterior edge no closer than 200 μ from the center of the FAZ, a limited amount of blood associated with the lesion, and relatively good visual function. Follow-up after 1 year revealed that 14% of treated patients and 42% of untreated patients had visual acuity of 20/200 or worse. After an additional 6 months, 25% of the treated eyes and 60% of the untreated eyes lost another six lines of visual acuity.

A second component of the clinical trial included krypton red laser photocoagulation for lesions located as close as 1 μm from the center of the FAZ, even if associated with significant hemorrhage and exudate and poor visual acuity. The Age-Related Macular Degeneration

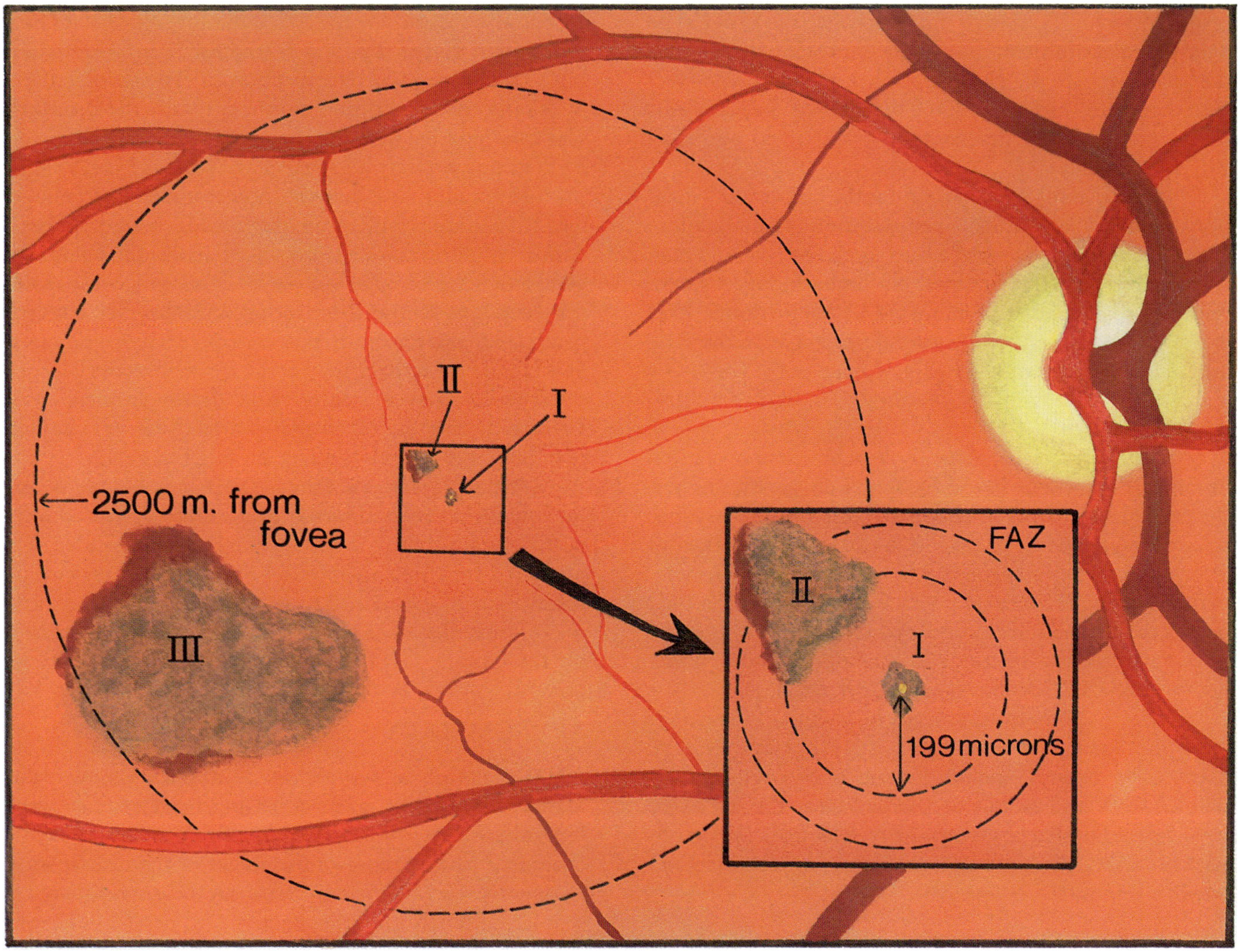

FIGURE 12.12. Illustration demonstrating criteria for Macular Photocoagulation Study Group treatment guidelines in exudative macular degeneration. Well-defined lesions located 199–2,500 μ (II, III) from the center of the foveal avascular zone (II) are most amenable to treatment and, when treated, help to prevent severe vision loss during the first 2 years after treatment. Subfoveal lesions (I) have the poorest prognosis and are currently being treated with the krypton laser. (FAZ = foveal avascular zone.)

Study—Krypton was convened to determine if treating lesions within this zone helped to prevent or postpone vision loss. Laser treatment either delayed or prevented a further decrease in visual acuity.

A third clinical trial was undertaken in 1986 to determine the effectiveness of treating well-demarcated subfoveal lesions. This study revealed that in patients with subfoveal neovascular membranes, visual acuity immediately after treatment was significantly reduced compared with untreated eyes. However, after 24 months of follow-up, treated eyes had slightly better visual function.

Retinal Pigment Epithelial Detachments

PED may be serous or hemorrhagic, and the latter is an accompanying finding in AMD in approximately 10% of cases. Serous PED is a prognosticator for the development of CNVM; up to 50% of patients who present with PED and no neovascularization eventually develop new vessels. Serous AMD may occur in the absence of CNVM, for example, in idiopathic central serous choroidopathy (ICSC), accompanying congenital optic pit, or Harada's disease. PED occurs most often in patients over age 50 years, whereas ICSC is more prevalent in the under 55-year-old population. PED occurs more often in women, and almost half of those demonstrating detachment develop CNVM. A hemorrhagic PED usually leads to a poor prognosis for preservation of vision and because of its appearance must be differentiated from a choroidal melanoma.

There may be two forms of vascularized PED: one type is actively vascularized, leaks, and is probably responsible for exudative maculopathy; the other type may represent infiltration of new choroidal vessels into the space beneath the pigment epithelium. This latter version demonstrates late staining with ICGA and contains fibrovascular tissue that is hypovascularized and may enlarge over time.

PEDs usually appear as smooth, blister-like elevations with regular borders. The elevation is usually more than 1 DD in size and may be surrounded by a yellow ring. Although PEDs transilluminate on fundus biomicroscopy, the subretinal fluid may be turbid. A hemorrhagic PED is obvious because blood accumulates between the RPE and the outer segments of the photoreceptors. The lesion is dark, and breakthrough bleeding may lead to a vitreous hemorrhage.

The FA pattern in a serous detachment shows rapid uniform filling of the lesion with mild progressive hyperfluorescence. However, the area of hyperfluorescence does not significantly change in size or shape, and the dye does not leak beyond the borders of the lesion. In hemorrhagic PED, the elevated dark mound within the PED produces blocked fluorescence. When suspecting a malignant melanoma, ultrasonography helps to differentiate hemorrhagic PED from a space-occupying lesion.

RPE tears or rips can occur following PED or after laser photocoagulation of neovascular membranes. RPE tears are a more constant finding with occult or ill-defined CNV and usually occur adjacent to the site of the new choroidal vessels. Occasionally, RPE tears are detected with disciform scars and are almost always associated with significant vision loss.

Vitreous Hemorrhage

A vitreous hemorrhage can occur with exudative AMD. When the patient reports a sudden vision loss, it is sometimes a result of the breakthrough hemorrhage. Other causes of vitreous hemorrhage should be considered when managing the patient. Retinal tears, vascular occlusive disease, and diabetic retinopathy are common causes of blood in the vitreous cavity. The vitreous hemorrhage resolves in 75% of patients; ultrasonography and stereoscopic fundus examination are indicated to rule out other etiologies.

End Stage of Age-Related Macular Degeneration

The final stage of the degenerative process in age-related maculopathy yields a variable outcome depending on the nature of the disease. In atrophic macular disease the RPE is absent, and the overlying photoreceptors are nonfunctional; visual function is impaired, and the patient reports scotoma and dysmorphopsia. The involved area is usually more confined compared with the disciform scar in exudative macular degeneration, and visual acuity is not as severely affected.

In exudative macular degeneration, a circular or disc-shaped scar results from the fibrous changes and exudation resulting from the neovascularization. There may be hemorrhage or other subretinal exudate accompanying this yellow or yellow-white lesion. Visual acuity is severely affected, and the entire posterior pole may be involved. Subretinal hemorrhage may break through to the vitreous, resulting in an even greater visual deficit. In these cases, vitrectomy may be recommended to preserve whatever remaining peripheral vision is left (see Figure 12.5).

Patients with end-stage AMD may be candidates for low vision rehabilitation. Referral to an optometrist with special training in low vision is recommended. The primary care clinician should be prepared to declare the patient legally blind and to offer information regarding the resources of local services, including the Commission for the Blind.

SUMMARY

AMD remains a significant threat to vision. With increased longevity and increasing numbers of elderly individuals, the primary care clinician is likely to encounter one or more of the stages of the disease more frequently. Identification of risk factors, careful stereoscopic examination of the macula, and patient education will help to identify those patients who are more likely to suffer visual loss. Routine surveillance and monitoring by the clinician and the patient are important factors in early treatment of sight-threatening neovascular lesions.

SUGGESTED READING

Bressler NM, Bressler SB, Fine SL. Age-related macular degeneration. Surv Ophthalmol 1988;32:375–413.

Gibson JM, Rosenthal AR, Lavery J. A study in the prevalence of eye disease in the elderly in an English community. Trans Ophthalmol Soc UK 1985;104:196–203.

Kahn HA, Liebowitz HM, Ganley JP, et al. Framingham Eye Study. I. Outline and major prevalence findings. Am J Epidemiol 1977;106:17–32.

Klein BE, Klein R. Cataracts and macular degeneration in older Americans. Arch Ophthalmol 1982;100:571–573.

CHAPTER

13

Presumed Ocular Histoplasmosis Syndrome

Anthony A. Cavallerano

Presumed ocular histoplasmosis syndrome (POHS), now sometimes referred to as *ocular histoplasmosis syndrome*, is an interesting if somewhat puzzling ocular malady that, because of the propensity to form choroidal neovascular membrane (CNVM), can lead to a significant loss of visual function. Often classified as a multifocal choroidopathy, POHS has been the subject of intense clinical interest for some time, especially since many of those afflicted are in the younger age groups. The introduction of laser photocoagulation for treatment of choroidal neovascularization (CNV) that may be associated with POHS has improved the prognosis for preservation of vision, but a definitive diagnosis is crucial to proper treatment and prevention of substantial visual loss.

Histoplasmosis is a systemic infection caused by the fungus *Histoplasma capsulatum*. This dimorphic fungus can produce an acute or chronic pulmonary infection and has been associated with multifocal choroidopathy. The designation of "presumed" ocular inflammation is used because it has been impossible to isolate *H. capsulatum* in ocular tissue. The incidence of disseminated choroiditis is 1.6% of the population in the Midwest, and the ocular form of the disease usually occurs between the ages of 20 and 50 years. POHS is rare in blacks, and it seems that the fundus lesions are apparent only after a patient develops a positive reaction to the skin test.

A majority of systemic histoplasmosis infections are benign and often go undetected. The patient may be asymptomatic or may complain of chills, fever, malaise, and fatigue, sometimes lasting days to weeks. The primary route of infection is through the lungs, and the organism is encountered in the mold form in soil and the yeast form in animals. Histoplasmosis has a worldwide distribution, but is particularly indigenous to river valleys throughout the midwestern, eastern, and southeastern United States and comparable areas throughout the rest of the world. In the United States, patients with histoplasmic ocular disease are found chiefly in the Midwest. Histoplasmic infection also is found to a lesser degree in Central and South America and southern Canada but is rarely encountered in Europe and Australia.

The histoplasmin skin test was introduced almost 50 years ago but is not employed universally in practice because almost two-thirds of the population in endemic regions have positive test results. In addition, the skin test may trigger a maculopathy in susceptible patients.

POHS is a condition that undergoes periods of remission and exacerbation throughout a lifetime. It appears that the *Histoplasma* fungus has an affinity for the choroid, in contrast to the toxoplasma parasite, which seems to seek out the retina (see Chapter 20). There is some evidence that in addition to other stimuli, macular involvement is brought on by emotional or physical stress.

CLINICAL PRESENTATION

POHS is characterized by findings that comprise an unmistakable triad: disseminated peripheral choroiditis consisting of choroidal infiltrate or scar, sometimes referred to as the punched-out spots of histoplasmosis; a parafoveal subretinal neovascular membrane; and peripapillary scarring represented by atrophic pigmented lesions (Figure 13.1). There are often flat, whitish lesions surrounding this rim of pigment. The characteristic punched-out lesions may be located anywhere in the fundus, but most are in the midperiphery, posterior to the equator. The syndrome is usually bilateral, and the pathophysiology of the lesions may be explained by areas of focal loss of the choriocapillaris,

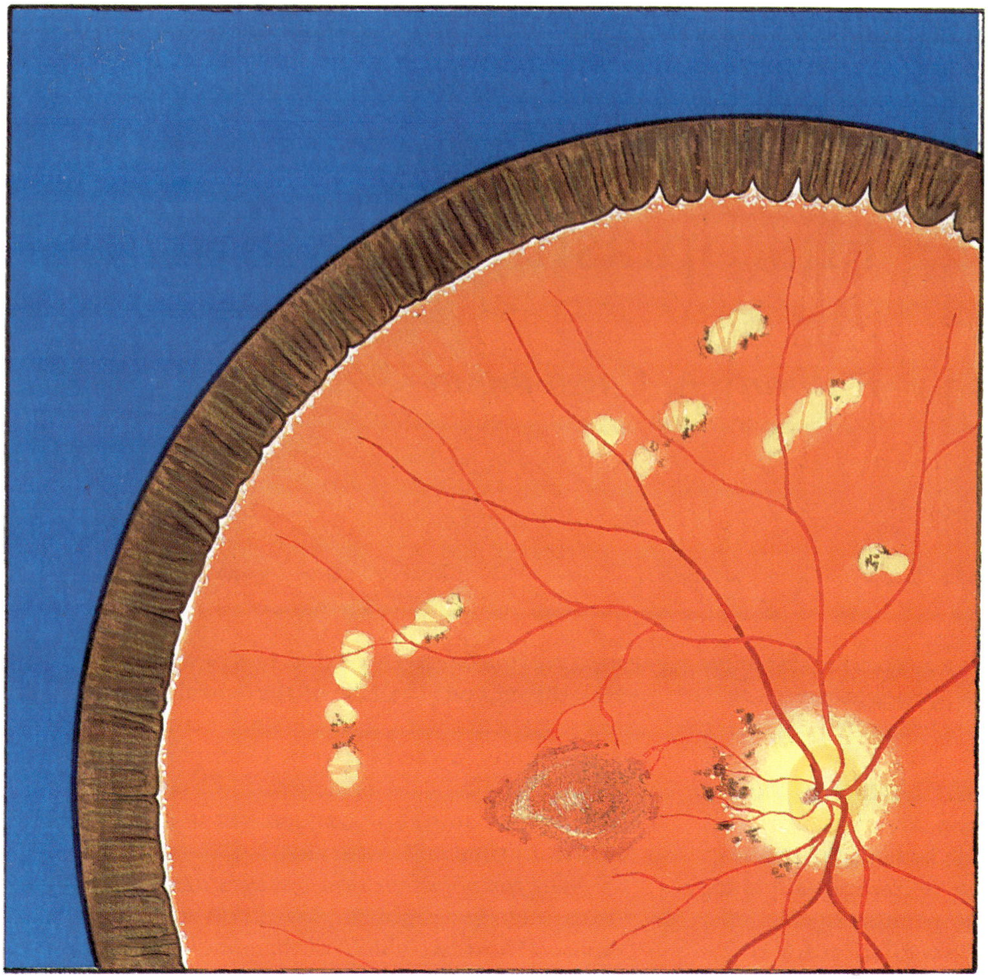

FIGURE 13.1. Composite illustration depicting the various lesions of presumed ocular histoplasmosis syndrome, including disseminated choroiditis with punched-out spots, a parafoveal choroidal neovascular membrane with a subretinal hemorrhage, and peripapillary atrophy. (Reprinted with permission from AA Cavallerano. Presumed ocular histoplasmosis syndrome. Clin Eye Vis Care 1990;3:150–154.)

lymphocytic infiltration of the choroid, disruption of the retinal pigment epithelium (RPE), and compromise to the outer retinal layers. The vitreous and anterior chamber are clear, but on rare occasions, blood enters the vitreous after breaking through the retina. Optic disc edema has also been reported as an uncommon finding in POHS.

Most patients with POHS are asymptomatic unless a choroiditis or a CNVM develops around scars in the macula area. Increased activity in histoplasmic retinal scars is manifested by detectable changes in the size, shape, and distribution of the lesions. A break in Bruch's membrane is necessary for a subretinal net to develop, and a break in the RPE can result in an ingress of fluid and a sensory retinal detachment. Dysmorphopsia as determined by the Amsler grid is present, and there is often a reduction of central visual acuity with macular involvement. The neovascular net develops around punched-out lesions, more as a result of the scar than of the lesions that caused the scar. The scars are bilateral 60% of the time, and there seems to be a greater number in areas of retinal vessels. A patient is totally asymptomatic unless a scar is in the macular area.

The pathophysiology of the retinal findings is demonstrated by the evaluation of the fluorescein angiogram (FA). The process and pathogenesis of the development of the subretinal neovascular net can be elicited by angiography. RPE changes, CNVM, retinal hemorrhage, and inactive scar are depicted in the clinical photographs and the accompanying red-free photograph identifying the various lesions in a patient with POHS shown in Figure 13.2. This patient has three types of lesions: quiet "histo" spots that fluoresce early but fade later in the transit, indicating transmitted fluorescence due to pigment epithelial window defects (Figure 13.3); an active subretinal neovascular membrane formation with associated sensory retinal detachment (Figure 13.4); and finally, an older CNVM that is converting to a disciform scar and chorioretinal scars (Figures 13.5 and 13.6). Other lesions present in the angiogram are a focus of the chronic choroidopathy without producing a break in Bruch's membrane or subsequent CNVM.

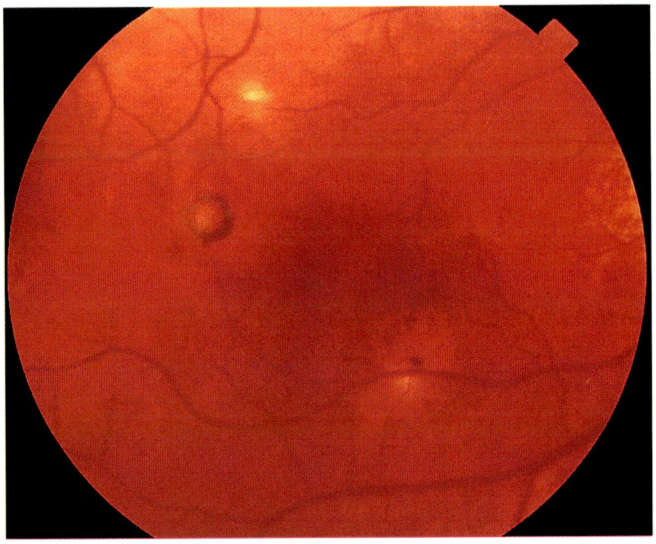

FIGURE 13.2. A hemorrhage surrounds a choroidal neovascular membrane temporal and superior to the fovea. Chorioretinal scars and retinal pigment epithelial window defects are also apparent. (Courtesy of AR Bell, CRA.) (Reprinted with permission from AA Cavallerano. Presumed ocular histoplasmosis syndrome. Clin Eye Vis Care 1990;3:150–154.)

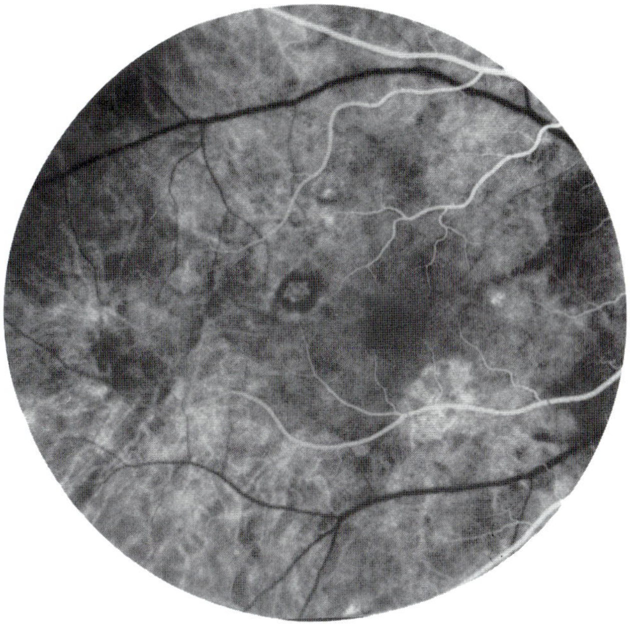

FIGURE 13.3. Early arteriovenous phase of the fluorescein angiogram depicting a lacy, irregular hyperfluorescence of a choroidal neovascularization lateral to the macula. (Courtesy of AR Bell, CRA.) (Reprinted with permission from AA Cavallerano. Presumed ocular histoplasmosis syndrome. Clin Eye Vis Care 1990;3:150–154.)

DIFFERENTIAL DIAGNOSIS

The differential diagnosis of POHS includes both inflammatory and noninflammatory chorioretinal diseases. Toxoplasmosis, sarcoid, angioid streaks, lacquer cracks, and toxocariasis are but a few of the entities that need to be considered in the differential diagnostic process. Multifocal choroidopathy from any cause, including punctate inner choroiditis, acute posterior multifocal placoid pigment epitheliopathy, birdshot retinochoroidopathy, and diffuse unilateral subacute neuroretinitis, must also be considered. Some of the previously mentioned causes are represented by atrophic lesions in the retina similar to the scars produced by histoplasmosis.

MANAGEMENT

Treatment of POHS is important, especially in the early stages of asymptomatic retinal changes. High doses of systemic corticosteroids are sometimes used to help prevent further damage to the macula. The role of steroids in treating POHS is debatable and their efficacy in preventing CNV has not been proven. A prophylactic dose of corticosteroids may be instituted if the patient is compliant and can be depended on to

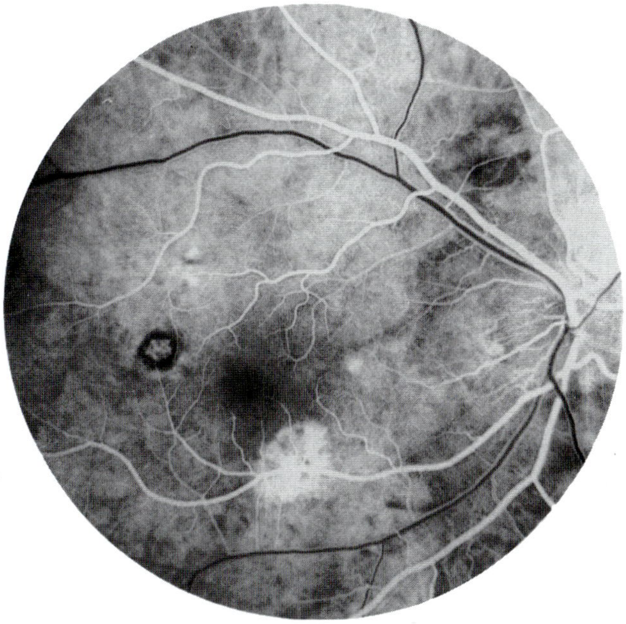

FIGURE 13.4. Subretinal hemorrhage blocks choroidal fluorescence. Hyperfluorescence of the choroidal neovascularization is blurred, indicating leakage. (Courtesy of AR Bell, CRA.) (Reprinted with permission from AA Cavallerano. Presumed ocular histoplasmosis syndrome. Clin Eye Vis Care 1990;3:150–154.)

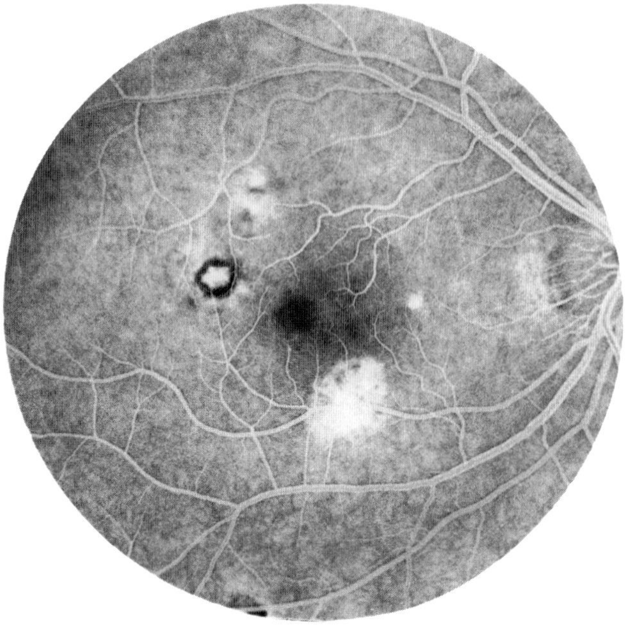

FIGURE 13.5. The venous phase of the angiogram indicating increased fluorescence of the subretinal lesion. There is increased hyperfluorescence of the lesion with indistinct borders. One lesion, temporal and inferotemporal, demonstrates intense staining by no fuzzy borders. (Courtesy of AR Bell, CRA.) (Reprinted with permission from AA Cavallerano. Presumed ocular histoplasmosis syndrome. Clin Eye Vis Care 1990;3:150–154.)

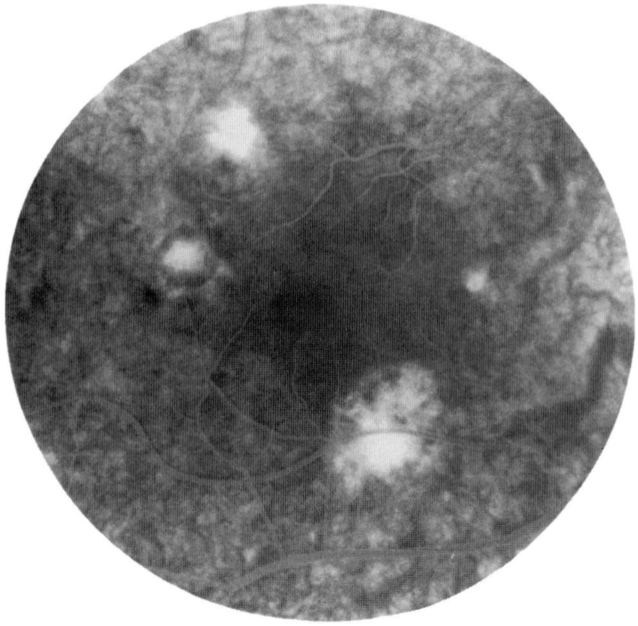

FIGURE 13.6. The late phase of the angiogram depicting a decrease in fluorescence, indicating a pigment epithelial window defect. (Courtesy of AR Bell, CRA.) (Reprinted with permission from AA Cavallerano. Presumed ocular histoplasmosis syndrome. Clin Eye Vis Care 1990;3:150–154.)

detect changes in the appearance of foveal vision by performing the home Amsler grid test regularly. Systemic and periocular steroids may be administered for long-term therapy, but there is always the risk of inducing serious ocular side effects.

Argon-green photocoagulation is used when CNVMs are detected. The entire membrane must be destroyed, and treatment must be undertaken only after evaluation with an FA, usually performed within 72 hours of treatment. Neither corticosteroids nor photocoagulation prevent recurrences of the macular form of POHS. Successful obliteration of the CNV does not safeguard against further visual loss, and the success of this treatment is dependent on such factors as location of the CNV and the formation of neovascular nets at other scar sites.

Careful evaluation and accurate diagnosis of patients presenting with the typical clinical findings of POHS is critical to proper management. Periodic examination and photodocumentation of the patient with scars and fundus lesions are imperative, and patient compliance is also important. Because the prognosis is often guarded, patients should be advised to evaluate the vision in each eye daily and to perform the home Amsler grid test frequently. They should be advised to return immediately for an evaluation if there is any question of a change in vision. Careful examination accompanied by an FA will help to determine the significance of any changes detected by the patient.

SUGGESTED READING

Beck RW, Sergott RC, Barr CC, et al. Optic disc edema in the presumed ocular histoplasmosis syndrome. Ophthalmology 1984;2:183–185.

Cavallerano AA. Punctate inner choroidopathy. Clin Vis Eye Care 1989;2:75–80.

Damato BE, Trope GE, Dudgeon J. Presumed ocular histoplasmosis. Trans Ophthalmol Soc UK 1981;101:403–408.

Deutsch TA, Tessler HH. Inflammation pseudohistoplasmosis. Ann Ophthalmol 1985;8:461–465.

Feman SS, Tilford RH. Ocular findings in patients with histoplasmosis. JAMA 1985;17:2534–2537.

Johnston RL, Mitchell PC, Berman AM. Presumed ocular histoplasmosis syndrome. J Am Optom Assoc 1988;5:401–405.

Kranian G. Vitreous hemorrhage secondary to presumed ocular histoplasmosis syndrome. Ann Ophthalmol 1985;5:295–298, 302.

Singerman LJ. Important points in management of patients with choroidal neovascularization. Ophthalmology 1985;5:610–614.

Smith RE. Studies of presumed ocular histoplasmosis syndrome. Trans Ophthalmol Soc UK 1981;101:328–334.

Thimons JJ. Presumed ocular histoplasmosis. Am J Optom Physiol Opt 1983;12:999–1002.

CHAPTER

14

Angioid Streaks

Anthony A. Cavallerano

Angioid streaks are noteworthy fundus findings occurring in a specific segment of the general population. When present, they may be the harbinger of underlying systemic disease and in fact have a close association with a number of constitutional maladies. At one time strictly associated with vascular disease, this fundus entity has the potential to cause significant vision loss due to the development of choroidal neovascular membrane (CNVM) and subsequent hemorrhage and scarring of the macula.

The moniker *angioid streaks* was first established by Knapp in 1891, a term he applied to a fundus condition reported by Doyne. Early investigators commented on the relationship between angioid streaks and choroidal hemorrhage, and they soon recognized the association with pseudoxanthoma elasticum (PXE) (Grönblad-Strandberg syndrome). Angioid streaks have been associated with numerous other systemic conditions, and although often idiopathic, almost one-half of patients with the fundus condition have one of three systemic disorders: PXE, Paget's disease of the bone (osteitis deformans), or sickle hemoglobinopathy. Other systemic diseases have been associated with angioid streaks, but these parallels may be coincidental.

Angioid streaks result from changes occurring in Bruch's membrane that render the lamina brittle and predisposed to linear cracking. Extensive calcification of Bruch's membrane (and other parts of the body in PXE) and extensive basophilia combined with the questionable effects of stress factors may play a role in the pathogenesis of the streaks. Iron deposition in Bruch's membrane, as seen in sickle cell disease, has also been implicated in the process. In addition, changes in the capillaries and retinal pigment epithelium (RPE) can result in the ingrowth of fibrovascular tissue into the subretinal space.

CLINICAL PRESENTATION

- Elevated linear lesions radiating from disc
- Red to light brown to dark brown
- Parallel or perpendicular to disc
- Bilateral, convoluted course
- Posterior polar region
- CNVM/serous maculopathy

Angioid streaks present a unique visage, and the clinical characteristics render this condition highly identifiable. The linear streaks radiate in a peripapillary ring or spider web pattern in all directions from the optic disc. The streaks are both parallel and perpendicular to the disc, and there is a slight predilection to the temporal aspect of the optic nerve. The streaks are narrow and taper in their course from the disc. Although confined to the posterior polar territory, they have been reported in the more anterior regions of the fundus and are invariably bilateral (Figure 14.1).

Angioid streaks derive their color from the surrounding fundus and the pigment of the choroid and RPE. They may appear red in a blonde fundus and range from light to dark brown in heavily pigmented eyes. Mottling of the RPE, referred to as *peau d'orange*, is frequently the first observable sign of the disease when associated with PXE and is seen in the temporal equatorial to midperipheral region of the retina. This appearance is attributed to microfolds in Bruch's membrane forging a fragile area under the basal lamina. Numerous other fundus findings are common with angioid streaks, including drusen, and atrophic punched-out spots similar to those found in presumed ocular histoplasmosis syndrome (POHS) have been observed (Figure 14.2).

Angioid streaks usually are not detected in children but first begin to appear in early adulthood. Fibrovascular

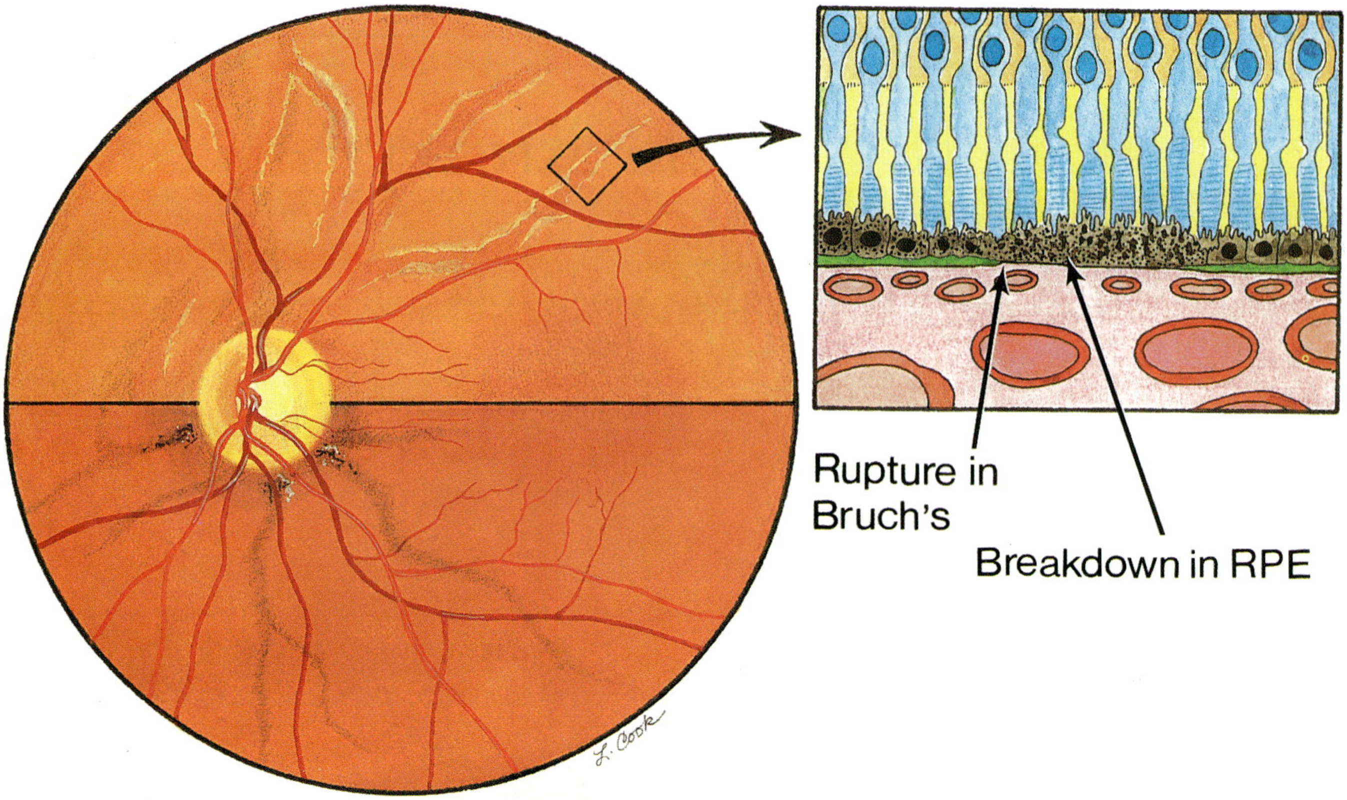

FIGURE 14.1. Illustration depicting the distribution and clinical appearance of angioid streaks. Variations in color are due to normal pigment differences in blonde versus darker fundi. The inset demonstrates the clinicopathologic change in which Bruch's membrane ruptures; there is a subsequent breakdown in the retinal pigment epithelium (RPE), thus allowing communication with the choriocapillaris and the potential for choroidal neovascularization.

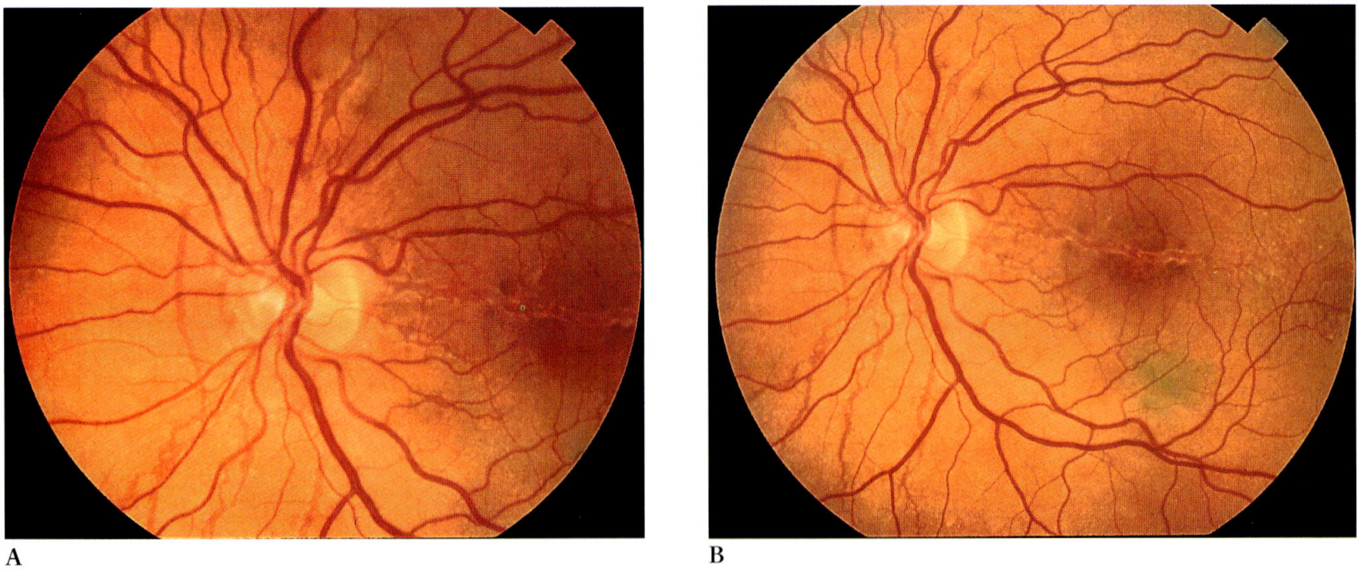

FIGURE 14.2. Angioid streaks in (A) the left eye, blonde fundus of a 40-year-old woman with no evidence of systemic disease, (B) with a streak running through the foveal area. There is an incidental choroidal nevus inferior to the macula. (Courtesy of A.R. Bell, CRA.)

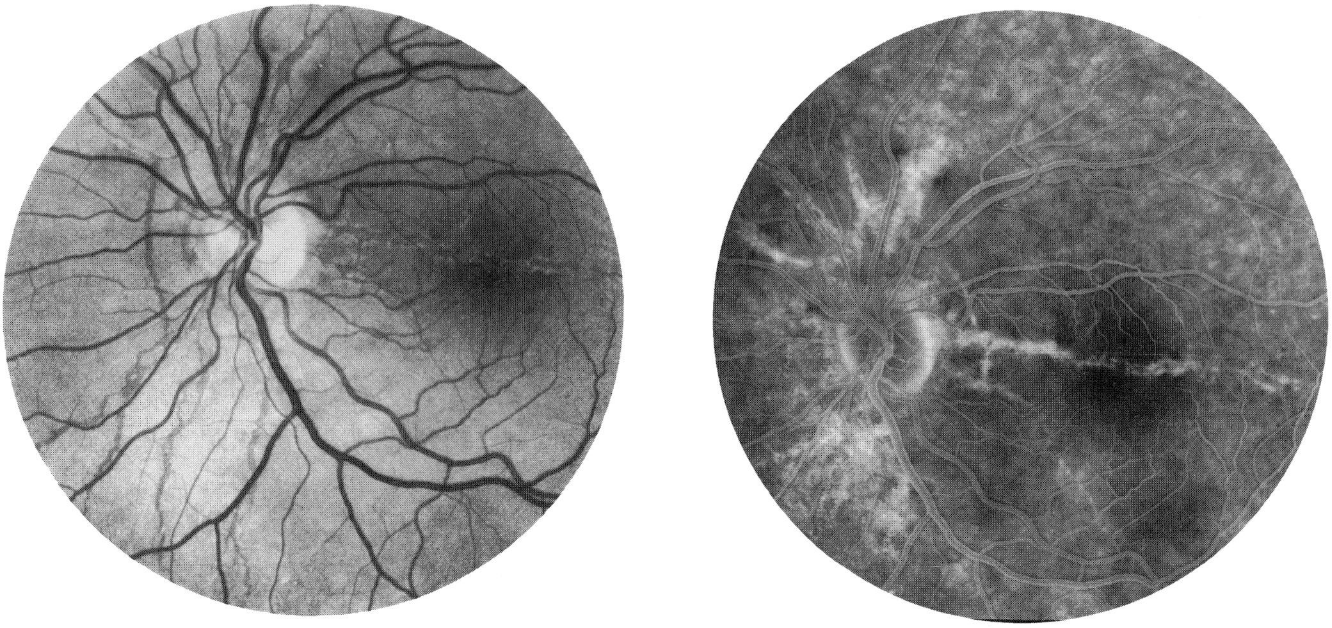

A B

FIGURE 14.3. A. Red-free photograph of the patient shown in Figure 14.2 with the angioid streak through the foveal area. B. The arteriovenous recirculation phase of the fluorescein angiogram showing hyperfluorescence. (Courtesy of A.R. Bell, CRA.)

ingrowth and CNVM formation will not usually develop until the fourth or fifth decade. The genesis of the choroidal neovascularization (CNV) may lead to exudative detachment of the overlying retina or RPE; if this occurs in the macular region, significant loss of vision may result. When observed in angioid streaks, these neovascular membranes have been reported to be fast growing but may be treatable with argon green laser photocoagulation if far enough removed from the center of the foveal avascular zone. Lesions in the area of the optic disc have been reported, many of which are treatable, if they represent a threat to vision. Angioid streaks may result in retinal hemorrhage in patients with PXE and, due to increased fragility of Bruch's membrane, can occur with relatively minimal trauma to the globe. Other macular changes include central areolar atrophy of the RPE and disciform scar secondary to a serous or hemorrhagic detachment of the macula.

Fluorescein angiography is useful in verifying the presence of a CNVM and to determine the suitability for treatment of the lesion depending on the location. The characteristic appearance of the transit reveals early hyperfluorescence if the choriocapillaris is intact, with persistent staining as the dye is removed from the retinal circulation. RPE detachment and CNV are represented by early hyperfluorescence and late staining, with continued leakage throughout the transit (Figures 14.3 and 14.4).

DIFFERENTIAL DIAGNOSIS

- Myopic degeneration and lacquer cracks
- POHS
- Traumatic rupture of Bruch's membrane
- Retinal vasculitis
- Choroidal sclerosis and choroidal folds
- Toxoplasmosis
- CNV from other causes

The medical survey for patients with angioid streaks should include radiologic evaluation and serologic testing, including serum alkaline phosphatase.

MANAGEMENT

- Diagnostic survey to rule out systemic disease
  - PXE
  - Paget's disease
  - Sickle hemoglobinopathy
- Fluorescein angiography to confirm CNVM when indicated
- Argon green laser photocoagulation
- Home Amsler grid testing

There is no treatment for angioid streaks unless the lesions are associated with CNVM, especially in the presence of a serous detachment of the macula. Prophylactic

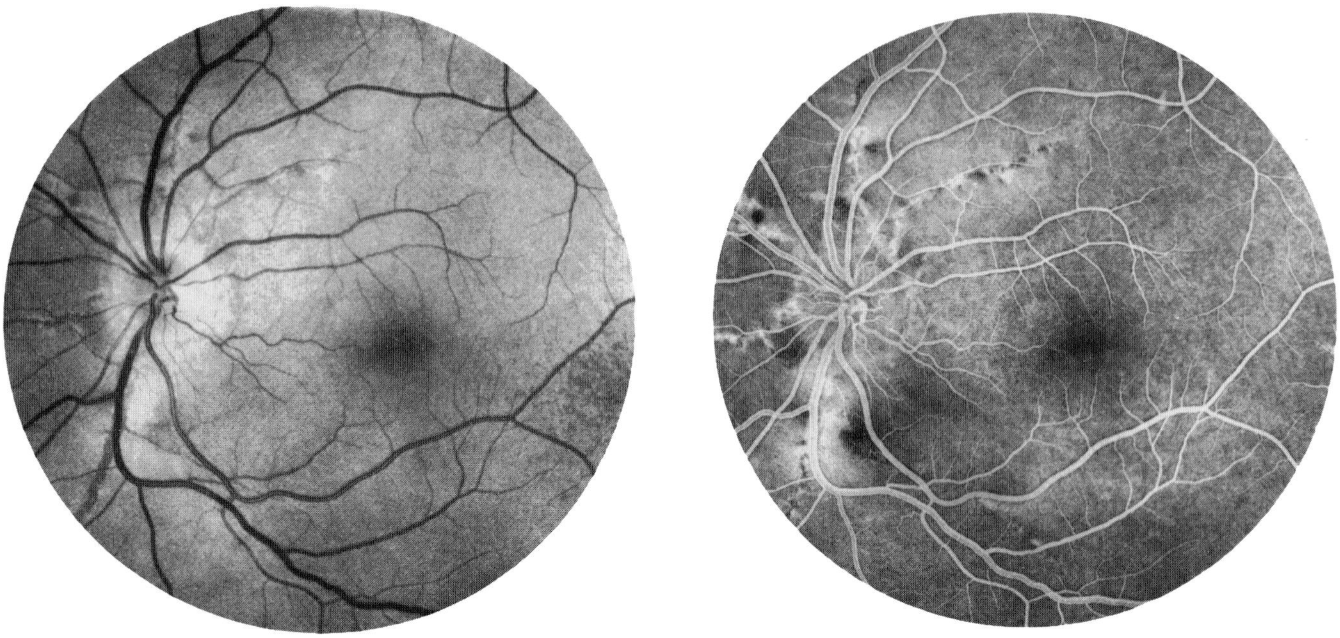

A B

FIGURE 14.4. A. Red-free photograph of the left eye of a patient demonstrating the radial peripapillary distribution of the streaks. Note the appearance of peau d'orange temporal to the macula in the extreme right edge of the photograph. B. Laminar flow phase of fluorescein transit demonstrating early hyperfluorescence of streaks. (Courtesy of A.R. Bell, CRA.)

treatment with the laser is not indicated since it can result in iatrogenic neovascular membrane formation.

SYSTEMIC DISEASE REPORTED WITH ANGIOID STREAKS

Most Common

- Paget's disease
- Pseudoxanthoma elasticum
- Sickle hemoglobinopathy

Others Reported

- Acromegaly
- Ehlers-Danlos syndrome
- Familial polyposis
- Hemochromatosis
- Hypercalcinosis
- Hyperphosphatemia
- Lead poisoning
- Phakomatoses
- Senile elastosis

Angioid streaks are a curious ocular finding that require careful evaluation and an estimation of importance based on the patient's systemic history. Fifty percent of patients with the streaks have systemic disease, and 85% of all patients with PXE eventually develop the streaks. Ten to 15% of patients with Paget's disease also manifest the fundus findings. The association with serous maculopathy warrants careful surveillance and appropriate patient self-assessment with the home Amsler grid test. Careful diagnosis, coupled with an understanding of risk factors, patient education, and appropriate referral to the patient's primary care physician to rule out the presence of systemic conditions, are important aspects in maintaining a discriminating standard of care.

SUGGESTED READING

Aessopos A, Stametelos G, Savvides P, et al. Angioid streaks in homozygous beta thalassemia. Am J Ophthalmol 1989;108:356–359.

Brown R, Raines MF. The blood retinal barrier in angioid streaks. Eye 1988;2:547–551.

Clarkson JG, Altman RD. Angioid streaks. Surv Ophthalmol 1982;26:235–246.

Federman JL, Shields JA, Tomer TL, et al. Angioid Streaks. In LA Yannuzzi, KA Gitter, HG Schatz (eds), The Macula: A Comprehensive Text and Atlas. Baltimore: Williams & Wilkins, 1978;218–231.

Fine SL. Angioid streaks. Int Ophthalmol Clin 1977;17:173–182.

Gelisken O, Hendrikse F, Deutman AF. A long-term follow-up study of laser coagulation of neovascular membranes in angioid streaks. Am J Ophthalmol 1988;105:299–303.

Grand MG, Isserman MJ, Miller CW. Angioid streaks associated with pseudoxanthoma elasticum in a 13-year-old patient. Ophthalmology 1987;94:197–200.

Johnson BW, Oshinskie L. Diagnosis and management of angioid streaks. J Am Optom Assoc 1988;59:704–711.

Kinsella FP, Mooney DJ. Angioid streaks in beta thalassaemia minor. Br J Ophthalmol 1988;72:303–304.

Mansour AM, Shields JA, Annesley WH, et al. Macular degeneration in angioid streaks. Ophthalmologica 1988;197:36–41.

Piro PA, Scheragen D, Fine SL. Angioid Streaks: Natural History and Visual Prognosis. In S Fine, S Owens (eds), Management of Retinal Vascular and Macular Disorders. Baltimore: Williams & Wilkins, 1983;136–139.

Pruet RC, Weiter JJ, Goldstein RB. Myopic cracks, angioid streaks and traumatic tears in Bruch's membrane. Am J Ophthalmol 1987;103:537–543.

Singerman LJ, Hatem G. Laser treatment of choroidal neovascular membranes in angioid streaks. Retina 1981;1:75–83.

CHAPTER

15 Lacquer Cracks

Anthony A. Cavallerano

Lacquer cracks represent breaks in Bruch's membrane sometimes observed in the posterior pole in a highly myopic eye. These distinctive fundus changes are quite common in axial myopia and may prognosticate hemorrhage from choroidal neovascularization (CNV) in the macular area. The condition is often associated with a pathologic or progressive form of myopia and most often occurs concurrently with posterior staphyloma.

Degenerative fundus changes have been known to occur in progressive myopia since posterior staphyloma and its attending complications were first described in 1806. If the distension of the globe leads to stretching of the underlying choroidal and scleral tissue, vascular changes can occur, leading to retinal and choroidal hemorrhage. Fuch's spot, subretinal hemorrhage, or exudative detachment of the retinal pigment epithelium (RPE) or neurosensory retina, results from serosanguinous leakage from choroidal neovascular membrane (CNVM) into the subretinal space. This characteristic lesion is also associated with lacquer cracks or pathologic changes in Bruch's membrane, as seen in high myopia, often when the axial length exceeds 30 mm. Often mistaken for angioid streaks, lacquer cracks are not associated with any underlying systemic disease.

Lacquer cracks are seen in 4.3% of highly myopic eyes. They are significant in that the reported incidence of CNVM associated with these lesions ranges from 4–11%. Conversely, lacquer cracks are found in over 80% of myopic eyes with CNV. The prevalence is probably higher since both the cracks and the neovascularization may go undetected in early stages without the aid of fluorescein angiography (FA).

There are two theories to explain the etiopathogenesis of lacquer cracks. Early studies hinted at sclerosis of choroidal vessels as the root cause for the cracks. More recently it has been postulated that lacquer cracks are caused by stretching of the retina and choroid in the staphylomatous globe. Continued growth of the globe exceeds the elastic resistance of Bruch's membrane, and a linear rent becomes obvious. These fissures in the Bruch's membrane and choriocapillaris complex can allow communication between the underlying choroid and the subretinal space and thus the plausibility exists for CNV. Some association seems to exist with tilted disc syndrome, another condition associated with ectasia of the posterior globe.

CLINICAL PRESENTATION

- Fine, irregular pale yellow or white lines
- Macular involvement
- Mottled pigment at borders
- Branching, crisscross, or reticular distribution
- Bruch's membrane–choriocapillaris complex
- Tesselated fundus
- Temporal crescent
- Chorioretinal atrophy in posterior segment
- Round, dense, and deep choroidal hemorrhage
- CNV
- Thinned, stretched posterior segment
- Decreased visual function, including color and visual field deficit

Visual function in pathologic myopia, and therefore patients with lacquer cracks, is often affected. An anatomically deformed globe is a constant finding, and the visual field and color discrimination may also be reduced. The clinical appearance of lacquer cracks is somewhat unique. The lesions are fine, irregular-shaped, pale yellow or white lines radiating in a stellate or reticular pattern in the posterior pole (Figure 15.1). The lesions may be single or branching, and they tend

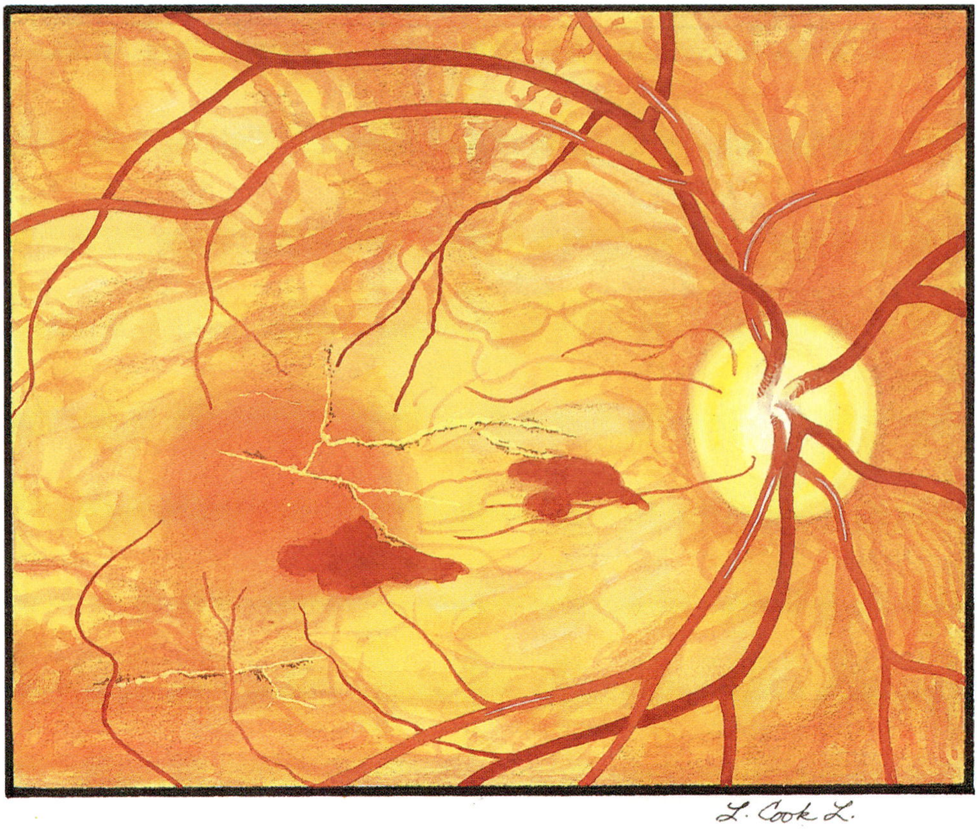

FIGURE 15.1. Illustration depicting the clinical appearance of lacquer cracks, with the tesselated, pale fundus, reticular distribution of pigmented linear lesions, and associated retinal hemorrhage. (Reprinted with permission from AA Cavallerano. Lacquer cracks. Clin Eye Vis Care 1991;3:190–195.)

to crisscross with one another. Almost always associated with a temporal crescent of the optic nerve head, the lesions are continuous with the crescent in 17% of cases. Most lacquer cracks traverse the macula and lie in the deeper layers of the retina. The Bruch's membrane–choriocapillaris complex is affected, but the overlying neurosensory retina, the inner retina, and the retinal vessels are unaffected. The fundus is often tesselated and may appear pale in the posterior polar region (Figure 15.2).

Choroidal hemorrhage in the absence of CNV is a frequent coexistent finding (Figure 15.3). These hemorrhages are dense in appearance and often resolve spontaneously. They may occur in younger age groups, are deep in the retina, and have been referred to as coin lesions. The hemorrhages occur along the linear aspect of the lesion, and the prognosis for retention of vision is often good. Chorioretinal atrophy eventually develops in the posterior pole, and the lacquer cracks become enfolded into these larger areas. As is often the case in pathologic myopia, CNVM formation can occur and may lead to significant vision loss (Figure 15.4).

FA results are characterized by early pseudofluorescence and hyperfluorescence due to abnormal transmission of atrophic RPE and choriocapillaris. Fluorescence increases slightly throughout the transit,

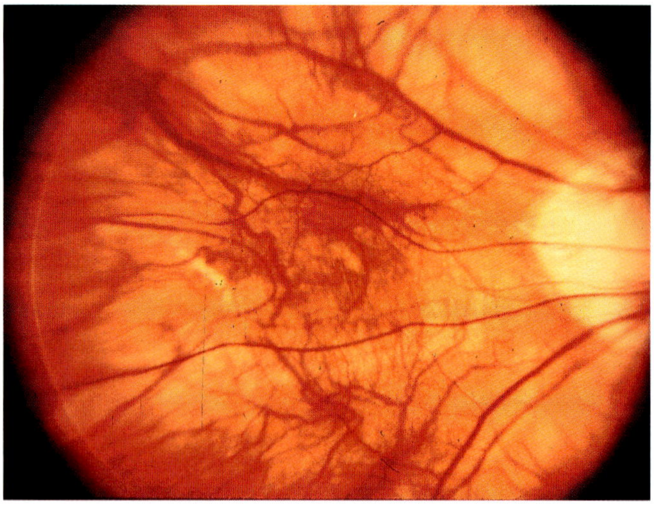

FIGURE 15.2. Fundus photograph of a highly myopic right eye showing tesselation, myopic crescent, and linear lesions characteristic of lacquer cracks.

and a faint hyperfluorescence remains in the late stage of the angiogram, probably due to scleral staining. A CNV elicits a characteristic irregular, lacy hyperfluorescence in the early phase, with increased staining and fuzzy fluorescence in the late phase of the transit.

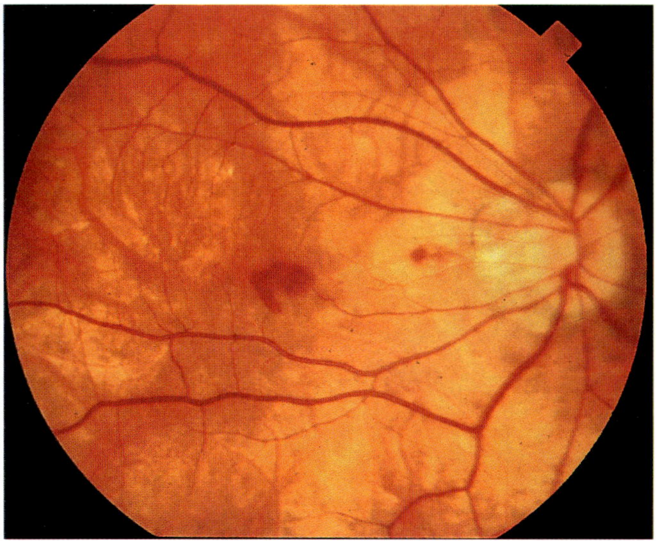

FIGURE 15.3. Right myopic fundus with lacquer cracks and hemorrhage in the absence of choroidal neovascular membrane.

DIFFERENTIAL DIAGNOSIS

- Angioid streaks
- Traumatic rupture of Bruch's membrane

The differential diagnosis of lacquer cracks includes traumatic rupture of Bruch's membrane, an event that usually follows contusive trauma to the globe (Figure 15.5). The lesion is linear or crescent shaped and often follows the contour of the optic disc. Additional consideration should be given to angioid streaks, linear lesions in Bruch's membrane that have a high degree of correlation with systemic disease. Angioid streaks radiate from the optic nerve head in all directions and range in color from gray to brown to red (Figure 15.6). Risk factors for lacquer cracks should be considered, and these include high myopia, usually greater than 6 diopters, in association with posterior staphyloma.

MANAGEMENT

- Explore family history
- Complete ocular examination, including color vision and visual fields
- FA
- Home Amsler grid testing
- Annual examination for high myopia
- Semiannual examination for lacquer cracks
- Immediate examination for sudden onset of dysmorphopsia
- Laser photocoagulation for CNVM when indicated
- Scleral reinforcement

Management of lacquer cracks includes a comprehensive ocular examination, including FA when CNV is suspected based on clinical findings or patient symptoms, especially new dysmorphopsia. Self-assessment with the home Amsler grid test should be done if there is an index

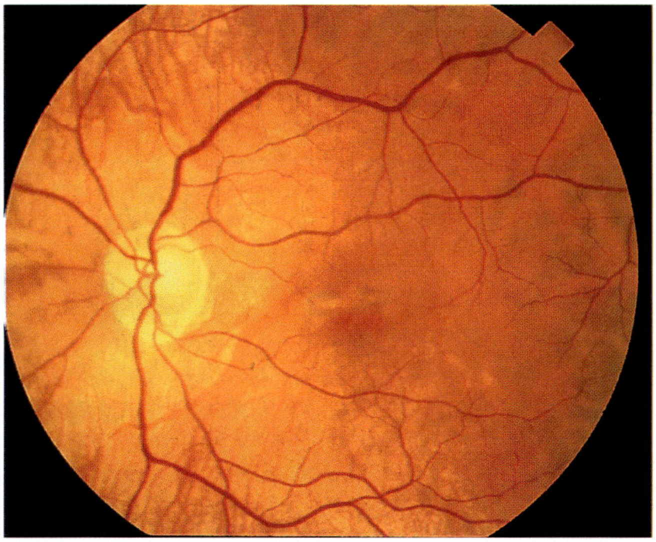

A

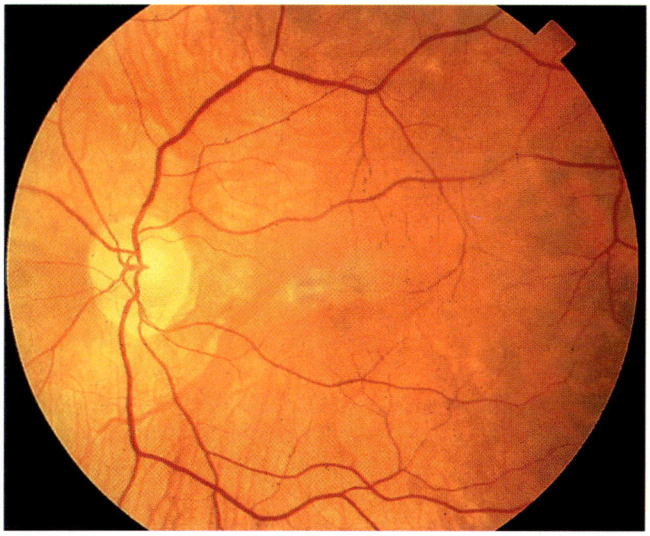

B

FIGURE 15.4. A. Lacquer crack with choroidal neovascular membrane in the left eye of a 40-year-old woman with visual acuity of 20/70. Late phase fluorescein angiogram reveals hyperfluorescence characteristic of choroidal neovascular membrane and subretinal leakage. B. Same patient after focal laser treatment for choroidal neovascular membrane. Mid-phase of fluorescein angiogram shows hypofluorescence indicating destruction of choroidal neovascular membrane.

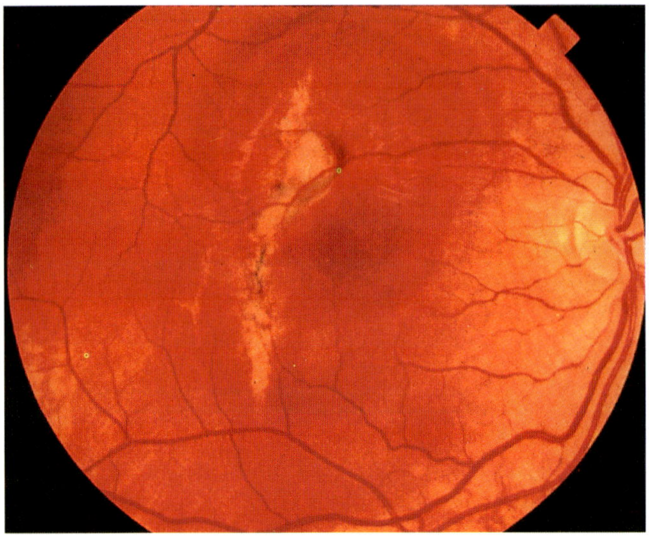

FIGURE 15.5. Ruptured Bruch's membrane in the right eye of a 13-year-old boy struck with a golf ball. Note the crescent-shaped orientation of the lesion.

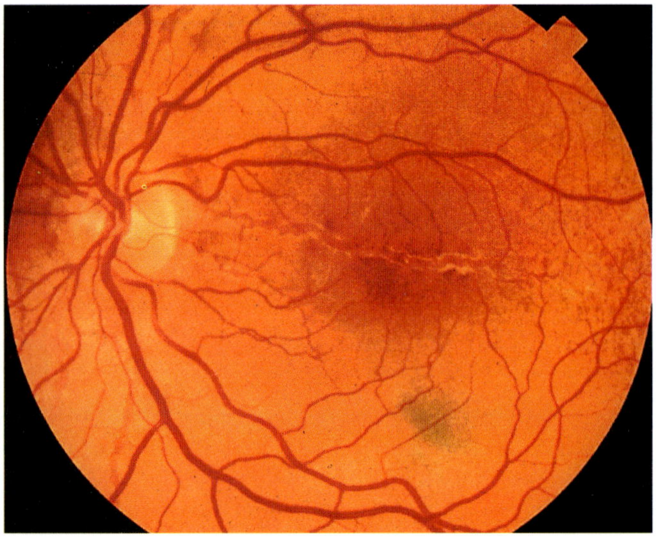

FIGURE 15.6. Example of angioid streaks in the left eye of a 40-year-old female patient radiating from the optic disc and traversing the macula. The reddish-brown color and radiation from the optic disc are distinctive and help to differentiate these lesions from paler lacquer cracks.

of suspicion for CNV. The detection of dysmorphopsia should alert the patient and the clinician to the possibility of ocular morbidity and visual loss.

Treatment has included an attempt at trying to reinforce the generalized thinning of the globe. This procedure, called *scleral reinforcement*, calls for scleral resection, and has been used in children. The procedure makes use of autologous fascia lata or animal tendon to strengthen the globe. Although there is evidence that it will halt the progression of myopia, it does not seem to arrest further degenerative changes.

SUMMARY

Lacquer cracks are typical clinical findings in a highly myopic fundus and should alert the clinician to the possibility of retinal hemorrhage with or without CNVM. Patients with high axial myopia warrant careful surveillance and regular ocular examination to rule out the development of fundus changes that may augur the onset of CNVM. If CNVM is suspected based on physical examination or a report of dysmorphopsia, then an FA should be obtained to determine if a treatable lesion is present.

SUGGESTED READING

Avila MP, Weiter JJ, Jalkh AE, et al. Natural history of choroidal neovascularization in degenerative myopia. Ophthalmology 1984;91:1573–1581.

Borley WE, Snyder AA. Surgical treatment of high myopia: The combined lamellar scleral resection with scleral reinforcement using donor eye. Trans Am Acad Ophthalmol Otolaryngol 1958;62:791–802.

Bottoni FG, Eggink CA, Cruysberg JR, et al. Dominant inherited tilted disc syndrome and lacquer cracks. Eye 1990;4:504–509.

Curtin BJ. The Etiology of Myopia. In The Myopias. Philadelphia: Harper & Row, 1985;61–64.

Curtin BJ. Myopia. In LA Yannuzzi, KA Gitter, H Schatz (eds), The Macula: A Comprehensive Text and Atlas. Baltimore: Williams & Wilkins, 1979;232–242.

Curtin BJ. The posterior staphyloma of pathologic myopia. Am Ophthalmol Soc 1977;75:67–86.

Curtin BJ, Karlin DB. Axial length measurements and fundus changes of the myopic eye. Am J Ophthalmol 1971;71:42–53.

Hotchkiss ML, Fine SL. Pathologic myopia and choroidal neovascularization. Am J Ophthalmol 1981;91:177–183.

Klein RM, Green S. The development of lacquer cracks in pathologic myopia. Am J Ophthalmol 1988;106:282–285.

Paton D. The relation of angioid streaks to systemic disease. Springfield, IL: Charles C. Thomas, 1972.

Pruett RC, Weiter JJ, Goldstein RB. Myopic cracks, angioid streaks, and traumatic tears in Bruch's membrane. Am J Ophthalmol 1987;103:537–543.

Vancea P. New concepts in the treatment of progressive myopia. Ann Ophthalmol 1971;3:1105–1108.

PART

IV

Miscellaneous Macular Disorders

CHAPTER

16

Cystoid Macular Edema

Anthony A. Cavallerano

Macular edema can result from numerous causes and is a relatively common cause for reduced visual function in various ocular disease states. A breakdown of the inner blood-retinal barrier results in leakage and a subsequent increase in thickness of the macula. The resulting edema can be diffuse or cystic in nature, and numerous complications can result in decreased visual function.

CONDITIONS AND SYNDROMES ASSOCIATED WITH CYSTOID MACULAR EDEMA

Common Causes

- Following intraocular surgery (including lensectomy, scleral buckling, penetrating keratoplasty)
- Venous occlusive disease (central retinal vein occlusion and branch retinal vein occlusion)
- Diabetes

Other Causes

- Following photocoagulation
- Cellophane maculopathy
- Intermediate uveitis
- Other uveitis
- Retinitis pigmentosa
- Following yttrium-aluminum-garnet (YAG) capsulotomy

Rare But Noteworthy Causes

- Medications such as acetazolamide
- Phototoxic retinopathy
- Epinephrine or dipivefrin use in aphakia or pseudophakia
- Coats' disease
- Radiation retinopathy

Cystoid macular edema (CME) is a relatively common cause for decreased visual function, especially in the elderly. It occurs secondary to certain ocular disease states and is characterized by thickening of the macula due to intraretinal edema. Often the cystic edema in the macular area occurs following intraocular surgery, especially lensectomy; other causes include vascular occlusive disease, retinal inflammatory disease, retinal phototoxicity, and diabetic retinopathy. Expansion of the extracellular space of the retina results from an accumulation of fluid within the retinal tissue due to abnormal leakage from the perifoveal capillaries. This abnormal leakage is also observed at the optic nerve and the peripheral retina. CME can significantly affect vision, and the prognosis is variable depending on the underlying cause of the edema.

CME was first described more than 40 years ago and later demonstrated angiographically. The syndrome was traditionally associated with intracapsular cataract surgery (Irvine-Gass syndrome) but is also observed in pseudophakic eyes following extracapsular procedures. Angiographic CME has been reported in 40–70% of eyes after cataract surgery and is quite common following uncomplicated lens extraction. The incidence is greater in the midphase of the postoperative period, i.e., after 4–7 months, rather than as an early postoperative complication. Seventy-five percent of CME following cataract surgery occurs within the first 6 months. However, in some instances the visual acuity remains unchanged because the leakage occurs in the perifoveal capillaries. In these cases, there is often a spontaneous resolution of the cystic changes and full visual function returns. There seems to be a lower incidence among those patients undergoing phacoemulsification, probably due to preservation of the posterior lens capsule, less disturbance of the vitreous, and implantation of a posterior chamber intraocular lens.

The etiopathogenesis of CME is debatable, but certain features of the entity are consistent. Common to all types of macular edema are disruption of the inner or outer blood-retinal barrier and subsequent incompetence of the retinal microvasculature. This breakdown leads to leakage and an accumulation of fluid with an expansion of the extracellular space of the retina, especially in the outer plexiform and inner nuclear layers. Leakage usually originates from the perifoveal capillaries, resulting in the formation of cystic changes. It has been postulated that the cystoid spaces might represent swollen Müller cells. Receptor cells are displaced, and in chronic CME, there may be permanent loss of neural tissue. Degenerative changes in the retinal pigment epithelium (RPE) have also been implicated.

Recently, the putative role of the mediator, prostaglandin, in the pathogenesis of CME has been studied. There is some evidence that prostaglandins lead to incompetence of the tight junctions of the perifoveal capillaries. Some theories point to the role of ultraviolet light in generating free radicals that promote the release of prostaglandins. Vitreoretinal factors have been associated with cystic edema of the macula since tractional forces seem to play a mechanical role in the pathogenesis of CME. This explanation is plausible since lamellar and full-thickness macular holes can accompany CME.

CME can result from any condition that disrupts the inner or outer blood-retinal barrier. Metabolic disease, especially diabetes mellitus, with focal or diffuse leakage from microaneurysms, can result in the formation of cystoid spaces. Retinal ischemia from any cause, including diabetes and retinal vascular occlusive disease, where venous obstruction causes leakage into the macular area, can cause macular edema. Other causes are collagen vascular disease, certain hereditary and familial diseases, retinitis pigmentosa, and acquired immunodeficiency syndrome. CME may be seen following intraocular surgery and is a common complication of penetrating keratoplasty and scleral buckle implantation for retinal detachment. It can follow neodymium-yttrium-aluminum-garnet capsulotomy and will occur with traction on the macula from epiretinal membrane formation. In fact, as CME subsides, an epiretinal membrane may develop, resulting in long-term complications, including macular hole formation. Retinal inflammatory disease, especially intermediate uveitis, is often associated with CME. It is thought that inflammatory mediators play a role in the development of the cystic changes in posterior and intermediate uveitis. Harada's disease, Leber's stellate maculopathy, and neoplastic disease are additional causes.

FACTORS INFLUENCING PSEUDOPHAKIC CYSTOID MACULAR EDEMA

- Vitreous traction
- Intraocular surgical trauma
- Posterior lens capsule rupture
- Surgical approach (phacoemulsification versus extracapsular extraction)
- Anesthetic solution containing hyaluronidase
- Retinal phototoxicity
- Absent ultraviolet filter in intraocular lens
- Release of prostaglandins
- Topical epinephrine
- Coexistence of systemic disease, especially diabetes mellitus and perhaps systemic hypertension

As a complication to cataract surgery, CME can reduce visual acuity from 20/50–20/100 even when initial postsurgical vision is normal. The patient reports decreased visual function in distance and near vision, occurring weeks to months following cataract surgery, including uncomplicated procedures. The decrease in vision is often gradual but is noticed suddenly by the patient. CME following cataract surgery may be related to inflammation or may be the result of mechanical factors, such as disruption of the vitreous contents. There is a greater risk if additional surgical factors come into play, such as iris tissue damage, vitreous incarceration in the surgical wound, posterior capsule rupture, or anterior chamber disorganization. The incidence of pseudophakic CME is 40–60%, as demonstrated by fluorescein angiography (FA), and 2–10% clinically. Eyes with the lowest risk seem to be those with less inflammation, namely those with a posterior chamber intraocular lens. CME may coexist with pseudophakic bullous keratopathy, a complication that may further decrease visual acuity. The obscured macula resulting from the corneal edema may add to the difficulty in observing the macula and diagnosing the CME. Fundus FA may be necessary to make or confirm the diagnosis with coexisting pseudophakic bullous keratopathy.

If the CME is secondary to other ocular conditions, the patient may notice an additional decrease in vision from the cystic maculopathy. However, patients with significant ocular disease such as retinal vascular disease may not notice additional visual loss. Similarly, a patient with posterior or intermediate uveitis may overlook visual changes due to the exceptional amount of debris or cells in the vitreous resulting from the inflammation.

CLINICAL PRESENTATION

- Decreased central visual acuity (20/50–20/100)
- Thickening of macula observed with fundus biomicroscopy

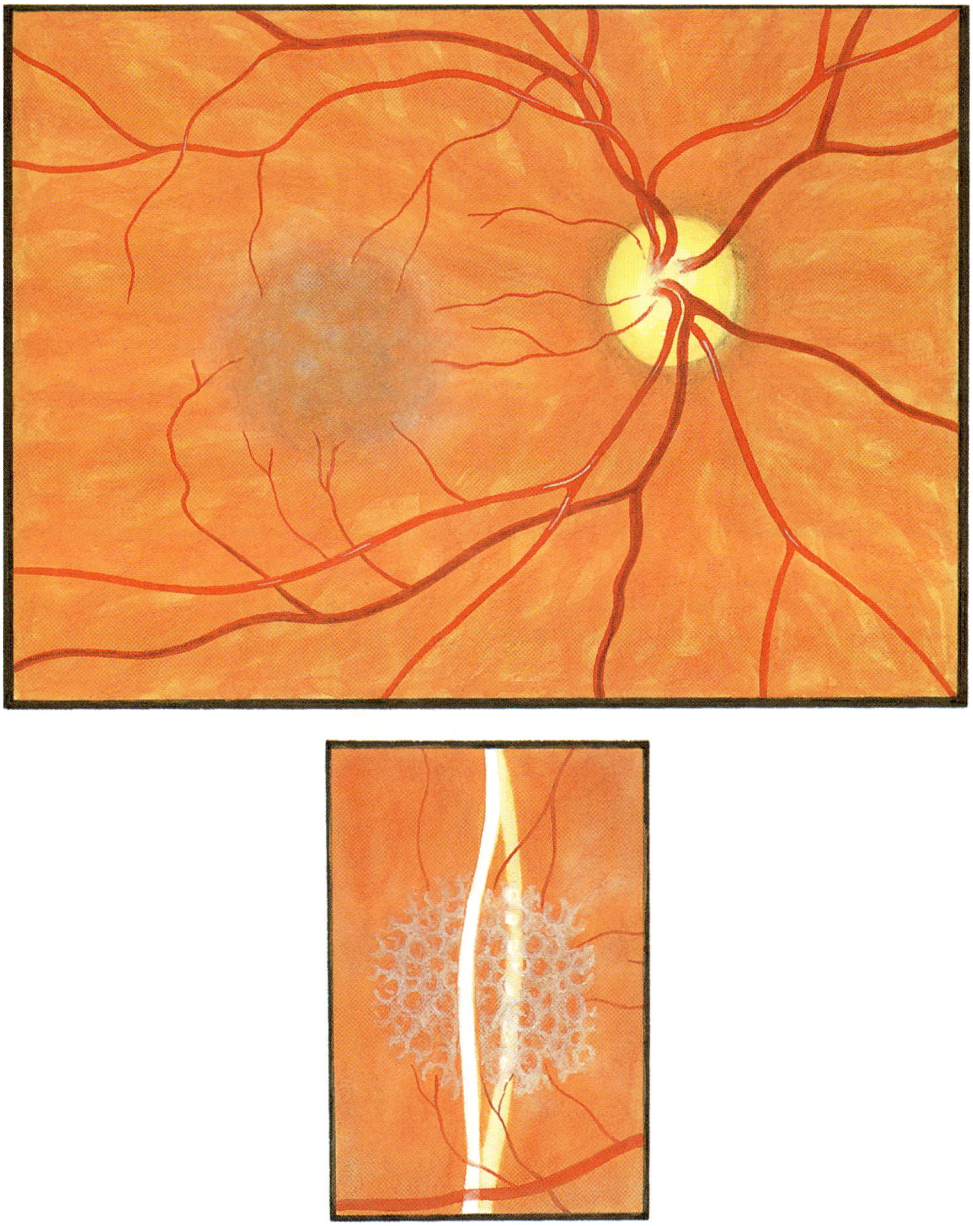

FIGURE 16.1. Illustration depicting the appearance of cystoid macular edema with loss of retinal transparency in the macular area and the slit-lamp view with evidence of macular thickening and the formation of cystic spaces.

- Loss of retinal transparency
- Loss of choroidal detail in macular area
- Optic nerve swelling
- Cells in vitreous and anterior chamber
- Fundus FA—early leakage progressing to late staining in petalloid or wreath-like pattern

Stereoscopic examination of the macula using fundus biomicroscopy is ideal for observing CME. Prominent cystic spaces may be observed, with the occasional appearance of subretinal fluid. Macular thickening is the most important finding and is detected with fundus biomicroscopy using the hand-held condensing lenses, the Hruby precorneal lens, or a fundus contact lens. Macular thickening is best observed by indirect illumination with the slit-lamp beam, looking for retro-illuminated cystic spaces. The spaces are subtle but obvious due to their light-scattering capabilities. The cystic spaces correspond to areas of perifoveal leakage, and macular thickening is a better indicator of predictable visual acuity than leakage. There is loss of retinal transparency, and the underlying choroidal detail is obscured (Figure 16.1). In severe cases, cells may be observed in the vitreous and the anterior chamber. Optic nerve swelling may occur and is more apparent by FA. FA typically demonstrates deep perifoveal capillary changes, with leakage in a petalloid or wreath-like pattern in the macular area. The leakage progresses in both directions and eventually forms a stellate arrangement due to the leakage following the orientation of Henle's layer. The outer borders of the leakage are irregular (Figures 16.2 and 16.3).

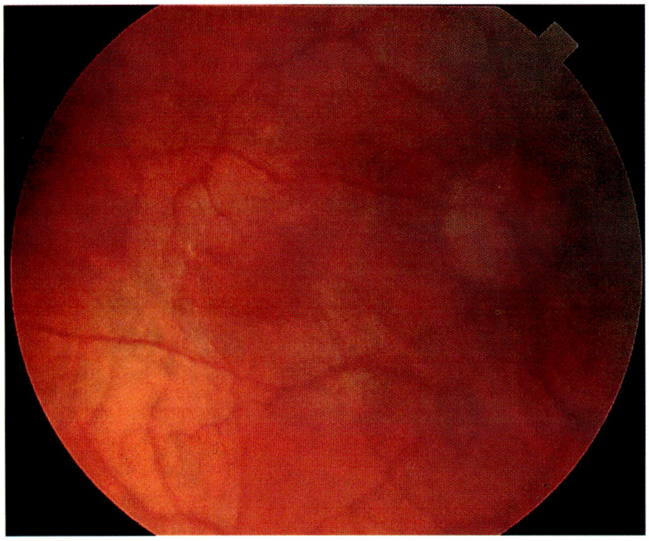

A

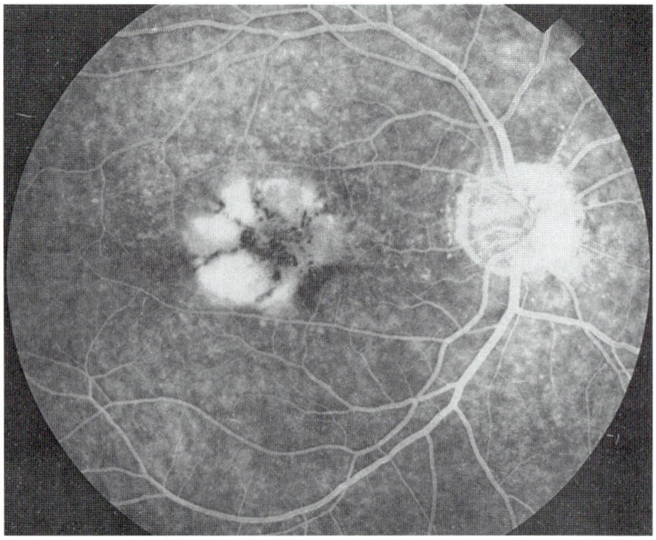

B

FIGURE 16.2. A. Cystoid macular edema in the right eye of a patient with pseudophakic cystoid macular edema following secondary anterior chamber lens implantation. B. Late phase of the fluorescein angiogram reveals the typical petalloid or wreath-like pattern of leakage from the perifoveal capillaries.

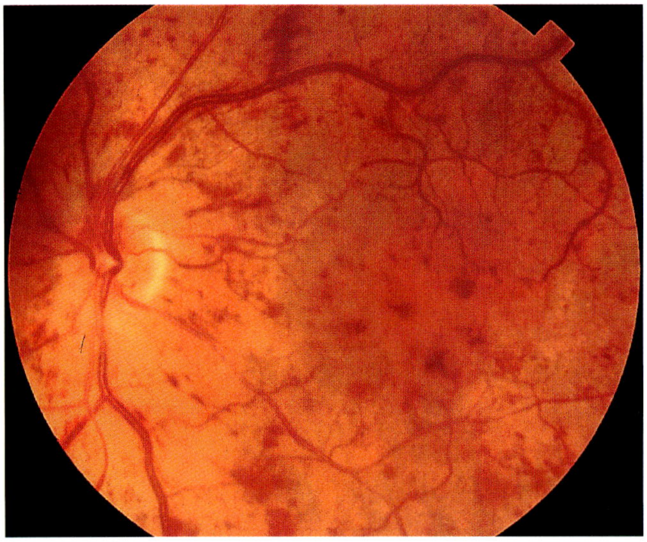

A

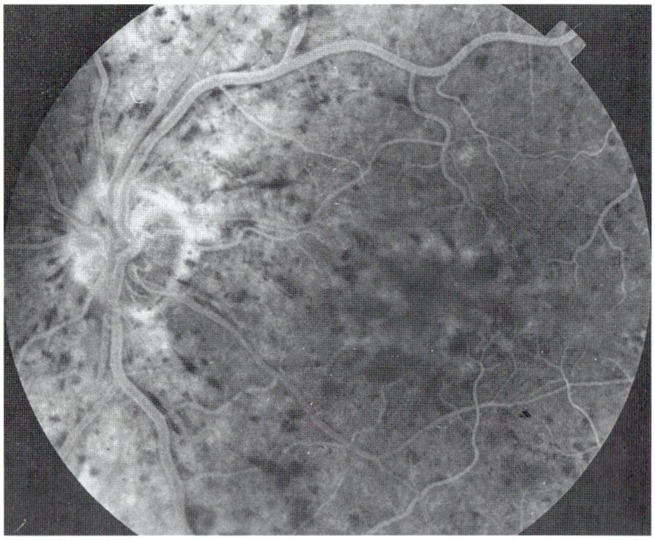

B

FIGURE 16.3. A. Mild cystic changes in the macula of a patient with nonischemic central retinal vein occlusion in the left eye. B. Cystic changes are apparent in the late phase of the fluorescein angiogram.

MANAGEMENT

- Explore history for recent ocular surgery
- Prescribe topical or systemic nonsteroidal anti-inflammatory drugs
- Prescribe topical, periocular, or systemic steroids
- Evaluate the retina stereoscopically to rule out posterior or intermediate uveitis
- Treat underlying ocular disease
- Use FA to confirm decreased vision and detect treatable causes of CME

Treatment for CME varies depending on the underlying etiology. Eliminating the underlying cause often restores the integrity of the inner and outer blood-retinal barrier. For example, in diabetes, focal or grid laser surgery is often effective. The exact mechanism has not been adequately explained, but it is thought that photocoagulation may disrupt the RPE, resulting in a drying of the edema. If caused by retinal inflammatory disease, treatment of the underlying cause with systemic steroids, photocoagulation, or cryosurgery often has some palliative effect on the cystic changes in the macula. CME uncovered by FA with normal visual function requires no treatment.

Aphakic and pseudophakic CME is treated with topical nonsteroidal anti-inflammatory agents such as flurbiprofen or diclofenac. Systemic nonsteroidal anti-inflammatory drugs such as indomethacin (Indocin) or diflunisal (Dolobid) have been employed. Topical, periocular, and systemic steroids have been used, and carbonic anhydrase inhibitors may be of some value in reducing the macular edema. Discontinuance of epinephrine compounds and replacement by other antiglaucoma medications by glaucoma patients usually results in resolution of the CME. Prophylactic treatment with topical nonsteroidal anti-inflammatory drugs prior to cataract surgery and during the initial postoperative period may be of some benefit in preventing CME. This may also be of benefit in treating the fellow eye since CME in the second eye is more common following an episode in the first eye.

SUMMARY

CME is a relatively common cause for diminished central vision in the elderly and is a common occurrence following uncomplicated cataract extraction. Those with concurrent risk factors may have a greater tendency toward CME and should be observed closely during the postoperative period. Patients with CME from intraocular disease or retinal vascular disease should be educated to look for the changes consistent with thickening and edema of the macula. FA will confirm the diagnosis and is useful in identifying ischemic retinopathy but should not be performed routinely. Early treatment may prevent the irreversible effects of chronic CME, and patients at risk should be kept under regular surveillance.

SUGGESTED READING

Durham DG. Three thousand YAG lasers in posterior capsulotomies: An analysis of complications and comparison to polishing and surgical discissions. Trans Am Ophthalmol Soc 1985;83:218–229.

Flach AJ, Stegman RC, Graham J, et al. Prophylaxis of aphakic cystoid macular edema without corticosteroids. A paired-comparison, placebo-controlled double-masked study. Ophthalmology 1990;97:1253–1258.

Gass JD, Norton EW. Cystoid macular edema and papilledema following cataract extraction: Fluorescein funduscopic and angiographic study. Arch Ophthalmol 1966;76:646–661.

Gass JD, Norton EW. Follow-up study of cystoid macular edema following cataract extraction. Trans Am Acad Ophthalmol 1969;73:665–671.

Hitchings RA, Chisolm IH. Incidence of aphakic cystoid macular edema. Br J Ophthalmol 1975;59:444–450.

Irvine AR, Bresky R, Crowder BM, et al. Macular edema after cataract extraction. Ann Ophthalmol 1971;3:1234–1240.

Irvine SR. A newly defined vitreous syndrome following cataract surgery. Interpreted according to recent concepts of the structure of the vitreous. Am J Ophthalmol 1953;36:599–619.

Jaffe NS, Clayman HM, Jaffe MS. Cystoid macular edema after cataract extraction with and without an intraocular lens. Ophthalmology 1982;89:23–29.

Jampol L. Pharmacologic therapy of aphakic and pseudophakic cystoid macular edema. Arch Ophthalmol 1985;103:1134–1135.

Milch FA, Yannuzzi LA. Medical and surgical treatment of aphakic cystoid macular edema. Int Ophthalmol Clin 1987;27:205–217.

Miyake K, Asakura M, Kobayashi H. Effect of intraocular lens fixation on the blood-aqueous barrier. Am J Ophthalmol 1984;98:451–455.

Nirankari VS, Richards RD. Complications associated with the use of the neodymium:YAG laser. Ophthalmology 1985;92:1371–1376.

Nussenblatt RB, Kauffman SC, Palestine AG, et al. Macular thickening and visual acuity: Measurement in patients with cystoid macular edema. Ophthalmology 1987;94:1134–1139.

Stark WJ, Worthen DM, Halladay JT, et al. The FDA report on intraocular lenses. Ophthalmology 1983;90:311–317.

Stern AL, Taylor DM, Dalburg LA, et al. Pseudophakic cystoid maculopathy. A study of 50 cases. Ophthalmology 1981;88:942–946.

Tso MO. Pathology of cystoid macular edema. Ophthalmology 1982;89:902–915.

Yannuzzi LA. A perspective on the treatment of aphakic cystoid macular edema. Surv Ophthalmol 1984;28:540–553.

Yanoff M, Fine BS, Brucker AJ, et al. Pathology of human cystoid macular edema. Surv Ophthalmol 1984;28:505–511.

CHAPTER

17

Idiopathic Central Serous Chorioretinopathy

Anthony A. Cavallerano

Idiopathic central serous chorioretinopathy (ICSC) is a relatively common, sometimes recurrent macular disorder affecting certain patient populations. It is characterized by choroidal exudation and localized neurosensory retinal detachment, resulting in a blister-like elevation of the macula, sometimes involving only the fovea. The retinal elevation is likely due to a focal defect in the retinal pigment epithelial (RPE) layer, allowing fluid to pass from the choroid under the neurosensory retina. Foveal involvement results in a visual disturbance.

ICSC was first recognized by von Graefe, who described the condition and assigned the designation *recurrent central retinitis*. Later it was referred to as *central angiospastic retinopathy* and *central serous retinopathy* before the current terms idiopathic central serous chorioretinopathy and central serous choroidopathy were finally adopted.

ICSC is rare under age 20 and affects men 9 to 1 over women; the incidence is twice as great in women aged 31–40 as compared with those aged 21–30. Stress appears to be a predisposing element, and certain personality characteristics seem to be an implicating factor. Migraine syndrome is sometimes associated with ICSC, and some patients report a headache as a prodrome to the maculopathy. Bilaterality seems to be comparable to the rate of recurrence, which is relatively common. One-third to one-half of patients with ICSC experience relapses, 50% of these during the first year. About 10% have a third episode, and the prognosis for full visual recovery decreases with each episode. When recurrent, more than 60% occur within 500 μ and 80% within 1,000 μ of the original leakage point. A majority of episodes spontaneously recover, usually within 4–8 weeks.

CLINICAL PRESENTATION

- Blurred vision
- Metamorphopsia (micropsia)
- Dyschromatopsia
- Positive central scotoma or dark spot
- Absent foveal reflex
- Transparent blister-like lesion in the macula with well-defined borders
- RPE changes (check fellow eye)

Alteration of central visual function is characterized by blur, dysmorphopsia, especially micropsia, and dyschromatopsia, particularly in the blue-yellow range. A positive central scotoma is sometimes reported, and the patient may notice a dark, cloudy, or dim area in the central field; there is a prolonged retinal recovery time after exposure to bright light. There is often a hyperopic shift in refraction, with a reported improvement in visual acuity with the addition of plus lenses. Although visual acuity may range from 20/30–20/200, the average effect is usually minimal, often in the 20/30–20/40 range.

The ophthalmoscopic features of ICSC demonstrate a neurosensory elevation of the retina. The foveal reflex is absent, and a well-defined elevated area, usually darker than the surrounding retina, is observed in the macula. This transparent round or oval blister has well-defined borders, and an annular reflex may be seen delineating the extent of the elevation (Figure 17.1). The elevation can exceed 2–3 DD in area and is observed as an increased distance separating the neurosensory retina from the underlying RPE with the slit beam during fundus biomicroscopy. The detached area of the retina maintains its normal thickness, and the posterior surface

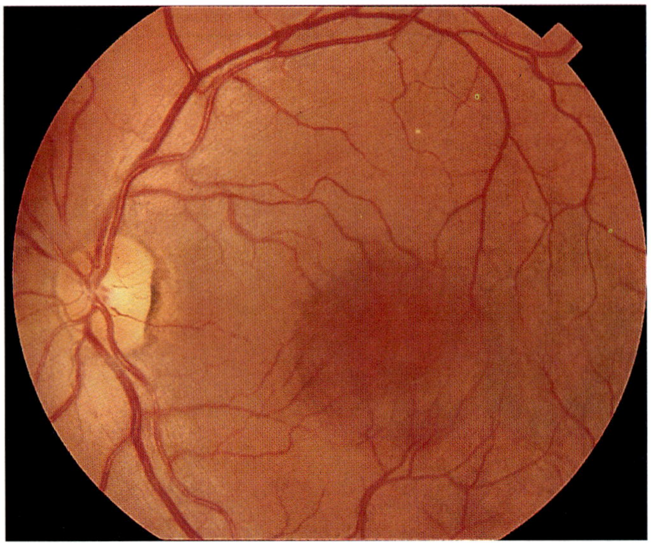

FIGURE 17.1. Active idiopathic central serous chorioretinopathy in the left eye of a 36-year-old man shows a blister-like elevation of the neurosensory retina darker than the surrounding retina. The foveal reflex is absent, and there is a mild disturbance of the retinal pigment epithelium. (Courtesy of AR Bell, CRA.) (Reprinted with permission from AA Cavallerano. Idiopathic central serous choroidopathy. Clin Eye Vis Care 1993;5:78–81.)

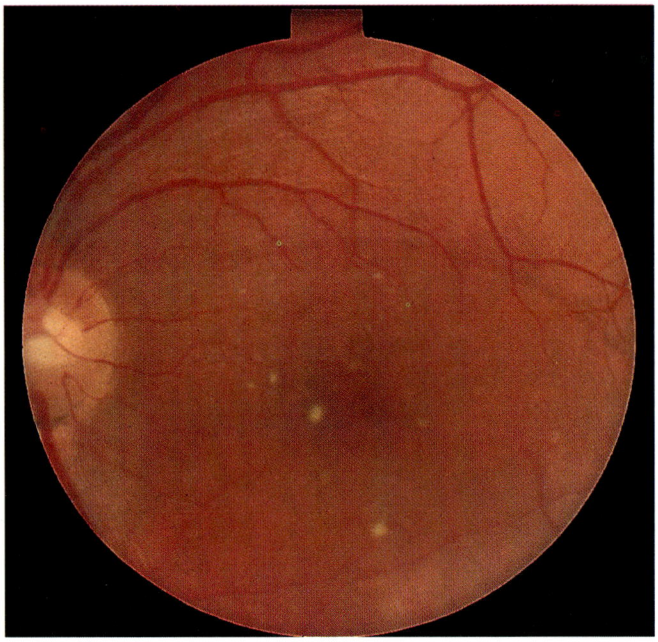

FIGURE 17.2. A patient with recurrent idiopathic central serous choroidopathy with yellow-white deposits in the deeper layers of the retina. This appearance may indicate chronic recurrence, and the deposits are probably comprised of fibrin. (Reprinted with permission from AA Cavallerano. Idiopathic central serous choroidopathy. Clin Eye Vis Care 1993;5:78–81.)

of the retina may contain yellow precipitates or a gray-white subretinal deposit, thought to be fibrin. A yellow spot in the center of the fovea is observed in chronic or recurrent cases and is thought to represent either exudative material or increased visibility of xanthophyll (Figure 17.2).

The expanse of the elevated area is limited by the tight junctions of the rods outside the macular area, which prevent the spread to the equatorial or peripheral retina. One-third of the leakage points in ICSC lie in the papillomacular bundle, and their incidence in the superior raphe is almost twice as great as in the inferior raphe. Most leaks appear to occur in the upper nasal quadrant of the foveal area.

An RPE disturbance often remains after the neurosensory retina flattens, which accounts for the residual RPE mottling, and depigmentation is suggestive of previous episodes. Visual function may return completely; however, a subjective difference in visual acuity is often noted by the patient.

Fluorescein angiography (FA) findings are characteristic of tiny points of leakage during the early phase. Subsequent phases of the transit reveal increased flow due to the attraction of the choroidal fluid. Diffusion of the dye reaches the borders of the blister after 20–30 minutes, and the fluorescein remains confined to the blister. Although fluorescein staining occurs within the blister, it never stains the borders of the elevated area. The dye ascends in what has been described as a "smokestack pattern" and expands laterally after reaching the upper limit of the blister to form a "mushroom-cap" or "umbrella-like" expression (Figures 17.3 and 17.4). This characteristic appearance during the angiogram occurs in up to 20% of the cases. Osmotic pressure due to different concentrations of protein in the blister versus that of the fluid entering the blister is responsible for this phenomenon. Angiographic findings may revert to normal following resolution.

The pathophysiology of ICSC relates to the disturbance of the RPE. The RPE serves as a barrier between the neurosensory retina and the circulating extravascular fluid in the choroid. Impairment of even a discrete number of RPE cells (even just one cell) can result in the movement of fluid in a choroidal to retinal direction. The breakdown of RPE cells and function may result from immunologic or circulatory disturbances or from neuronal or infectious causes. The breakdown results in a movement of fluid across the RPE into the neurosensory retina, forming a blister-like lesion. The borders of the blister are well defined, and fluid does not continue to increase the size of the blister despite continued flow.

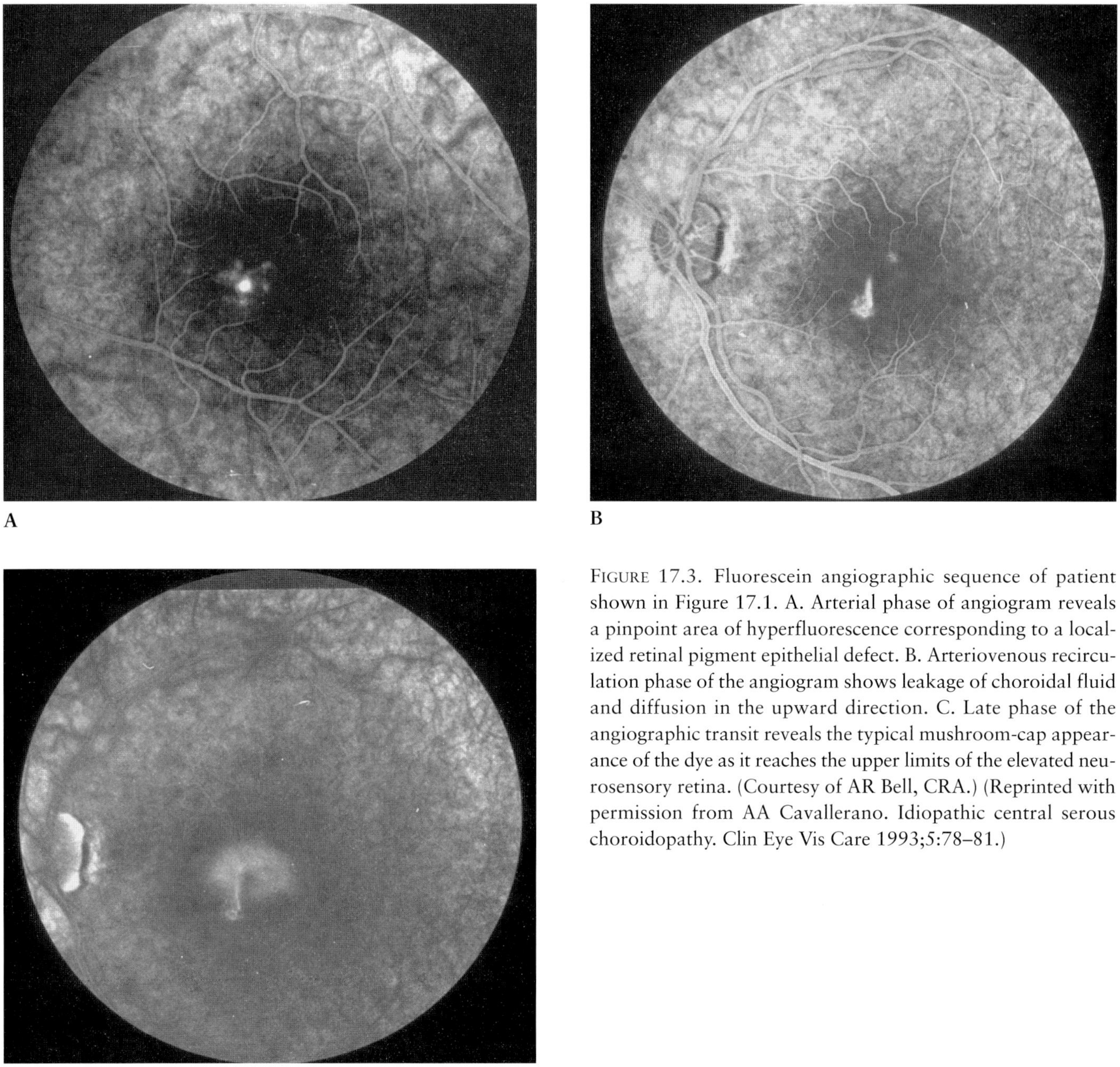

A B C

FIGURE 17.3. Fluorescein angiographic sequence of patient shown in Figure 17.1. A. Arterial phase of angiogram reveals a pinpoint area of hyperfluorescence corresponding to a localized retinal pigment epithelial defect. B. Arteriovenous recirculation phase of the angiogram shows leakage of choroidal fluid and diffusion in the upward direction. C. Late phase of the angiographic transit reveals the typical mushroom-cap appearance of the dye as it reaches the upper limits of the elevated neurosensory retina. (Courtesy of AR Bell, CRA.) (Reprinted with permission from AA Cavallerano. Idiopathic central serous choroidopathy. Clin Eye Vis Care 1993;5:78–81.)

The mechanism for removal of fluid is poorly understood, but fluorescein studies demonstrate that there is no flow through intercellular spaces. If this occurred, fluorescein would be visible in the vitreous and anterior chamber, and this is clearly not the case. Rather, the liquid remains confined within the blister and is transported back to the choroid by the intact RPE cells adjacent to the leak. There is a demonstrable increase in activity of these adjacent RPE cells. It is possible that this phenomenon damages the adjacent cells, thus accounting for the altered appearance of the macula after recovery. The scar that remains is always larger than the original leakage point. The site of the leakage may be beyond or within the extent of the foveal border, and a 1-mm ring is frequently observed around the fovea. Leakage almost always extends into the foveal area due to the paucity of rods, which are responsible for strong adherence. Leakage not impinging onto the fovea may not cause any visual disturbance.

ICSC has been classified based on the layer of retinal separation (Figure 17.5). Type I accounts for 94% of ICSC and refers to a condition in which there is clear fluid under the neurosensory retina. Type II occurs when the RPE is detached and is seen in about 3% of cases. In

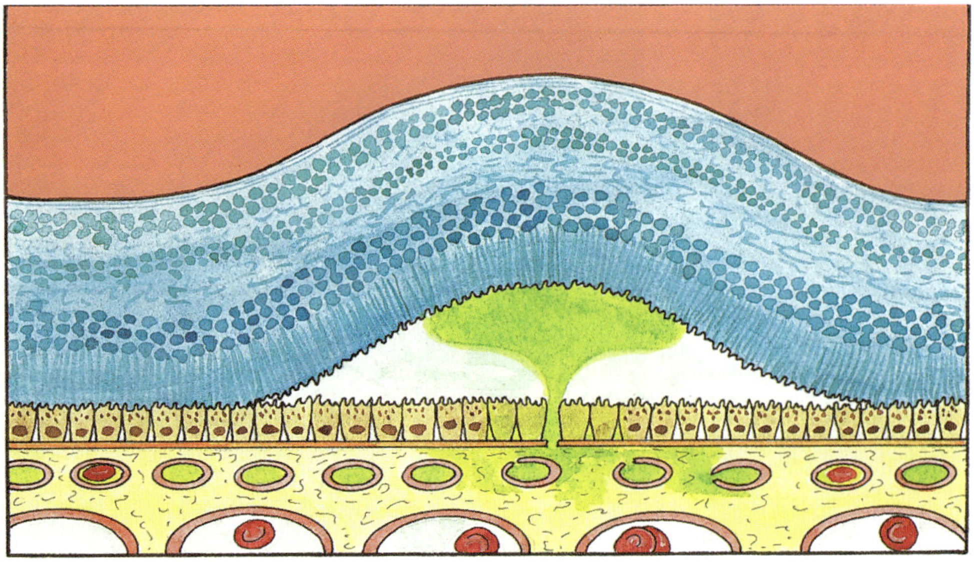

FIGURE 17.4. Demonstration of the mechanism of the mushroom-cap formation of hyperfluorescence. Fluorescein dye leaks through a retinal pigment epithelial defect and diffuses in the subretinal area until it reaches the elevated neurosensory retina. The more viscous nature of the choroidal fluid is responsible for this pattern of diffusion and distribution in the space.

a small percentage of cases, both the RPE and the neurosensory retina are detached. Referred to as the intermediate type, this is the least common of the three classifications.

DIFFERENTIAL DIAGNOSIS

- Presumed ocular histoplasmosis syndrome
- Age-related macular degeneration with pigment epithelial detachment (over age 50)
- Optic pit with serous retinal detachment
- Angioid streaks
- Idiopathic choroidal neovascular membrane
- Choroidal melanoma
- Choroidal metastasis (older patients)
- Posterior scleritis
- Harada's disease
- Choroidal hemangioma

The differential diagnosis for ICSC includes any retinal or macular condition resulting in neurosensory retinal detachment. Inflammatory and neoplastic disease must be excluded, and when doubtful, FA will confirm the diagnosis. Because ICSC occurs more often in those under age 50, exudative maculopathy in patients over age 50 may indicate age-related macular degeneration.

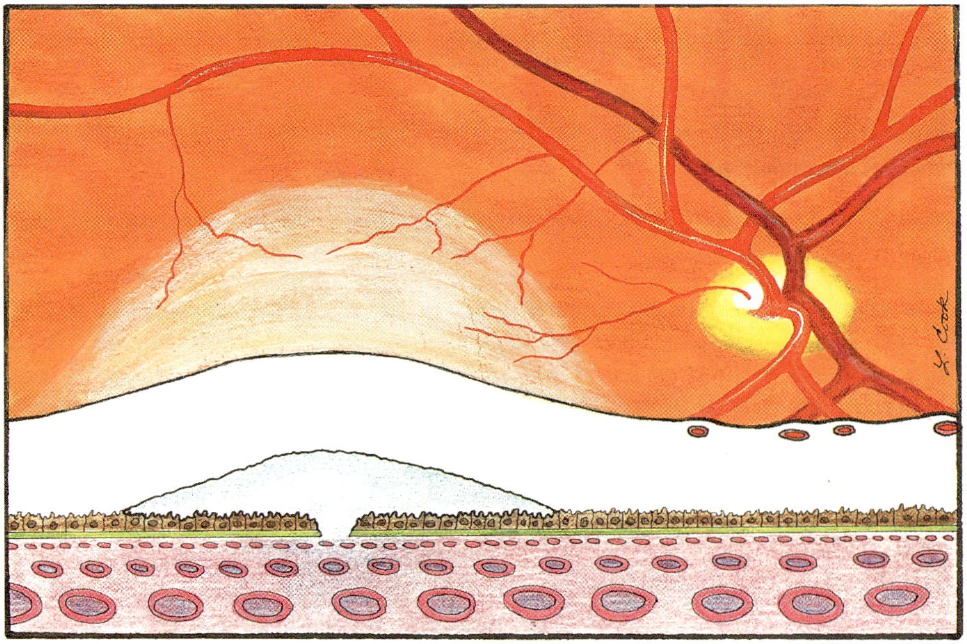

A

FIGURE 17.5. A. Illustration depicting type I idiopathic central serous chorioretinopathy with an elevation of the neurosensory retina due to a defect in the retinal pigment epithelium. *(continued)*

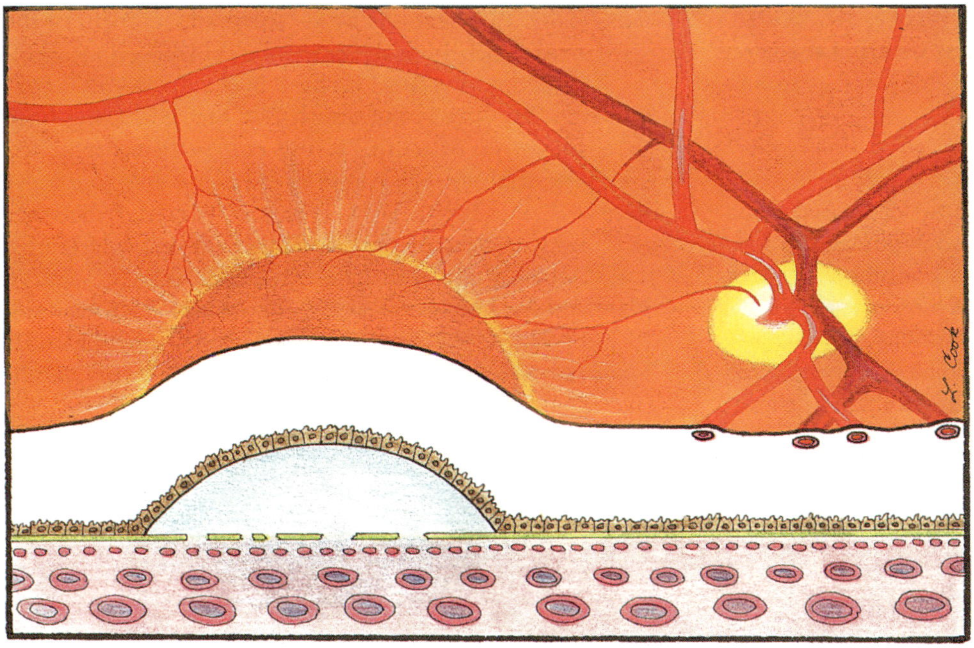

B

FIGURE 17.5. *(continued)* B. Illustration of type II idiopathic central serous chorioretinopathy showing a retinal pigment epithelial detachment with a defective Bruch's membrane. Note that the retinal pigment epithelium may remain intact in this form of detachment. C. Intermediate type of idiopathic central serous chorioretinopathy depicting a separation of the retinal pigment epithelium and concomitant detachment of the neurosensory retina. This type occurs when there is a defect in Bruch's membrane as well as the retinal pigment epithelial cells. (Reprinted with permission from AA Cavallerano. Idiopathic central serous choroidopathy. Clin Eye Vis Care 1993;5:78–81.)

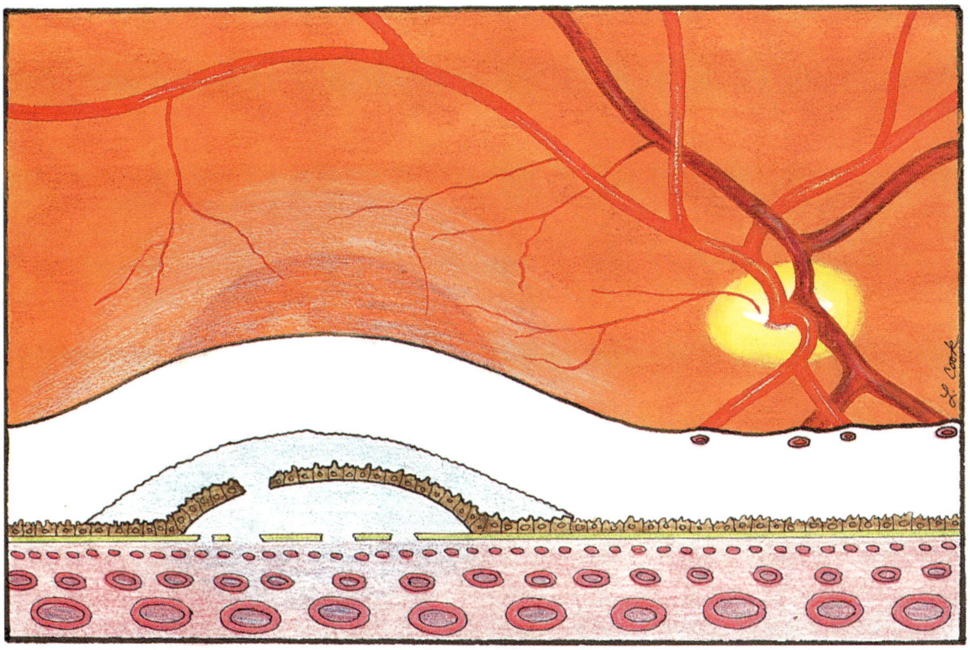

C

In these cases, the clinician should be alert for choroidal neovascular membrane.

MANAGEMENT

- FA in long-standing cases
- Laser surgery during acute phase or in recurrent situations for select cases
- Self-assessment with the home Amsler grid test

Treatment of ICSC is often conservative, and spontaneous recovery of good visual function is usually the rule. Patient education and self-assessment with the home Amsler grid test to monitor for recurrence and exacerbation are important components to patient management. Systemic corticosteroids have not proven to be effective. Photocoagulation has been employed to seal specific sites of leakage but should not represent the first line of treatment. Laser treatment is of benefit in recurrent cases of

ICSC since it seems to decrease the rate of recurrence and the duration of the episode, especially during the acute phase. FA helps to determine the suitability for treatment.

SUMMARY

ICSC is a relatively common cause for decreased visual function due to maculopathy in the adult population from 21–55 years of age. The distinctive symptoms of metamorphopsia, blur, and positive central scotoma should alert the clinician and the patient to the possibility of recurrence. Although the prognosis for visual recovery is usually very good, even without treatment, the patient should be monitored regularly and advised to look for the characteristic symptoms with home Amsler grid testing.

SUGGESTED READING

Bennet G. Central serous retinopathy. Br J Ophthalmol 1955;39:605–618.

Gass JDM. Pathogenesis of disciform detachment of the neuroepithelium I: General concepts and classification. Am J Ophthalmol 1967;63:573–585.

Gass JDM. Pathogenesis of disciform detachment of the neuroepithelium II: Idiopathic central serous chorioretinopathy. Am J Ophthalmol 1967;63:587–561.

Gilbert CM, Owens SL, Smith PD, Fine SL. Long-term follow-up of central serous chorioretinopathy Br J Ophthalmol 1984;68:815–820.

Klein ML, von Buskirk EM, Friedman E, et al. Experience with nontreatment of central serous choroidopathy. Arch Ophthalmol 1974;91:247–250.

Nanijiani M. Long-term follow-up of central serous retinopathy. Trans Ophthalmol Soc UK 1977;97:656–661.

Spitznas M. Central serous chorioretinopathy. Ophthalmology 1980;87:88–93.

Spitznas M. Pathogenesis of central serous chorioretinopathy: A new working hypothesis. Graefes Arch Clin Exp Ophthalmol 1986;224:321–324.

Spitznas M, Huke J. Number, shape and topography of leakage points in acute type I central serous retinopathy. Graefes Arch Clin Exp Ophthalmol 1987;225:437–440.

CHAPTER

18

Epiretinal Membranes

Anthony A. Cavallerano and
Rodney K. Gutner

Epiretinal membranes (ERMs) are an idiopathic age-related maculopathy or disorder that sometimes occurs secondary to ocular disease states. A cellophane-like membrane over the macula develops after glial cells communicate with the inner surface of the retina and proliferate, resulting in fibrocellular material. The disorder has been alternately referred to as preretinal fibrosis, retroretinal membrane, premacular gliosis, macular pucker, surface wrinkling maculopathy, and cellophane maculopathy. Classically, the designations have been based on the ophthalmoscopic appearance and are called *idiopathic ERM* when not associated with other ocular disease states.

Idiopathic ERMs have a direct association with posterior vitreous detachment and generally affect patients 50 years of age or older, although the condition has been observed in younger patients. When observed in children and younger patients, the membranes are usually nonprogressive and have a predilection for extending from the macula to major retinal vessels. ERMs are observed in 2% of patients at age 50 and in up to 20% by age 75; they are observed in 3.5–5.5% of autopsied eyes, and of this group, 2% are idiopathic. They are bilateral in 20–30% of cases, but marked asymmetry is often the rule.

ERMs arise from a proliferation of glial cells on the inner surface of the retina. The mechanism for the ERM formation purportedly relates to astrocytes that migrate through dehiscences in the internal limiting membrane of the retina. In addition to astrocytes, the membranes are most likely composed of fibrocytes, halocytes, retinal pigment epithelial cells, and macrophages. Pigmented and nonpigmented retinal pigment epithelial cells may be found attached to ERM. Formation of the membrane is predicated on one or more stimuli, but the exact mechanism is unknown. Posterior vitreous detachment (PVD) seems to play an important role in the pathogenesis of ERM, and 80–96% of cases are found in patients with PVD. A collagen scaffold affords communication of the vitreal surface and the inner retinal surface, and contraction of cells leads to a wrinkling of the internal limiting membrane of the retina. This contraction may be spontaneous and may lead to the mechanical dragging of the fovea.

CLINICAL PRESENTATION

- Mild to moderate to severe loss of central vision
- Diplopia, photopsia, and macropsia
- PVD
- Shimmering, irregular light reflex
- Wrinkling of internal limiting membrane
- Tortuosity of perifoveal net
- Angiographic evidence of perifoveal vessel leakage
- Ectopic fovea

The clinical findings of ERM are distinctive but vary depending on the severity and extent of the membrane. Many patients with idiopathic ERM report no symptoms or may notice mild blurring or distortion. A central photopsia is often noticed, indicating traction on the macular area, and patients may report a shimmering effect to their vision. Rarely is visual acuity worse than 20/70 with the idiopathic variety of ERM. However, if ERM progresses to severe pucker with distortion of the macula, central visual function will be affected.

If ERM is present, a translucent, cellophane-like membrane is observed in the macular area with careful fundus biomicroscopic examination (Figures 18.1 and 18.2). Wrinkling of the internal limiting membrane may be seen with membrane contraction (Figure 18.3). Sometimes the membrane is ectopic and may drag the

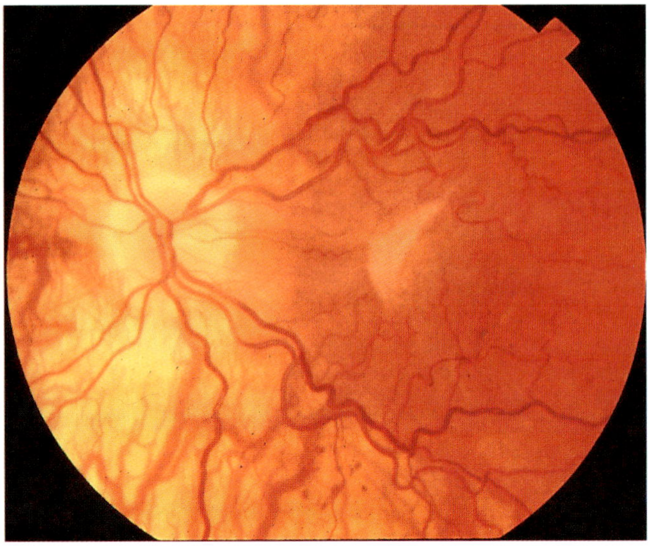

FIGURE 18.1. An epiretinal membrane in the left eye of a 14-year-old patient who underwent scleral buckling surgery for traumatic retinal detachment. (Reprinted with permission from AA Cavallerano, RK Gutner. Epiretinal membrane. Clin Eye Vis Care 1993;5:164–167.)

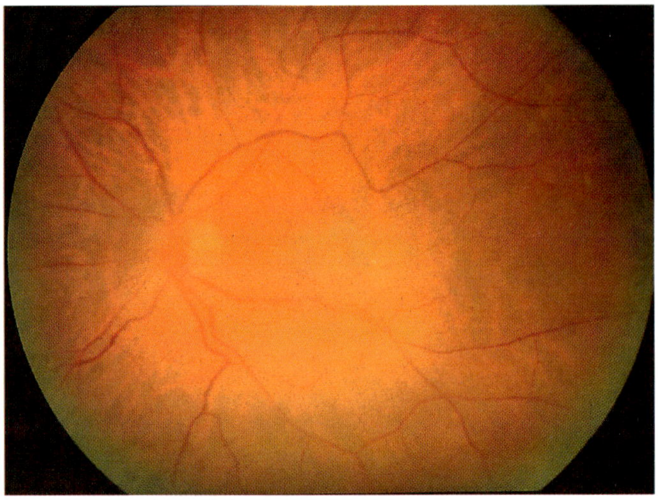

FIGURE 18.2. An epiretinal membrane in the left eye of a patient with vascular occlusive disease. Collateral vessels may be seen on the nasal aspect of the optic disc. (Reprinted with permission from AA Cavallerano, RK Gutner. Epiretinal membrane. Clin Eye Vis Care 1993;5:164–167.)

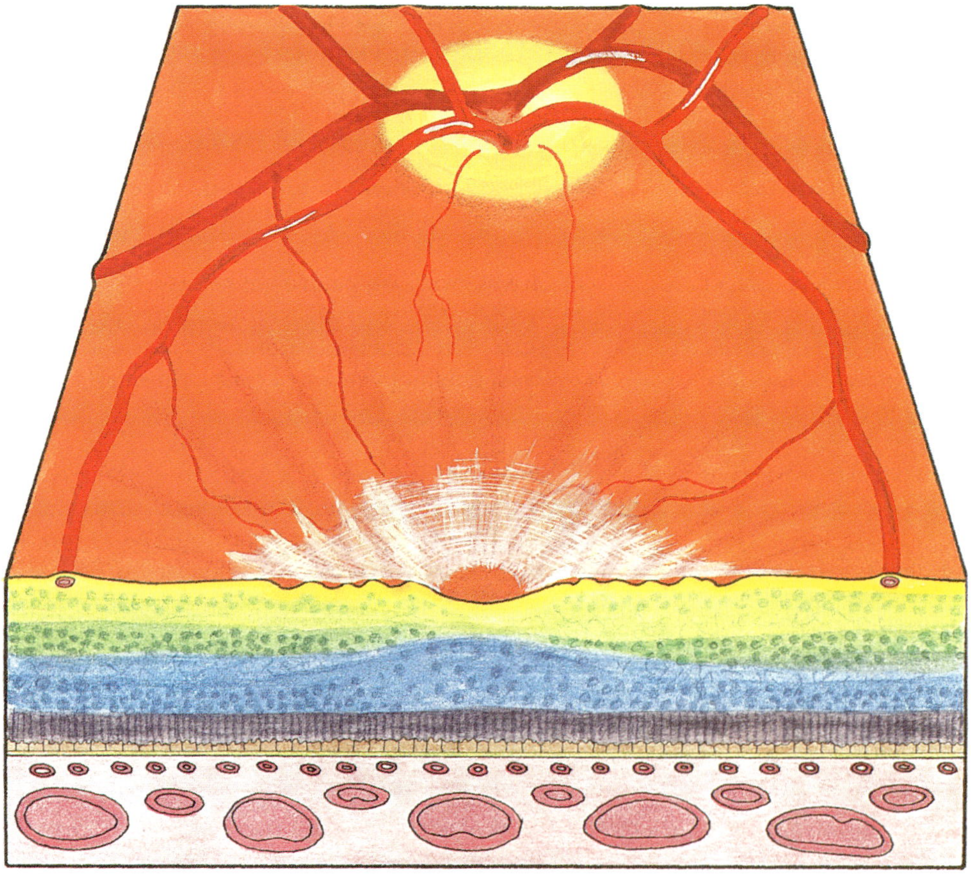

FIGURE 18.3. An illustration demonstrating the vitreomacular interaction at the level of the internal limiting membrane. Wrinkling of the membrane and macular pucker are also depicted. (Reprinted with permission from AA Cavallerano, RK Gutner. Epiretinal membrane. Clin Eye Vis Care 1993;5:164–167.)

macula, with an adverse effect on central vision. Tortuosity of the finer retinal vessels may be observed on one side of the membrane, with straightening of the vessels on the opposing side of the membrane (Figure 18.4). As the membrane progresses, punctate hemorrhages may be observed when the membrane becomes significant. When associated with retinal vascular disease, cotton wool spots are observed, especially along the membrane edge. The membrane is often dense and opaque when observed following retinal detachment. Posterior vitreous detachment is present in almost all patients with ERM and may occur in association with the membrane or as an independent event. Eyes with significant vitreal traction have a greater tendency for cystoid macular edema (CME).

Fluorescein angiographic findings in ERM are often obscure but are helpful in confirming the diagnosis and determining the etiology of the membrane. Retinal vascular tortuosity is apparent by observing the distortion of the perifoveal net. The extent of the membrane may be determined by the corresponding area of retinal vascular leakage and macular edema, producing areas of hyperfluorescence. The angiography also helps to confirm the presence of diffuse edema or CME.

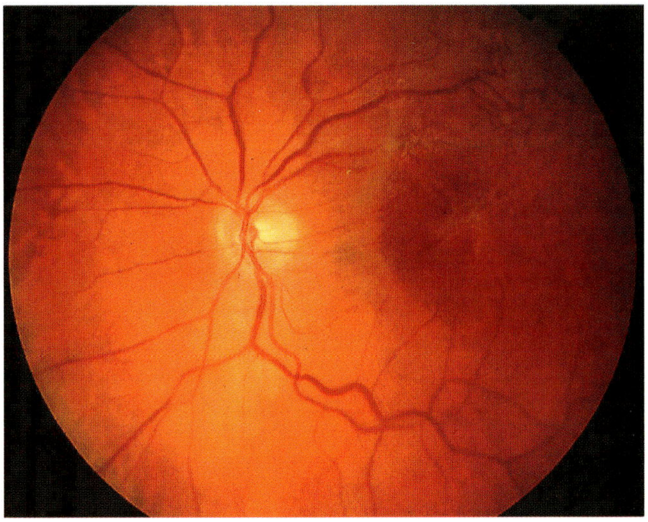

FIGURE 18.4. A dense, ectopic epiretinal membrane with dragging of the retinal vessels between the optic disc and the macula. Tortuosity of the finer retinal vessels in the superior and temporal aspect of the macula may be seen. (Reprinted with permission from AA Cavallerano, RK Gutner. Epiretinal membrane. Clin Eye Vis Care 1993;5:164–167.)

DIFFERENTIAL DIAGNOSIS

- Early proliferative vitreoretinopathy
- Macular pucker
- Macular hole
- Trauma
- Retinal vascular occlusive disease
- Sickle cell hemoglobinopathy
- Intraocular tumors
- Hamartomas
- Retinal angiomas, telangiectasis
- Retinitis pigmentosa

ERM and surface wrinkling of the macula can occur following any form of intraocular surgery; extracapsular cataract surgery is the most common surgical cause. Membranes have also been reported as a potential complication of trabeculectomy, and significant ERMs are prevalent following retinal detachment surgery. Macular pucker is reported in 3.0–8.5% of eyes following surgery for rhegmatogenous retinal detachment. These membranes tend to be denser and more opaque than idiopathic ERMs. Certain subgroups of patients are considered to be at high risk following scleral buckling for retinal detachment: those with rolled retinal edges, equatorial ridges, or star-pattern folds in the detached portion of the retina.

ERM may occur with retinal vascular occlusive disease, with vitreous hemorrhage, in diabetic and hypertensive retinopathy, in aphakic CME, and accompanying macular holes and rhegmatogenous retinal detachment. It has also been reported with sickle cell hemoglobinopathy, intraocular tumors, and hamartomas. Ocular trauma is the most common nonsurgical cause of ERM, and the mechanism is thought to be the development of a rent in the internal limiting membrane following PVD.

Gass has classified ERMs according to the clinical appearance and severity of retinal distortion. Cellophane maculopathy is classified as grade 0, resulting in a minimal tissue response and little or no effect on visual function. His system progresses from grade 0 to grade 2, which represents macular pucker and a marked reduction in vision (Table 18.1).

MANAGEMENT

- Home Amsler grid testing
- Treatment and elimination of underlying cause
- Membrane stripping and vitrectomy

The decision to treat ERM is predicated on the prognosis for retention of good visual function. Epiretinal membranectomy and vitrectomy are indicated when visual acuity is worse than 20/70–20/100. Patients with ERM often complain of dysmorphopisa and, in some instances, eliminating the distortion results in significant improvement from the patient's standpoint, even if the visual acuity does not improve. A postoperative visual acuity improvement has been reported in 83% of cases, with 32% having vision better than 20/40. Surgical removal of the membrane sometimes results in loss of the

TABLE 18.1. Classification of Epiretinal Membranes

Classification	*Designation*	*Features*
Grade 0	Cellophane maculopathy	Translucent membrane; cellophane light reflex ophthalmoscopically; usually no distortion of inner retinal surface
Grade 1	Crinkled cellophane maculopathy	Follows contraction of ERMs; irregular folds, irregular, iridescent light reflex; perifoveal area; PVD; acuity may be normal
Grade 2	Macular pucker	Dense grayish ERMs, retinal edema, small retinal hemorrhages, cotton wool spots, serous detachment, PVD; visual acuity often 20/200 or worse, metamorphopsia; fluorescein angiogram—leakage of dye from underlying vessels

ERMs = epiretinal membranes; PVD = posterior vitreous detachment.

internal limiting membrane of the retina and part of the nerve fiber layer due to the close approximation of the membrane to the retina. Other complications include peripheral retinal tears and detachment, endophthalmitis, and lenticular opacities. Tissue regrowth is also possible and occurs in a small number of cases. In spite of observable retinal edema in some cases of ERM, corticosteroids are not indicated.

SUMMARY

ERM is a potential cause for decreased visual function in the elderly population, especially as a postsurgical complication following intraocular procedures and in retinal detachment procedures. The idiopathic form of the disease is relatively benign, and in most instances, the patient will maintain good visual function. Those subgroups of patients with high-risk characteristics for progressive ERM should be monitored carefully. Surgery, when indicated, should be undertaken only when there is significant risk for progression and further loss of central visual function.

SUGGESTED READING

Appiah AP, Hirose T. Secondary causes of premacular fibrosis. Ophthalmology 1989;96:389–392.

Barr CC, Michels RG. Idiopathic nonvascularized epiretinal membranes in young patients: Report of six cases. Ann Ophthalmol 1982;14:335–341.

Chambers RB, Mendlovic DB, Davidorf FH. Epiretinal membranes: A clinically oriented review. Contemp Ophthal Forum 1986;4:131–136.

Clarkson JG, Green WR, Nassof D. A histological review of 168 cases of epiretinal membrane. Am J Ophthalmol 1977;84:1–17.

Detry-Morel M, Kittel B, Lemagne JM. Surface-wrinkling maculopathy as a potential complication of trabeculectomy: A case report. Ophthalmic Surg 1991;22:38–40.

Gass JDM. Stereoscopic Atlas of Macular Disease. St. Louis: Mosby, 1987;671–726.

Kampik A, Kenyon KR, Michels RG, et al. Epiretinal and vitreous membranes: A comparative study of 56 cases. Arch Ophthalmol 1981;99:1445–1454.

Kimmel AS, Weingeist TA, Blodi CF, et al. Idiopathic premacular gliosis in children and adolescents. Am J Ophthalmol 1989;108:578–581.

Lobes LA Jr, Burton TC. The incidence of macular pucker after retinal detachment surgery. Am J Ophthalmol 1978;85:72–77.

McDonald HR, Schatz H. Introduction to Epiretinal Membranes. In SJ Ryan (ed), Retina (Vol II). St. Louis: Mosby, 1989:789–795.

Michels RG. Vitrectomy for macular pucker. Ophthalmology 1984;91:1384–1388.

Noble KG, Carr RE. Idiopathic preretinal gliosis. Ophthalmology 1982;89:521–523.

Roth AM, Foos RY. Surface wrinkling retinopathy in eyes enucleated at autopsy. Trans Am Acad Ophthalmol Otolaryngol 1971;75:1047–1058.

Sidd RJ, Fine SL, Ownes SL, et al. Idiopathic preretinal gliosis. Am J Ophthalmol 1982;94:44–48.

Wiznia RA. Posterior vitreous detachment and idiopathic macular gliosis. Am J Ophthalmol 1986;102:196–198.

CHAPTER

19 Idiopathic Macular Holes

Rodney K. Gutner and
Anthony A. Cavallerano

A macular hole is a full-thickness opening in the posterior pole involving the foveola and resulting in substantial loss of central visual function. It is an affliction that predominantly affects otherwise healthy women over 60 years of age, who report a sudden and sometimes profound loss of central visual acuity, often preceded by photopsia and resulting in a central scotoma.

Macular holes are relatively rare and are most often unilateral. Long-term prospective studies have demonstrated a bilaterality of less than 10%, and the prevalence is significantly lower if there is posterior vitreous detachment in the fellow eye.

There is controversy regarding the role of the vitreous in the pathogenesis of idiopathic macular holes. There is reportedly an increased risk of hole formation when strong vitreous attachments are present at the macula. Complete posterior vitreous detachment may actually safeguard against formation of a macular hole. Macular hole formation may be attributed to tangential traction of the vitreous on the inner limiting membrane of the retina in the foveal area. Epiretinal membrane is present in 10% of patients with full-thickness macular holes, and vitreous contraction on the retinal surface may precipitate the break. This mechanism produces oval or irregularly shaped macular holes. In spite of this explanation, however, some authors suggest that idiopathic macular holes may be independent of posterior vitreous detachment.

A macular hole can form as a result of trauma, damage to a retinal cyst, or cystoid macular edema and has been reported in rhegmatogenous retinal detachment with peripheral retinal breaks. Macular holes have been reported in 0.5–1.0% of retinal detachment cases. Peripheral retinal breaks and detachment should be treated prior to directing treatment toward the macular hole. Gass divided idiopathic senile macular holes into various stages, which he thought reflected their natural history and development. The first stage is foveal detachment characterized by a loss of foveal depression and the appearance of a yellow spot or ring due to the distribution of xanthophyll. The second stage results in early hole formation with a full-thickness macular opening; vitreous separation in the macular area then leads to the third stage. Complete and obvious posterior vitreous separation along with a full-thickness macular hole constitutes stage IV of the process.

CLINICAL PRESENTATION

- Metamorphopsia
- Profound loss of central visual function
- Positive central scotoma
- Photopsia
- Floaters
- Dark round or oval red spot involving the foveola
- Gray halo surrounding full-thickness macular opening
- Slight increase in background hyperfluorescence on fluorescein angiography with full-thickness holes

Clinically, an idiopathic macular hole is often undetectable in its earliest formative stages. With progression, an approximately one-third disc diameter round hole forms in the foveola. A grayish halo, corresponding to a serous detachment, surrounds a darker, often red, area that contains an accumulation of xanthophyll, thus accounting for the yellow spot or ring. Yellow-white dots are often observed in the floor of the hole (Figures 19.1 through 19.3). Firm attachment of the vitreous to the macular area often precedes the development of a macular hole. This quickly gives rise to complete vitreous

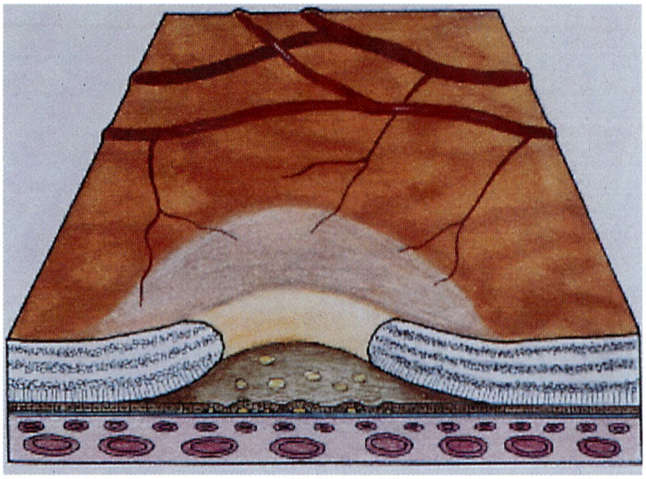

FIGURE 19.1. Illustration of full-thickness macular hole demonstrating grayish, elevated halo corresponding to localized serous detachment, retinal pigment epithelial changes, and yellow deposits on the bottom of the hole. (Reprinted with permission from RK Gutner, AA Cavallerano. Idiopathic macular holes. Clin Eye Vis Care 1993;5:82–85.)

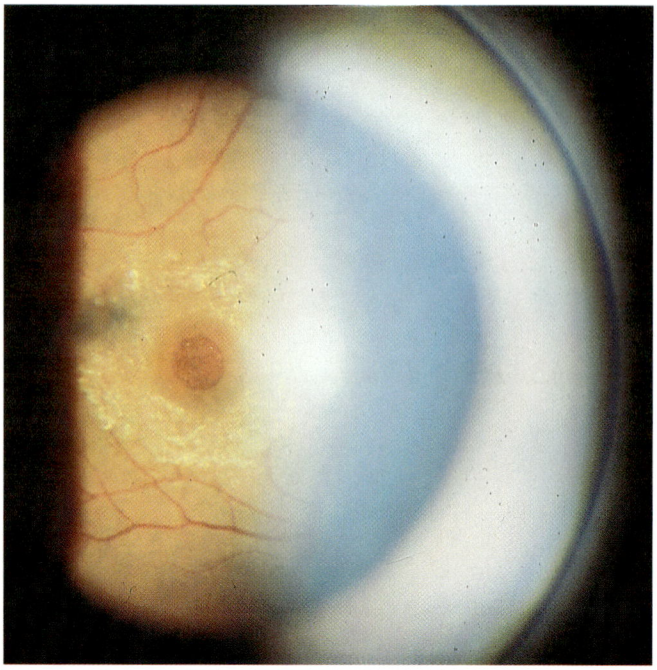

FIGURE 19.2. Clinical photograph through a universal fundus contact lens depicting a full-thickness macular hole with all of the characteristics described in Figure 19.1. Vitreoretinal traction and epiretinal membrane formation are apparent in the adjacent area surrounding the hole. (Reprinted with permission from RK Gutner, AA Cavallerano. Idiopathic macular holes. Clin Eye Vis Care 1993;5:82–85.)

detachment, and an operculum may be seen attached to the posterior hyaloid membrane of the vitreous. This may best be seen by a kinetic examination of the vitreous using fundus biomicroscopy. A biomicroscopic technique is available for better visualization of macular holes using a narrow laser beam that can be focused more precisely.

Unilateral decreased vision and metamorphopsia are reported by most patients. Occasionally, vitreomacular traction may result in entoptic symptoms, including photopsia and the sudden onset of new floaters. A positive central scotoma is detected on the Amsler grid test or macular studies using automated perimetry.

DIFFERENTIAL DIAGNOSIS

- Lamellar macular hole
- Macular cyst
- Solar macular burn
- Pseudohole

Macular holes, full thickness or lamellar, should be differentiated from macular cysts and solar burns. Visual acuity is almost always worse than 20/70 in full-thickness holes. Macular cysts and lamellar holes yield a central visual acuity of better than 20/70 in most cases, with noticeably less dysmorphopsia on Amsler grid testing (Figure 19.4). Patients with solar maculopathy may retain full or near normal visual function (Figure 19.5).

Red-free photographs are useful in identifying full-thickness macular breaks. Fluorescein angiography is

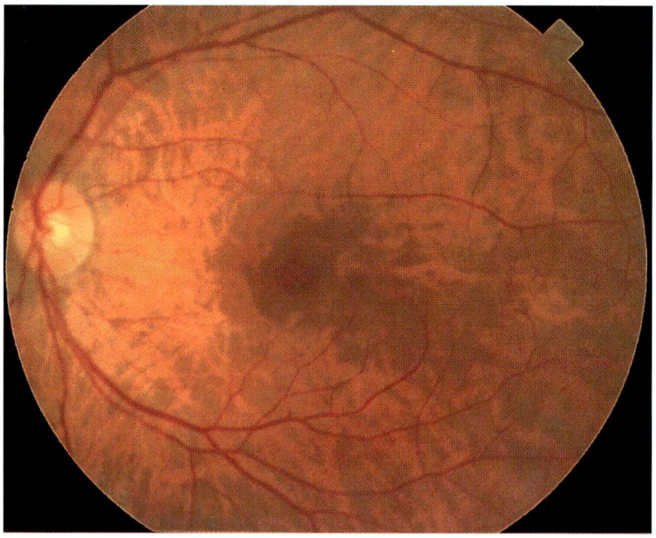

FIGURE 19.3. Macular hole with surrounding gray halo. (Reprinted with permission from RK Gutner, AA Cavallerano. Idiopathic macular holes. Clin Eye Vis Care 1993;5:82–85.)

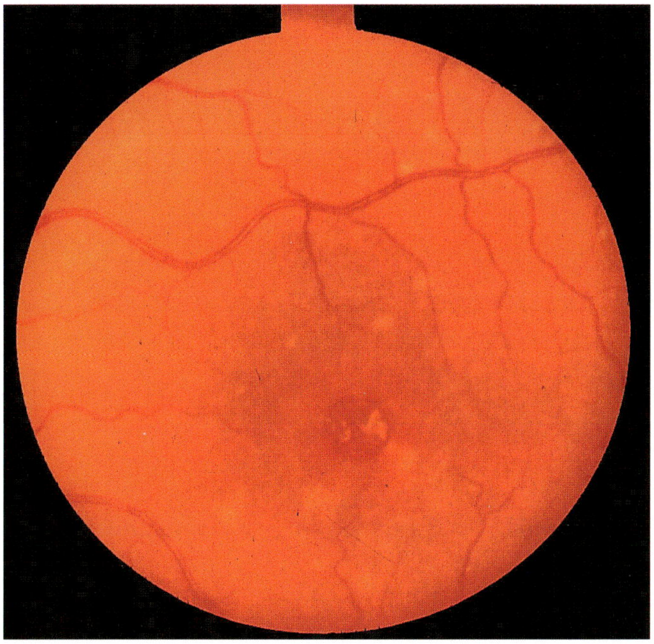

FIGURE 19.4. Partial thickness macular hole with accompanying finding of multiple drusen bodies. (Reprinted with permission from RK Gutner, AA Cavallerano. Idiopathic macular holes. Clin Eye Vis Care 1993;5:82–85.)

indicated when a macular hole is detected to rule out additional causes, including chronic cystoid macular edema (Figure 19.6). Angiographic findings reveal a modest increase in the background fluorescence in a full-thickness macular hole. This is likely due to dissemination of xanthophyll and the possible breakup of retinal pigment epithelium. In a lamellar hole, the xanthophyllic complexion remains intact, yielding a normal fluorescein appearance.

MANAGEMENT

- Home Amsler grid testing
- Laser photocoagulation
- Modified vitrectomy, including membrane peel
- Transforming growth factor β_2
- Low vision devices

Treatment of macular holes is often futile unless undertaken at the appropriate time. Treatment consists of two basic modalities: laser or vitreous surgery. Early intervention by photocoagulating the rim of the hole using the argon green or blue-green wavelength may prevent progression to a full-thickness hole and subsequent sealing of the opening. This technique has met with only limited success, however. Vitreous surgery, employing a modified vitrectomy technique, is a delicate procedure that relieves the vitreous traction in impending macular hole formation. Management must also include frequent home Amsler grid testing and routine surveillance. Low vision devices are helpful for those patients suffering severe bilateral visual loss due to full-thickness macular holes or additional causes. The most recent treatment modality, although controversial, is the local application of transforming growth factor β_2, which is injected directly into the retinal pigment epithelial cells with a syringe during macular surgery.

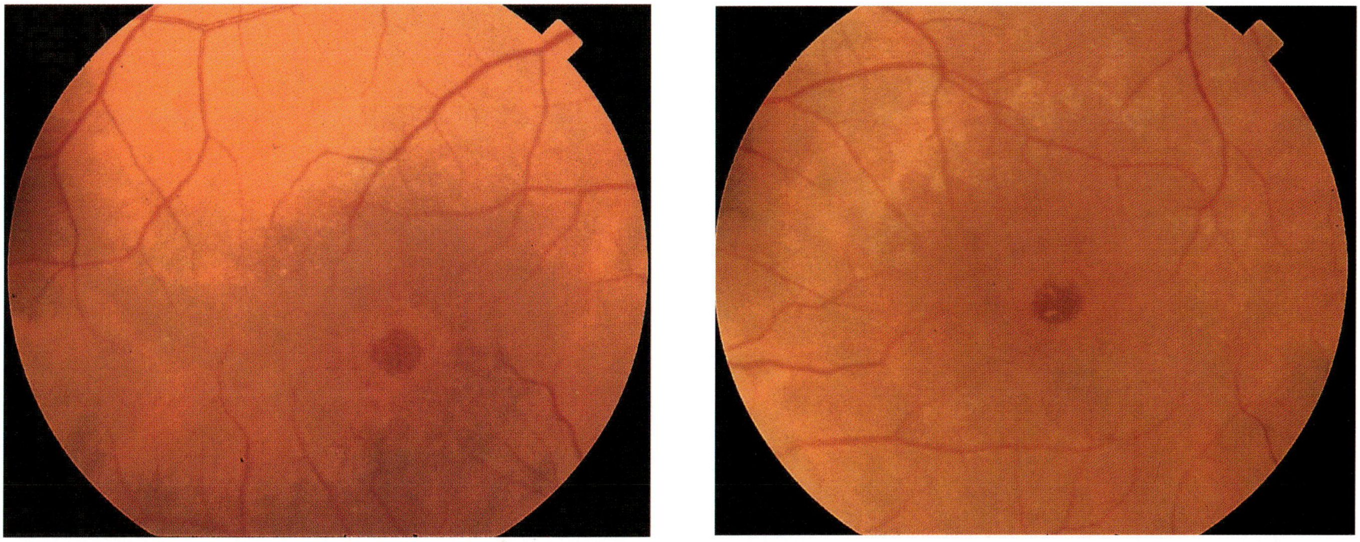

FIGURE 19.5. An example of bilateral solar maculopathy, a symmetrical finding, resulting from sungazing. Visual acuity was 20/25 in right and left eyes. (Reprinted with permission from RK Gutner, AA Cavallerano. Idiopathic macular holes. Clin Eye Vis Care 1993;5:82–85.)

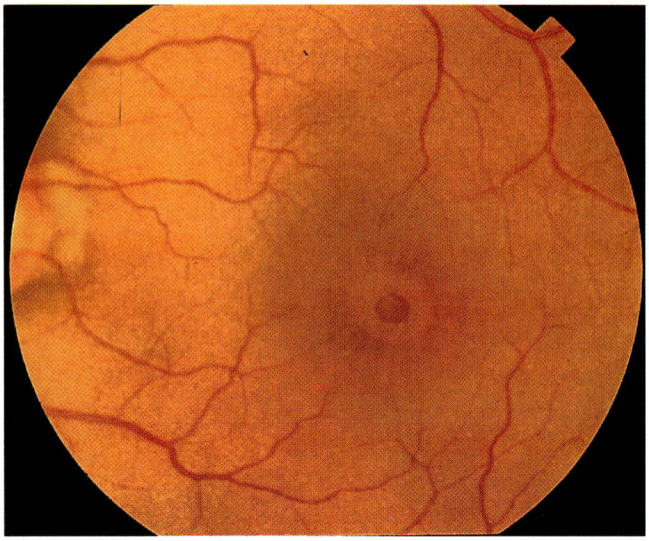
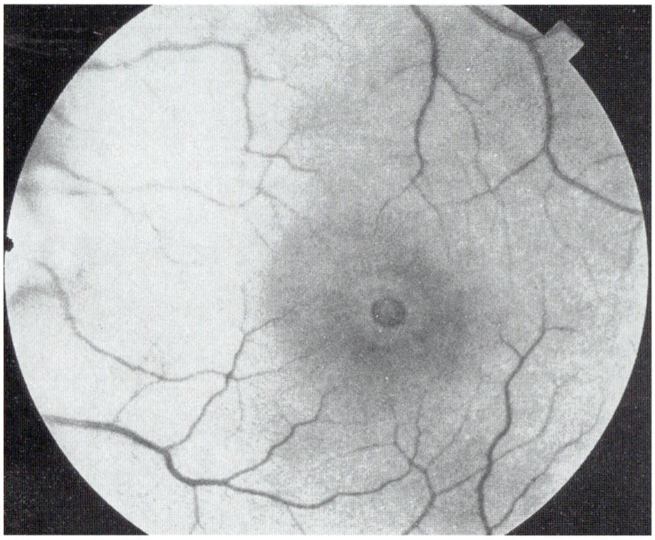

A B

FIGURE 19.6. A. A full-thickness macular hole in a 62-year-old woman. Visual acuity was 20/200 on initial presentation. B. Preinjection phase of fluorescein angiogram (left) and arteriovenous phase showing focal area of hyperfluorescence (right).

SUMMARY

Macular holes can cause devastating effects on central visual function. Full-thickness macular holes result in permanent damage to the foveal area. Firm vitreous adhesion and traction to the retina in the macular area, along with the appearance of a yellow ring, are high risk features for progression to a full-thickness macular hole, especially if the visual acuity is less than 20/50 and there is already a hole in the fellow eye. Patients with impending macular holes or holes in evolution should be evaluated for possible or suitable laser treatment or vitreous surgery.

SUGGESTED READING

Akiba J, Quiroz MA, Trempe CL. Role of posterior vitreous detachment in idiopathic macular holes. Ophthalmology 1990;97:1610–1613.

Bielinski MR, Muchnick BG. Transforming growth factor-beta: A treatment for macular holes. Clin Vis Eye Care 1993;5:26–28.

Chambers RB, Davidorf FH, Gresak P, et al. Modified vitrectomy for impending macular holes. Ophthalmic Surg 1991;22:730–734.

Gass JDM. Idiopathic senile macular holes: Its early stages and pathogenesis. Arch Ophthalmol 1988;106:629–639.

Glaser BM, Michels RG, Kuppermann BD, et al. Transforming growth factor-β_2 for the treatment of full-thickness macular holes: A prospective randomized study. Ophthalmology 1992;99:1162–1173.

Gutner RK, Cavallerano AA. Idiopathic macular holes. Clin Eye Vis Care 1993;5:82–85.

Howard GM, Campbell CJ. Surgical repair of retinal detachments caused by macular holes. Arch Ophthalmol 1969;81:317–320.

Kelly NE, Wendel RT. Vitreous surgery for idiopathic macular holes. Arch Ophthalmol 1991;109:654–659.

Ogura Y, Shahidi M, Mori MT, et al. Improved visualization of macular hole lesions with laser biomicroscopy. Arch Ophthalmol 1991;109:957–961.

Schocket SS, Lakhanpal V, Xiaoping M, et al. Laser treatment of macular holes. Ophthalmology 1988;95:574–581.

Smiddy WE, Michels RG, Green WR. Morphology, pathology and surgery of idiopathic vitreoretinal macular disorders: A review. Retina 1990;10:288–296.

Yannuzzi L, Gitter KA, Schatz H. The Macula: A Comprehensive Text and Atlas. Baltimore: Williams & Wilkins, 1979;264–265.

PART

V

Inflammatory Disease

CHAPTER

20

Toxoplasmosis Retinochoroiditis

Anthony A. Cavallerano

Chorioretinal inflammatory disease may affect the macula by direct invasion or may reduce vision through the secondary effects of the inflammation. Vitreous infiltration or hemorrhage, macular edema, and pigment degeneration or dispersion are some of the means by which the macula becomes secondarily involved in many inflammatory states.

Toxoplasmosis is a prevalent disease affecting both humans and animals and is one of the most common causes of retinal infection. The cat is the definite host for this parasitic organism, and its feces are the vector of transmission to humans. *Toxoplasma gondii* may affect any organ of the body, and it is the most predominant opportunistic infection in the immunocompromised host, including those with acquired immunodeficiency syndrome (AIDS) (see Chapter 23). This obligate intracellular parasite invades the posterior segment of the eye, and if the organism reaches the ocular structures via the blood system, it may enter retinal cells and produce a retinitis. It can produce devastating effects on vital ocular structures and, if left untreated, represents a serious threat to visual function.

The term *toxo*, meaning arc, is used to describe the configuration of the parasite, which was first described by Laveran in 1900. *T. gondii* was first identified by Nicolle and Manceaux from the North African rodent *Ctenodactylus gondi*, and it was long suspected that toxoplasmosis produced uveitis, a fact that was proven by Wilder in 1952. In 1965, Hutchinson uncovered evidence that the organism originated in feline feces.

The mode of transmission of toxoplasmosis can include ingestion of uncooked or undercooked meat, the drinking of raw milk, ingestion of the oocyte from contaminated hands, organ transplantation, and transplacental transmission. Although toxoplasmosis is one of the most common opportunistic infections occurring in immunocompromised hosts, it can occur in immunocompetent hosts. Most forms of acquired disseminated systemic infections are subclinical; however, some infections may manifest as a flulike illness. Other clinical entities have been described, including acute febrile toxoplasmosis, lymphadenopathy, encephalitis, and retinochoroiditis. The laboratory diagnosis is made with the dye test, direct agglutination test, indirect fluorescent antibody test, the complement fixation test, or the enzyme-linked immunosorbent assay.

There is no congenital predisposition to ocular toxoplasmosis, but most of those developing the disease are born to mothers infected during pregnancy. Intraretinal cyst formation results from transplacental transmission and eventually the cyst ruptures, probably initiating the disease process. Tissue destruction probably occurs as a result of local invasion, toxic effects of the organism, hypersensitivity response, active phagocytosis and cell lysis, or autoimmune mechanisms. In addition to transmission to the eye via the blood system, a body of evidence exists to suggest that the parasite may reach the retina through the optic nerve. Evidence exists to support all of these as possible causes of the retinal damage that occurs with the disease.

CLINICAL PRESENTATION

- White, fluffy retinal lesions in an active state
- Retinal edema
- Vitreous cells
- Vitreous hemorrhage
- Pigment epithelial hypertrophy
- Retinoblastoma
- Retinal detachment
- Cystoid macular edema
- Gray-white granuloma in retina

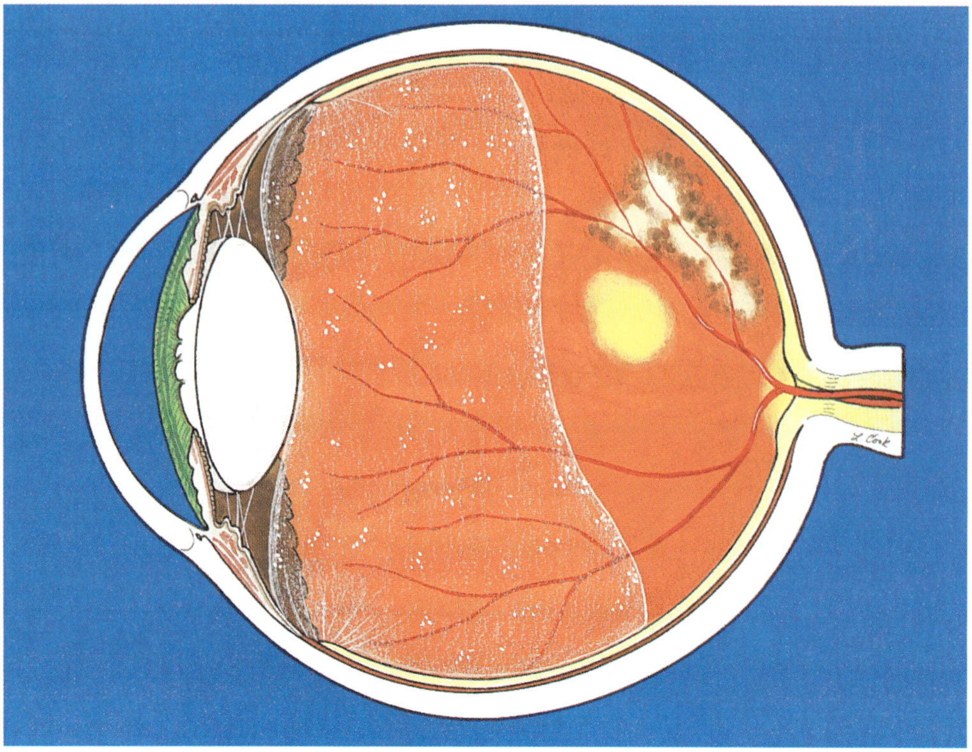

FIGURE 20.1. Illustration depicting various ocular manifestations of toxoplasmic retinochoroiditis, including an active lesion, pigment hypertrophy and inactive lesions, vitreous inflammation, and attachment of inflammatory cells to the posterior hyaloid face of the vitreous. (Reprinted with permission from AA Cavallerano. Toxoplasmosis retinochoroiditis. Clin Eye Vis Care 1990;2:213–216.)

- Punctate lesions at the level of retinal pigment epithelium
- Pigment hyperplasia
- Optic neuritis
- Anterior uveitis

Toxoplasmosis retinochoroiditis produces a focal necrotizing infection associated with white, fluffy lesions surrounded by retinal edema. Cells are seen in the vitreous and may attach to the posterior hyaloid face of the vitreous (Figure 20.1). The retina is the primary site of infection, but the choroid and sclera also may be involved. The retinal lesions are characterized by small to large single or multiple areas of gray-white granulomas (Figure 20.2). Some patients develop punctate retinal involvement at the level of the retinal pigment epithelium, and these lesions may be observed in the macular area. Other causes of multifocal chorioretinopathy must be considered in these cases. These patients do not develop a vitritis, and the lesions may resolve, leaving a granular appearance to the retinal pigment epithelium. If the macula becomes involved, an exudative retinal detachment may occur. As the lesion heals, pigment hyperplasia produces a permanent scar that may harbor the toxoplasma cysts. Lesions in the macular area are thought to be the result of free-swimming parasites, and cystoid macular edema occurs when the lesions are in close proximity to the macula. Recurrent retinochoroiditis often produces new lesions close to these scars (Figure 20.3).

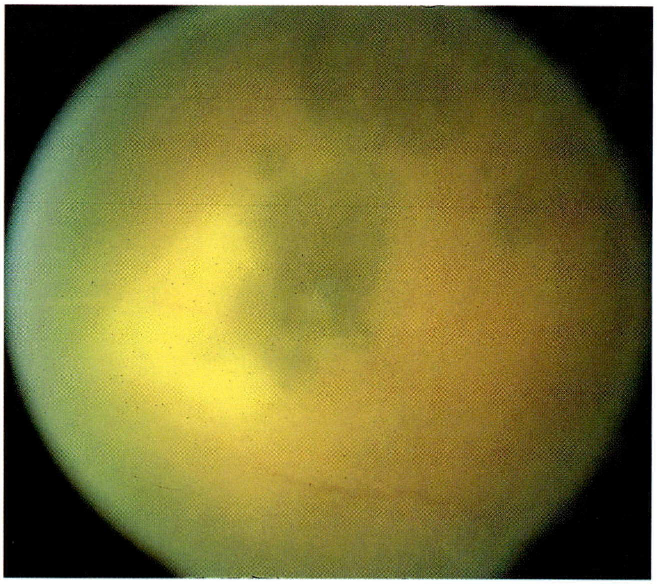

FIGURE 20.2. An active toxoplasmosis retinochoroiditis with fluffy retinal lesions, pigment hypertrophy, and a murky vitreous obscuring fundus detail.

Hypersensitivity reactions seem to play an important role in the pathogenesis of ocular toxoplasmosis. Optic neuritis may be seen with toxoplasmosis ocular infections and can occur in the absence of retinal or choroidal involvement. The obligate parasite does not invade the vitreous, but accumulations of inflammatory

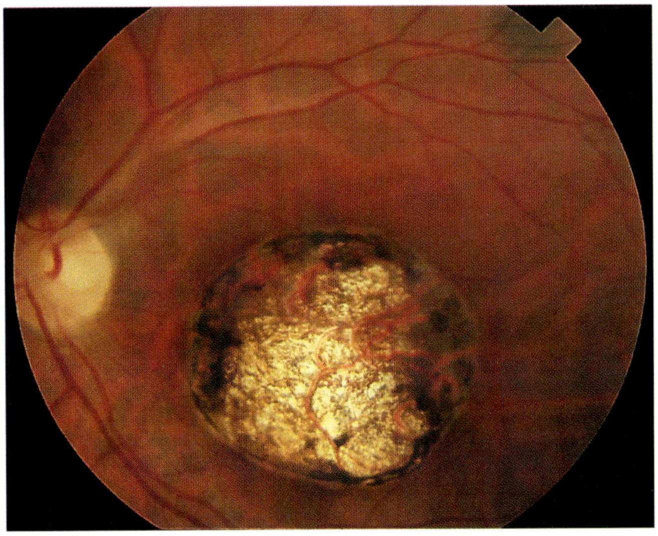

FIGURE 20.3. Inactive retinal lesion of toxoplasmosis. (Courtesy of AR Bell, CRA.)

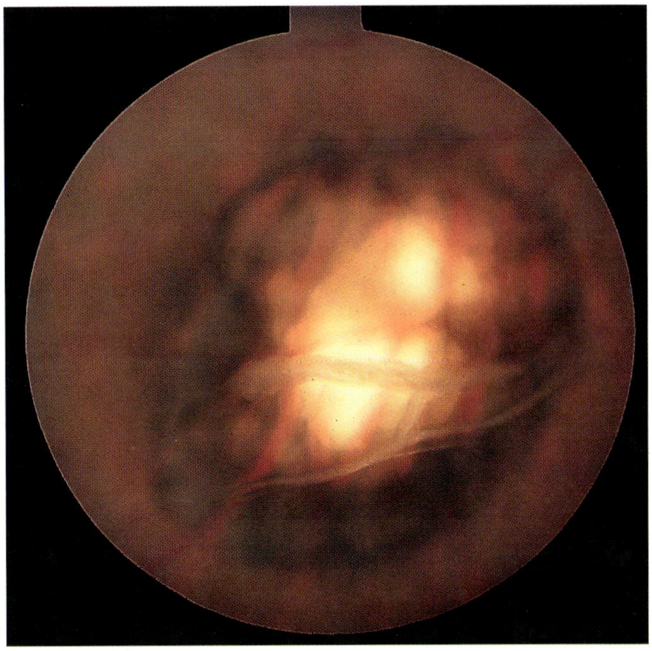

FIGURE 20.4. A large vitreous floater superimposed over an inactive retinal lesion.

cells may be found in the vitreous and on the posterior vitreous face. A vitreous hemorrhage can occur, and a sudden increase in the appearance of floaters sometimes indicates a reactivation of the retinochoroiditis (Figure 20.4). Anterior uveitis occurs, possibly as a result of a hypersensitivity reaction, and secondary glaucoma and its attendant complications may be seen with *Toxoplasma* infection. Fuch's heterochromic iridocyclitis has been described in patients with necrotizing retinochoroiditis. Subretinal neovascularization and neovascularization of the optic nerve can occur during the course of toxoplasmosis retinochoroiditis. Extraocular muscle involvement, nystagmus, and optic atrophy have all been reported as ocular manifestations of the disease.

DIFFERENTIAL DIAGNOSIS

- Viral infections with cytomegalic inclusion
- Herpes simplex retinitis
- Toxocariasis
- Acute retinal necrosis
- Rubella
- Measles
- Coats' disease
- Pigment epithelial hypertrophy
- Retinoblastoma
- Familial macular coloboma

The differential diagnosis of ocular toxoplasmosis should include the divergent disease of the posterior segment, including viral infections with cytomegalic inclusion, herpes simplex retinitis, rubella, measles, and acute retinal necrosis. Additionally, noninfectious disorders include Coats' disease, pigment epithelial hypertrophy, retinoblastoma, and familial macular coloboma. Multifocal choroidopathies, especially those with a predilection to the macular area, should also be considered.

The diagnosis of toxoplasmosis may be made by observing the typical clinical picture of necrotizing retinochoroiditis and can be confirmed by serologic testing, including the Sabin-Feldman dye test, indirect fluorescent antibody test, indirect hemagglutination test, complement fixation test, and enzyme-linked immunosorbent assay, and by detection of antigens. Once the diagnosis is confirmed, prompt treatment is indicated due to the potentially devastating effects of the disease and potential loss of visual function caused by ocular toxoplasmosis.

MANAGEMENT

- Spiramycin
- Sulfadiazine
- Sulfamethazine
- Sulfamerazine
- Pyrimethamine
- Clindamycin
- Corticosteroids
- Cryotherapy
- Photocoagulation
- Vitrectomy

There is no effective treatment against the encysted form of *T. gondii*. Trisulfapyrimidines, including sulfadiazine and sulfamethazine, pyrimethamine, spiramycin, and clindamcyin, have all been shown to be effective in the treatment of ocular toxoplasmosis in humans. Systemic corticosteroids and subtenon injection of steroids are usually added to the regimen of therapy if vision-threatening lesions are present. Their benefit lies with the effect that steroids have on the hypersensitivity component of the infectious process, but it is recommended that they should not be used without the concomitant use of at least one antitoxoplasmic agent. There is no need to treat small peripheral lesions that are not at risk of causing loss of visual function. Vitrectomy, photocoagulation, and cryotherapy have been used in the treatment of ocular toxoplasmosis.

SUMMARY

Ocular toxoplasmosis can be a destructive disease that occurs without warning and produces a necrotizing retinitis. Awareness is an important aspect of preventing this common disease affecting humans, and simple measures such as adequate cooking of meat and avoidance of sandboxes and cat litter boxes are important in prevention. Food handlers should exercise care and should wear gloves when handling food products. Early detection, definitive diagnosis, and prompt institution of treatment can prevent serious loss of vision.

SUGGESTED READING

Chowdhury MN. Toxoplasmosis: A review. J Med 1986;17:373–397.

Dutton GN. The causes of tissue damage in toxoplasmic retinochoroiditis. Trans Ophthalmol Soc UK 1986;105:404–412.

Dutton GN. Toxoplasmic retinochoroiditis—A historical review and current concepts. Ann Acad Med 1989;18:214–221.

Frenkel JK. Ocular toxoplasmosis: Pathogenesis, diagnosis and treatment. Arch Ophthalmol 1986;59:260–279.

Holland GN, Engstrom RE, Glasgow BJ, et al. Ocular toxoplasmosis in patients with acquired immune deficiency syndrome. Am J Ophthalmol 1988;106:653–667.

Smith RE. Toxoplasmic retinochoroiditis as an emerging problem in AIDS patients. Am J Ophthalmol 1988;106:738–739.

CHAPTER

21

Multifocal Chorioretinopathy

Leonard J. Oshinskie

Several unique and less common conditions known as *multifocal chorioretinopathies* or *choroidopathies* have been identified during the last two decades. These conditions are found in young adults, and an association with a viral-like prodrome has been reported in some of the entities. In their active stage, these conditions present with creamy or white fundus lesions of various size. Symptoms of decreased visual acuity, scotomata, or photopsia have been reported, along with a vitritis or anterior chamber reaction. Retinal pigment changes such as mottling, dispersion, dropout, and clumping have been described as a sequela to the active inflammatory process. The prognosis for vision recovery varies; choroidal neovascularization (CNV) and its associated findings have been reported with several of these conditions. Conditions in this category of diseases include:

- Acute posterior multifocal placoid pigment epitheliopathy (APMPPE)
  - Young adults
  - Bilateral
  - Viral prodrome
- Multiple evanescent white dot syndrome
  - Female > male subjects
  - Bilateral
- Punctate inner choroidopathy (PIC)
- Vitiliginous ("birdshot") choroidopathy
- Serpiginous (geographic helicoid) choroidopathy
- Punctate outer retinal toxoplasmosis
- Diffuse unilateral subacute neuroretinitis (DUSN)
  - Children and young adults in the southern United States
  - Nematode infection (parasite visible in vitreous)
    - Transient multiple gray-white lesions
    - Papillitis, vitritis
    - Optic atrophy, retinal pigment epithelial (RPE) changes, vascular changes
    - Severe loss of vision and visual field in late stages

ACUTE POSTERIOR MULTIFOCAL PLACOID PIGMENT EPITHELIOPATHY

APMPPE usually occurs in patients from the second to fourth decade. Most patients with this condition are white, and there is no sex predilection. Patients complain of a sudden onset of decreased vision, scotoma, photopsia, and floaters. A viral-like illness has been reported in 25–30% of patients, including an upper respiratory infection, headache, malaise, and fever. The macular response consists of bilateral, multifocal, yellowish-white placoid lesions of various sizes with indistinct borders at the level of the RPE or choroid (Figure 21.1).

An anterior uveitis and vitritis are sometimes present, with choroidal neovascularization membrane (CNVM) occurring only rarely. Recurrence is unusual, and the lesions usually resolve in 7–10 days, resulting in characteristic pigment changes.

MULTIPLE EVANESCENT WHITE DOT SYNDROME

Multiple evanescent white dot syndrome occurs predominantly in women in the second to fourth decade of life, and there is no racial predilection. The disease is usually unilateral and is characterized by a sudden decrease in vision that resolves within 1–16 weeks in most cases. As in APMPPE, a history of a viral-like illness is often elicited. The macular lesions consist of transient, multiple, small, white dots at the level of the RPE and granular pigment changes (Figure 21.2). The lesions are often

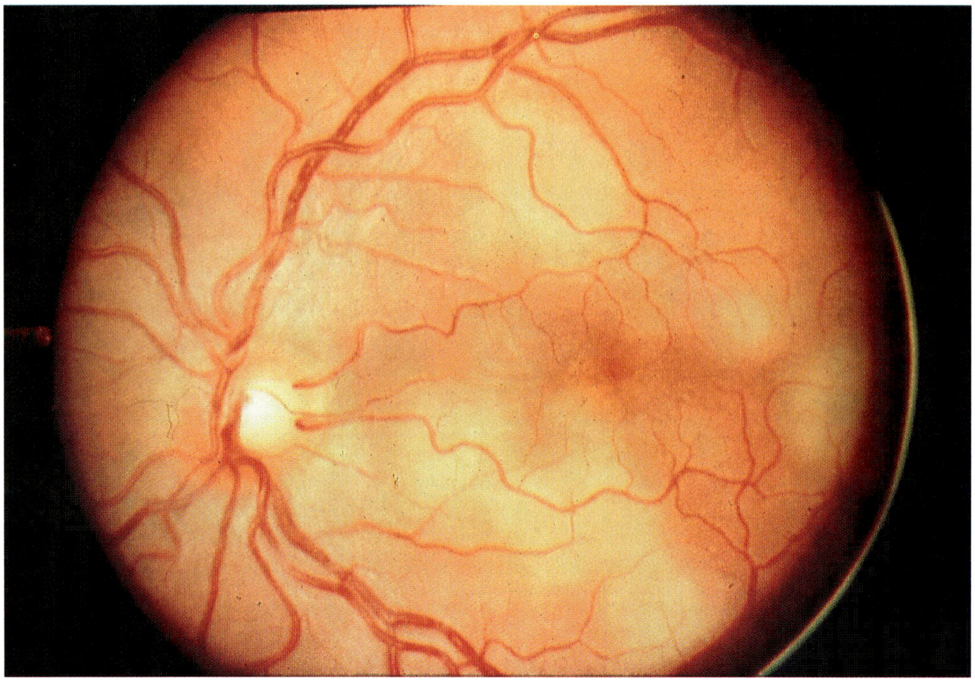

FIGURE 21.1. Yellow-white placoid lesions in the left eye of a young adult with acute posterior multifocal placoid pigment epitheliopathy.

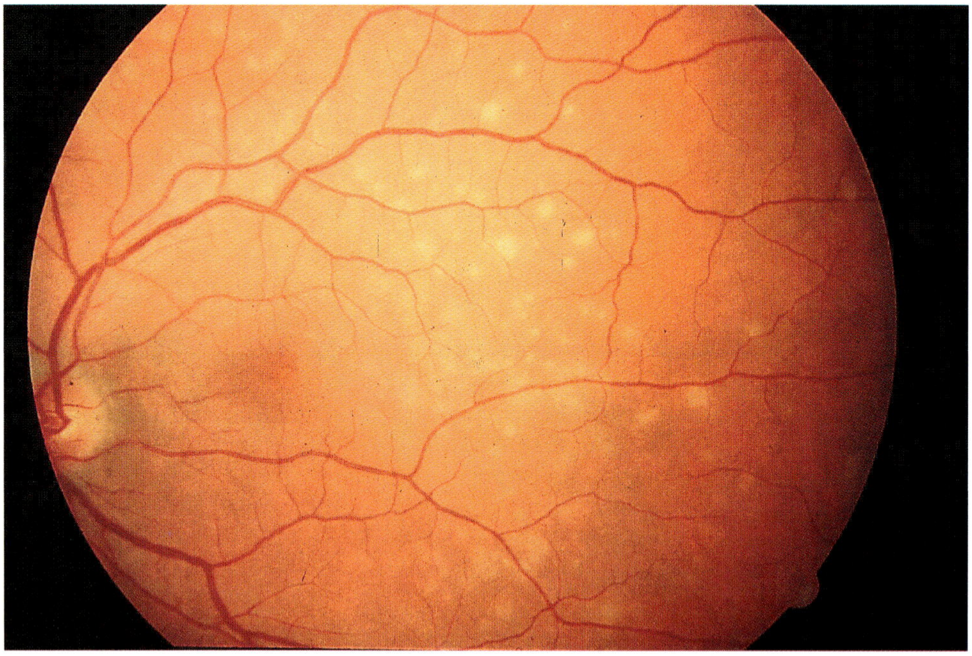

FIGURE 21.2. Small white lesions at the level of the retinal pigment epithelium in a patient with multiple evanescent white dot syndrome.

located near the retinal vessels. Disc hyperemia, venous sheathing, and a posterior vitritis can occur. In spite of a significant reduction in acuity in the early stages of the disease, recovery of visual function is expected.

PUNCTATE INNER CHOROIDOPATHY

PIC occurs most commonly in myopic women in their third and fourth decades; there is usually no preceding viral illness. Symptoms include decreased vision, scotoma, and photopsia. Ocular signs include the appearance of numerous gray-white or yellow puncate lesions (100–300 μ) at the level of the inner choroid and RPE, usually confined to the posterior pole (Figure 21.3). The lesions are sometimes found in linear streaks or clumps and are bilateral in 80% of cases. The prognosis is uncertain due to the possibility of an overlying serous neurosensory detachment or CNVM, which usually occurs

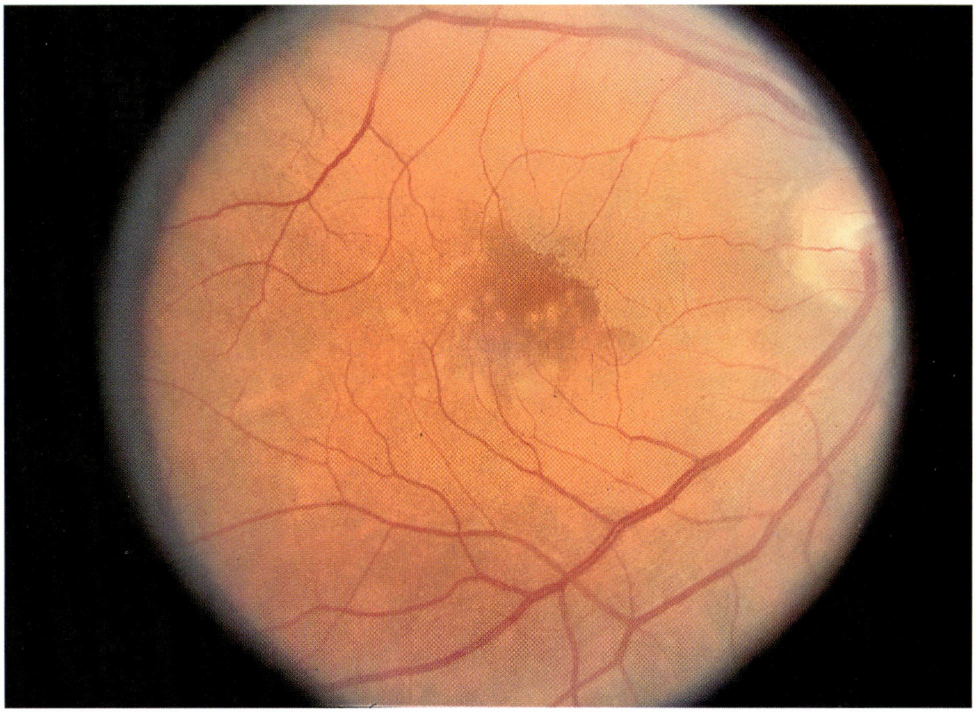

FIGURE 21.3. Punctate inner choroidopathy, with the characteristic small white lesions in the macular area.

during the first 6 months. PIC should be differentiated from ocular histoplasmosis syndrome, which manifests larger and fewer lesions and has no sex predilection. Inner choroidopathy may also be confused with multifocal choroiditis (MFC); however, vitritis, which is unusual with PIC, is common with other multifocal choroidopathies. Referral to an internist to rule out systemic conditions associated with chorioretinitis, i.e., histoplasmosis, toxoplasmosis, syphilis, sarcoidosis, and tuberculosis, is appropriate.

VITILIGINOUS CHOROIDOPATHY

Vitiliginous choroidopathy is also known as birdshot chorioretinitis since fundus pigmentation is lost in patches, similar to the dermatologic condition vitiligo. Patients are generally middle-aged, with women affected twice as often as men, and symptoms include floaters and blurred vision. In this condition, numerous bilateral, yellow-white or faint pink or orange depigmented patches at the level of the choroid are observed posterior to the fundus equator, with minimal macular involvement (Figure 21.4). Vitritis is a universal finding, and disc edema and cystoid macular edema, which require treatment, are also commonly seen.

SERPIGINOUS CHOROIDITIS

Serpiginous choroiditis (giant helicoid choroidopathy) exhibits a geographic peripapillary atrophy with juxtapapillary, cream-colored lesions. Pigment changes often accompany the retinal findings, and the condition progresses in a serpentine confluence, hence the name serpiginous choroiditis. Bilaterality is common; however, the fellow eye often remains uninvolved until years later. Patients are usually young to middle-aged, and unlike many patients with other forms of MFC, they do not have a preceding viral-like illness. Recurrence is common, and therefore the prognosis for retaining useful vision is guarded. There is a variation of this disease that begins in the central macula and then extends toward the optic disc (Figure 21.5).

DIFFUSE UNILATERAL SUBACUTE NEURORETINITIS

DUSN demonstrates multifocal lesions similar to those observed in other multifocal choroidopathies. However, DUSN is caused by a nematode and is generally seen in young patients, with a mean age of 16 years. Whites are affected more commonly than others, and there is no sex predilection. Patients are usually from endemic areas, including the southeastern United States and the Caribbean. Symptoms include decreased vision, which is often insidious in nature, as well as scotoma. The fundus lesions are almost always unilateral and are located deep in the retina. They are transient, multiple, gray-white or yellow-white lesions, approximately 300–1,500 μ in size, and are found in aggregates in the macular and paramacular regions. Optic nerve head

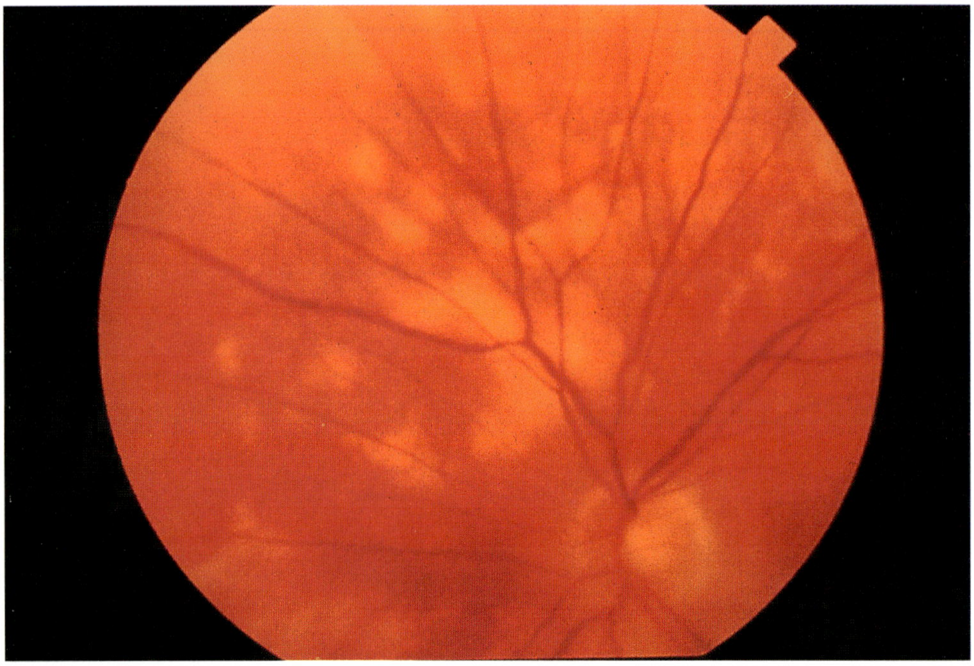

FIGURE 21.4. Birdshot choroidopathy with multiple areas of depigmentation superior to the optic nerve.

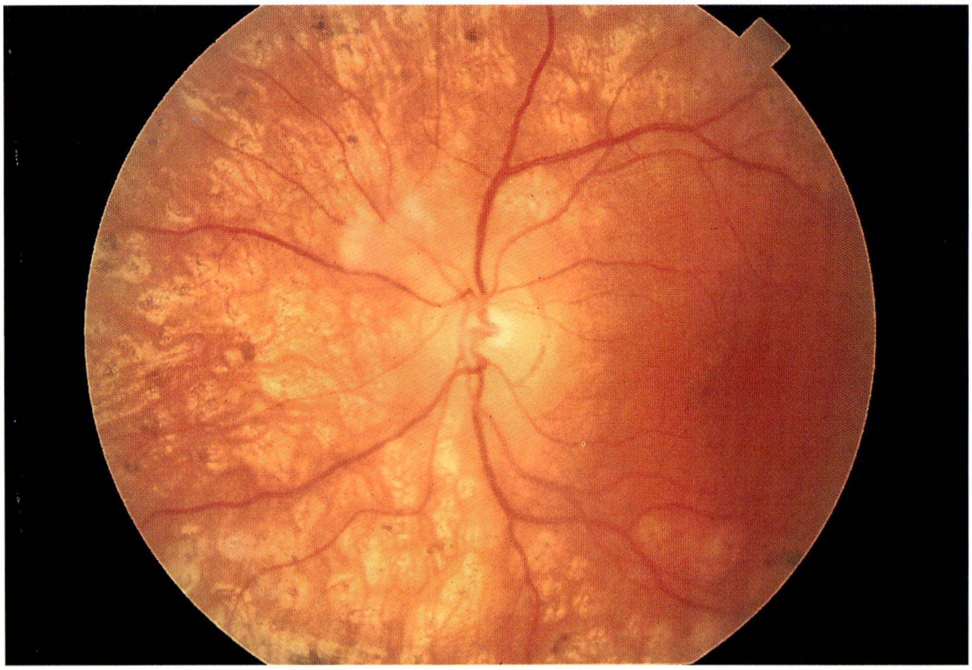

FIGURE 21.5. Giant helicoid choroiditis demonstrating the juxtapapillary pigment changes and creamy white lesions typical of one form of the disease.

edema or atrophy is often present, and vitritis is a consistent finding. The causative nematode can be isolated in the vitreous of some patients. Complications from this infection can include CNV (10%) and cystoid macular edema (5%). Referral to a retinologist for oral corticosteroids, antihelminthics, or laser ablation of the nematode is indicated.

PUNCTATE OUTER RETINAL TOXOPLASMOSIS

Puncate outer retinal toxoplasmosis differs from the typical cases of toxoplasmosis chorioretinitis in that only the outer layers of the retina are involved. A vitritis is rarely seen, and the macular lesions occur in younger patients and are small, gray-white, and deep, with fluffy borders. Chorioretinal scarring is seen adjacent to the active lesions.

SUMMARY

Multifocal chorioretinopathies are unusual presentations often resulting in a macular response. Lesions from these disorders are variegated in size and appearance and are usually located deep to the retina. Preservation of visual function is dependent on the location of pigment changes and on the variability of CNV formation. Patients should be educated as to the signs and symptoms of neurosensory or RPE elevation of the macula and should return immediately for evaluation if dysmorphopsia is noted.

SUGGESTED READING

Doft BH, Gass JDM. Punctate outer retinal toxoplasmosis. Arch Ophthalmol 1985;103:1332–1336.

Dreyer RF, Gass JDM. Multifocal choroiditis and panuveitis. Arch Ophthalmol 1984;102:1776–1784.

Eldem B, Sener C. Punctate inner choroidopathy and its differential diagnosis. Ann Ophthalmol 1991;23:153–158.

Gass JDM, Gilbert WR, Guerry RK, et al. Diffuse unilateral subacute neuroretinitis. Ophthalmology 1978;85:521–545.

Jampol LM, Sieving PA, Pugh D, et al. Multiple evanescent white-dot syndrome. Arch Ophthalmol 1984;102:671–674.

Mansour AM, Jampol LM, Packo KH, et al. Macular serpiginous choroiditis. Retina 1988;8:125–131.

Schatz H, Johnson RN, McDonald HR. Differential diagnosis of dots, spots, flecks, and specks of the fundus. Retina 1992;12:67–69.

Watzke AJ, Packer AJ, Folk J, et al. Punctate inner choroidopathy. Am J Ophthalmol 1984;98:572–584.

CHAPTER

22 Ocular *Toxocara Canis*

Rodney K. Gutner and
Anthony A. Cavallerano

Toxocara canis is a nematode whose infestation often causes a devastating retinal inflammatory response, sometimes involving the macula. This roundworm, an ascarid, is common in cats and dogs, and the larvae find their way into soil via animal feces. After human ingestion, the eggs hatch, penetrate the intestinal wall, and migrate throughout the body. The vector for human ingestion is through oral–fecal transmission from puppies or through contaminated food.

The importance of human *T. canis* invasion, or toxocariasis, was first described in the early 1950s when it was found to produce two human disease states, visceral larva migrans and intraocular *T. canis*. Ocular *T. canis* was first described by Wilder when she examined eyes that had been enucleated for suspected retinoblastoma. Her findings were corroborated almost 10 years later when histologic verification of the various ocular forms of the disease was recognized.

Ocular *T. canis* can cause severe uveal and retinal inflammation that is usually limited to pediatric age groups. Some studies show that almost one-third of asymptomatic children in specific demographic groups may demonstrate positive serologic test results. Although systemic infection is relatively common, ocular findings are considered rare.

Systemic findings range from eosinophilia to potentially fatal pulmonary and cardiac involvement. Ocular lesions, including granuloma surrounding the optic nerve and macula, peripheral choroidal lesions, and diffuse endophthalmitis, with accompanying tractional retinal detachment, manifest months to years following the initial ingestion of the organism. The panocular nature of the ocular inflammation often yields a poor visual prognosis.

CLINICAL PRESENTATION

- Decreased visual function
- Anterior segment often "white and quiet"
- Granulomatous anterior uveitis
- Peripheral anterior synechiae
- Posterior synechiae
- Leukokoria
- Hypopyon
- Strabismus
- Hazy vitreous due to cellular infiltration and fibrous response
- Ill-defined, hazy, white or gray granuloma in posterior pole
- Localized, well-defined white mass in retinal periphery
- Disseminated chorioretinitis
- Optic neuritis

The clinical presentation of ocular *T. canis*, although not pathognomonic, is highly distinctive. There are four classifications of inflammatory response in intraocular *T. canis*. The first is *chronic endophthalmitis*, or vitreous abscess, which produces a significant cellular response in the vitreous, along with tractional retinal detachment. A granulomatous anterior chamber reaction may be observed, and hypopyon is often present.

The second classification of the inflammatory response is termed *posterior pole granuloma*. Ill-defined white or gray-white, hazy intraretinal and subretinal lesions, ranging in size from 0.5–4.0 DD, may be observed through hazy media (Figures 22.1 and 22.2). However, the vitreous may clear after the inflammation subsides; these lesions frequently occur in the macula, often accompanying vascular anastomoses. Central vision is markedly diminished by the time the diagnosis is made, and the child may present with a strabismus. *Toxocara* infection is also a cause of leukokoria, or white pupil, and the disorder needs to be differentiated from a

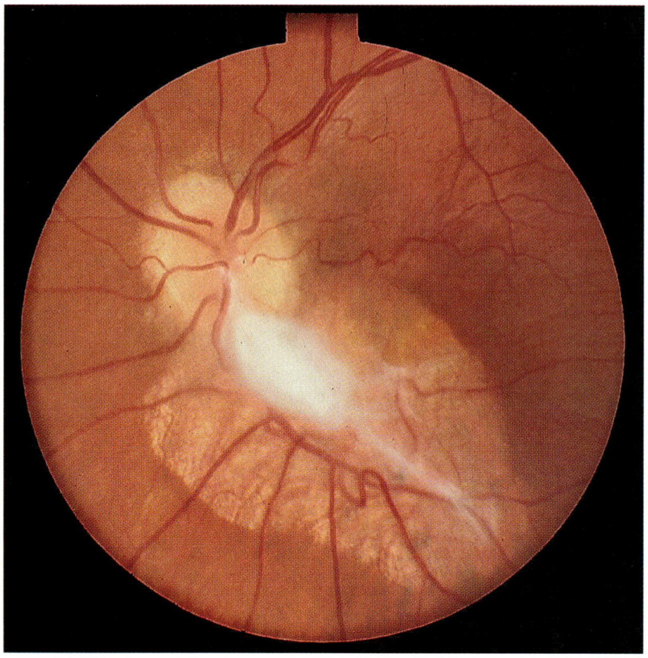

A

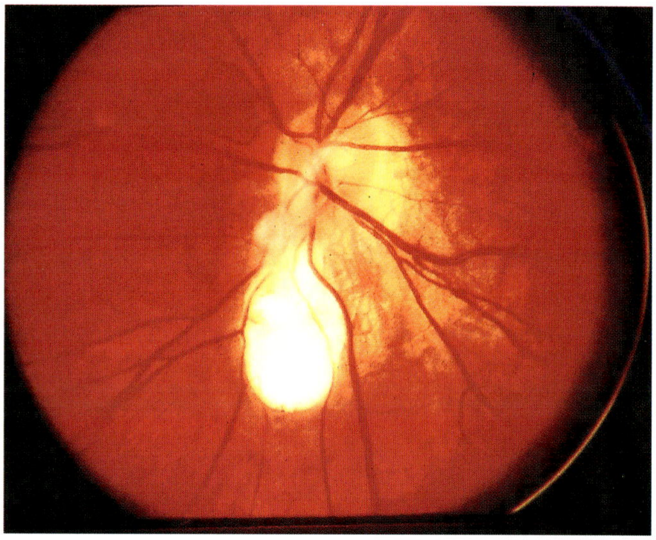

B

FIGURE 22.1. A. Central inflammatory mass in posterior pole with minimal macular traction in a patient with *Toxocara canis*. B. An example of posterior pole granuloma in toxocariasis. (Reprinted with permission from RK Gutner, AA Cavallerano. Ocular *Toxocara canis*. Clin Eye Vis Care 1993;5:29–32.)

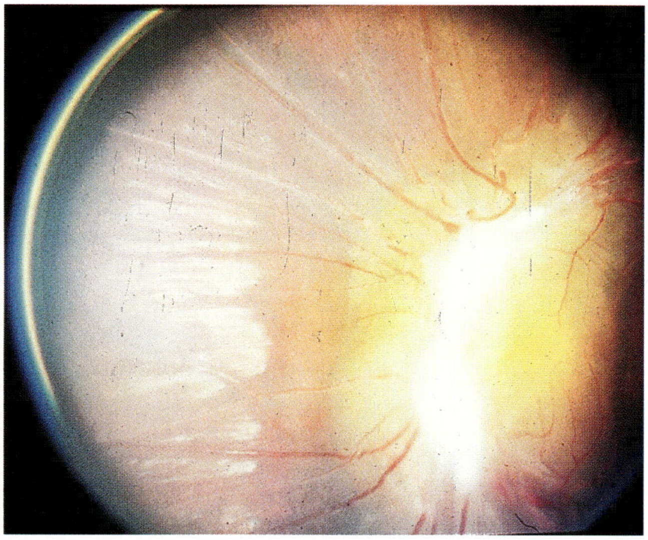

FIGURE 22.2. An example of severe macular traction in toxocariasis. (Reprinted with permission from RK Gutner, AA Cavallerano. Ocular *Toxocara canis*. Clin Eye Vis Care 1993;5:29–32.)

retinoblastoma since both conditions affect the pediatric population.

The third response is a *peripheral inflammatory mass* or *granuloma*, which is characterized by a dense, well-defined mass in the retinal periphery. Retinal traction can result from the fibrous response, and dragging of the macula toward the lesion is common (Figure 22.3).

Additional findings have been reported that are not characteristic of the nematode infestation but represent a fourth category of response that is atypical. These findings include inflammation of the optic nerve head, diffuse chorioretinitis, and active subretinal nematode.

Visual acuity in all types of endophthalmitis is dependent on the extent and location of the inflammatory reaction. A low-grade iritis with peripheral anterior synechiae can occur, along with hypopyon, leukokoria, and iris nodules. Chronic endophthalmitis is present, along with posterior polar granuloma with retinochoroiditis. Secondary effects can include vitreous opacification, membrane formation with vitreoretinal traction, and progressive cyclitic membrane formation.

The macula is particularly vulnerable to the effects of inflammatory and tractional damage. Vitreous traction in the macular area disposes to macular hole formation; chronic inflammation can lead to cystic changes in the macula. The retinal vasculitis can cause sheathing of the perimacular vessels.

Although the diagnosis is primarily clinical, *Toxocara* must be considered part of the differential diagnosis in any patient presenting with leukokoria. The enzyme-linked immunosorbent assay (ELISA) may be used as an adjunct laboratory test but is not specific enough to be used for definitive diagnosis. Direct testing of intraocular fluids by the ELISA method or cytology

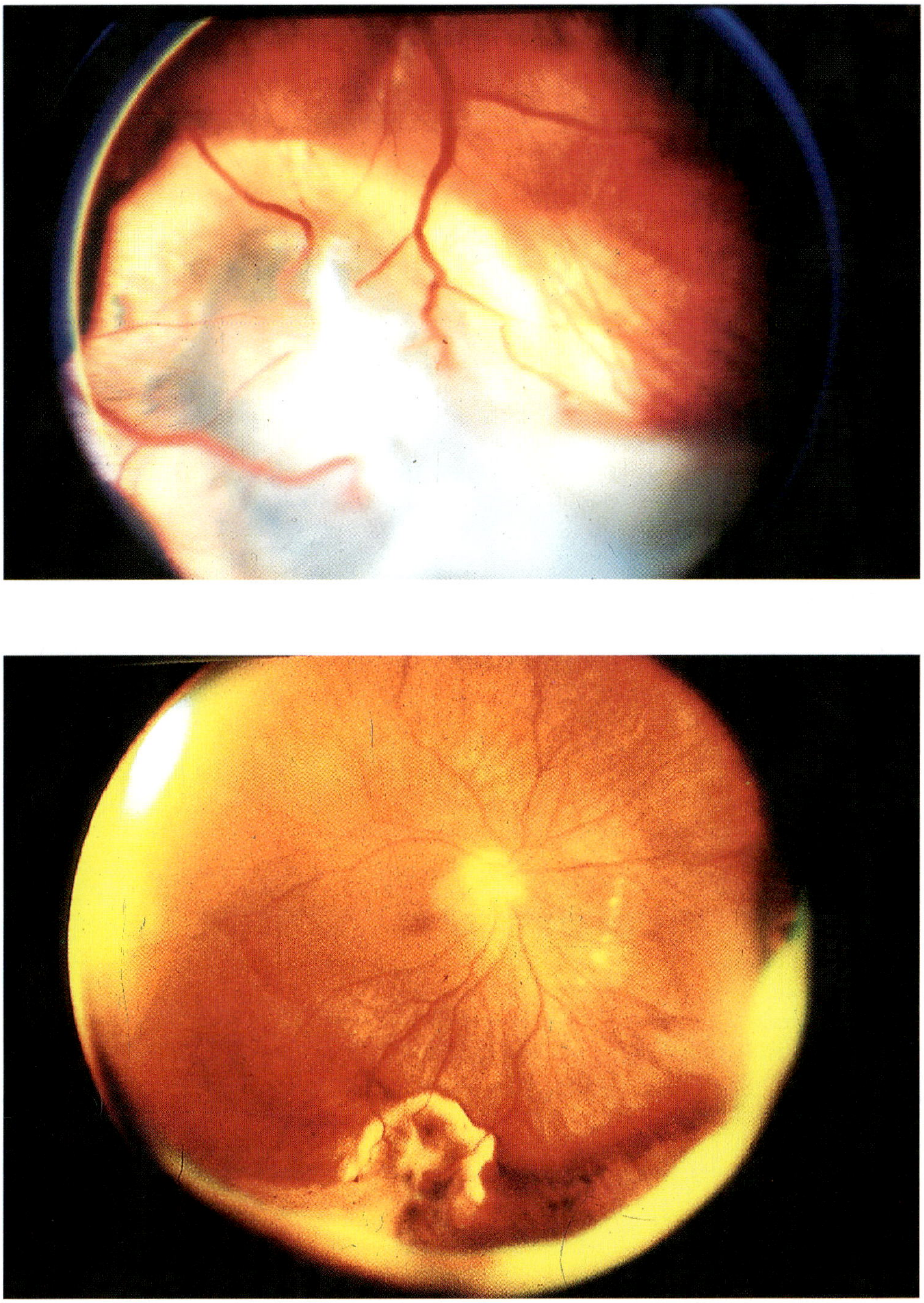

FIGURE 22.3. Examples of peripheral granulomas in a patient with toxocariasis. (Reprinted with permission from RK Gutner, AA Cavallerano. Ocular *Toxocara canis*. Clin Eye Vis Care 1993;5:29–32.)

has proven to be more promising. Computed tomography scanning has been used in patients with leukokoria to detect a mass lesion, but it too is not specific enough to differentiate various types of posterior pole tumors. Beta-scan ultrasonography can sometimes be useful in differentiating various retinal lesions.

DIFFERENTIAL DIAGNOSIS

- Retinoblastoma
- Any cause of granulomatous uveitis
- Other causes of endophthalmitis
- Retinopathy of prematurity (retrolental fibroplasia)
- Familial exudative vitreoretinopathy
- Persistent hyperplastic primary vitreous
- Any cause of optic neuritis

The differential diagnosis should include any entity causing leukokoria, especially retinoblastoma. The differential diagnosis should also include any cause of endophthalmitis. The diagnosis is rendered more difficult, however, if there are significant media opacities. Other conditions that should be considered include Coats' disease, persistent hyperplastic primary vitreous, retinopathy of prematurity (retrolental fibroplasia), familial exudative vitreoretinopathy, and tuberous sclerosis. The diagnostic scheme should also include clinical entities that cause optic neuritis.

MANAGEMENT

- ELISA and cytologic testing including intraocular fluids
- Topical and systemic corticosteroids
- Antihelminthics
- Laser photocoagulation
- Vitrectomy
- Retinal detachment surgery

Primary care management of *T. canis* requires proper identification of the complex of clinical findings. Prevention is the best measure. Medical treatment, using anti-inflammatory agents, is directed toward reducing inflammation-induced injury and secondary fibrotic damage. Cycloplegics are indicated for the uveitis, and topical and systemic corticosteroids can help to reduce the inflammation. Antihelminthic agents are another modality that has been used with varying degrees of success. It is of questionable benefit to kill intraocular organisms since there may be a concomitant exacerbation of the inflammation with the death of the larva.

Surgical management has been attempted with laser and other forms of photocoagulation to destroy the nematode directly. Vitrectomy with membrane peeling has been employed to reduce the transvitreal and epiretinal membrane vitreoretinal traction. Scleral buckle procedures aid in the reattachment of the retina. Prognosis for visual outcome is directly related to preoperative vision. Preoperative tractional folds in the macula can lead to a poor visual outcome.

SUMMARY

Intraocular *T. canis* is a relatively rare manifestation of a ubiquitous ascarid. Prevention is an important component in primary care patient management. Since it predominantly affects children, any patient with leukokoria should be evaluated for intraocular tumors, especially retinoblastoma.

SUGGESTED READING

Ashton N. Larval granulomatosis of the retina due to *Toxocara*. Br J Ophthalmol 1960;44:129–148.

Beaver PC, Snyder CH, Carrera GM, et al. Chronic eosinophilia due to visceral larva migrans. Pediatrics 1952;9:7–19.

Clemmett OS, Williamson HJE, Hidajat RR, et al. Ocular *Toxocara* infections: Diagnosis by enzyme immunoassay. Aust N Z J Ophthalmol 1987;15:145–150.

Edwards MG, Pordell GR. Ocular toxocariasis studied by CT-scanning. Radiology 1985;157:685–686.

Ellis GS Jr, Pakalnis VA, Worley G, et al. *Toxocara* infestation: Clinical and epidemiological associations with seropositivity in kindergarten children. Ophthalmology 1986;93:1032–1037.

Irvine WC, Irvine AR Jr. Nematode endophthalmitis: *Toxocara*—Report of one case. Am J Ophthalmol 1959;47:185–191.

Maguire AM, Green WR, Michels RG, et al. Recovery of intraocular *Toxocara* by pars plana vitrectomy. Ophthalmology 1990;97:675–680.

Richer SP, Stiles WR. Presumed *Toxocara canis* with peripheral retinal granuloma and secondary macular hole. J Am Optom Assoc 1987;58:404–407.

Shields JA. Ocular toxocariasis: A review. Surv Ophthalmol 1984;28:361–381.

Small KW, McCuen BW II, de Juan E Jr, et al. Surgical management of retinal traction caused by toxocariasis. Am J Ophthalmol 1989;108:10–14.

Wilder HC. Nematode endophthalmitis. Trans Am Acad Ophthalmol Otolaryngol 1950;109:99–109.

Zinkham WH. Systemic Visceral Larval Migrans. In SJ Ryan, RE Smith (eds), Selected Topics on the Eye in Systemic Disease. New York: Grune & Stratton, 1974;167–175.

CHAPTER

23

Macula in Acquired Immunodeficiency Syndrome

Timothy Harkins

Because of their underlying immune suppression, patients with acquired immunodeficiency syndrome (AIDS) are at risk for opportunistic infections that rarely affect the immune-normal population. It is this increased risk of infection, specifically retinal infection, that can ultimately affect the macula. Macular disease alone is not an expected complication of AIDS, rather it is seen as part of the clinical picture of infectious retinitis. Cytomegalovirus (CMV) retinitis is the only common retinal infection in AIDS and must be considered first in the differential diagnosis of a patient with suppressed immunity. Other retinal infections seen in AIDS are toxoplasmosis, syphilis, tuberculosis, herpes simplex, and herpes zoster. In all of these cases, involvement of the macula is possible and may be observed ophthalmoscopically. Immune suppression is, of course, not protective, and AIDS patients can manifest any maculopathy seen in the immune-normal population.

CYTOMEGALOVIRUS

CMV retinitis is the most common ocular infection and the leading cause of blindness in AIDS patients. Ten to 34% of AIDS patients develop this condition. It is almost always accompanied by systemic CMV infection, and its diagnosis carries a dim prognosis; if left untreated, the median life expectancy after diagnosis is 2–4 months.

Patients with CMV retinitis may be asymptomatic or may complain of blur, decreased visual field, or floaters. The diagnosis is made ophthalmoscopically, and the disease classically manifests as white granular lesions accompanied by exudates, hemorrhages, and overlying mild vitritis (Figure 23.1). Less frequently, CMV can present simply as granular or necrotic retinopathy without hemorrhage and vitritis (Figure 23.2). This is consistent with a profoundly suppressed immune system's inability to mount a response to the virus.

The differential diagnosis for early CMV retinitis includes any vascular disease that can cause hemorrhage or cotton wool spots (CWS). More progressive cases must be differentiated from other infectious causes of retinitis (although CMV is statistically far more likely than all other retinal infections in AIDS), peripheral vascular disease, and metastasis.

The presumed retinal diagnosis can be corroborated by positive blood, urine, or throat culture results. Serum antibodies are not helpful since they only indicate previous exposure, and 50–70% of American adults are seropositive. The definitive test would be retinal biopsy, but this high-risk procedure is rarely indicated. The most reliable and practical method of diagnosis remains observation of the characteristic retinal lesions.

CMV is not more likely to affect or to spare the macula than any other part of the retina. If the macula is involved, it will be apparent ophthalmoscopically, and visual acuity will be reduced. The visual acuity loss is permanent because of the retinal necrosis that accompanies the infection.

Peripheral infection results in an absolute visual field defect corresponding to the area of affected retina. Because of thinning and atrophy of infected peripheral retina, the eye is at risk for rhegmatogenous retinal detachment, which can ultimately involve the macula.

Presently, there are two approved therapies for CMV retinitis: ganciclovir and foscarnet. Each are approximately 65–90% effective at halting retinitis, and they prevent monocular infection from becoming binocular in 85–100% of cases. Because ganciclovir and foscarnet are virustatic, reactivation of retinitis after discontinuing therapy occurs in 90–100% of the cases.

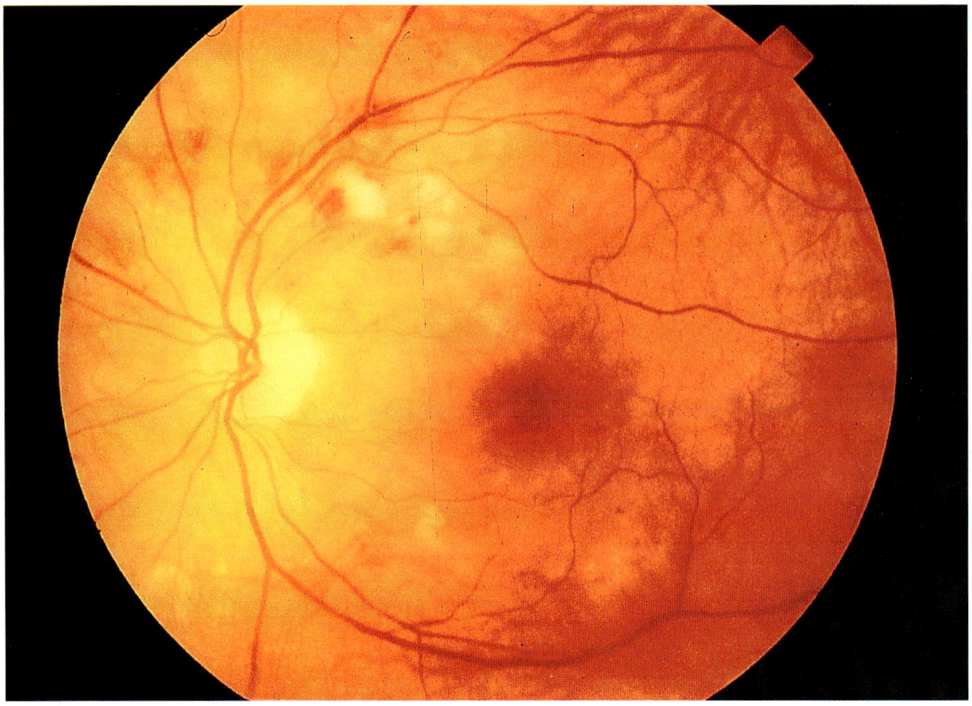

FIGURE 23.1. The ophthalmoscopic appearance of cytomegalovirus retinitis, which classically manifests as white granular lesions accompanied by exudates, hemorrhages, and overlying mild vitritis.

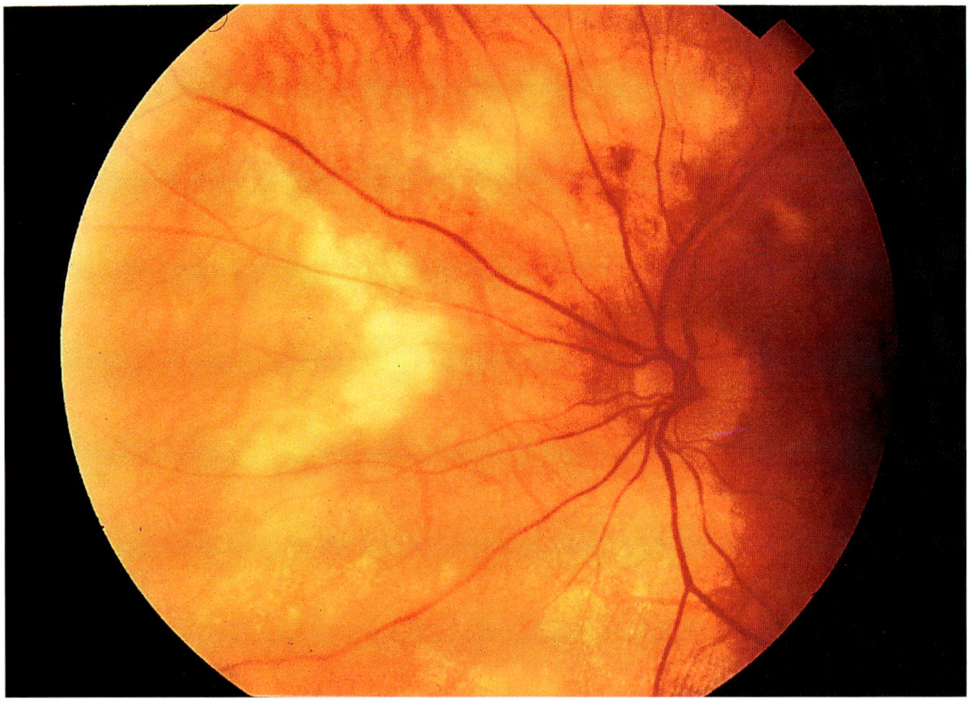

FIGURE 23.2. Cytomegalovirus can present simply as granular or necrotic retinopathy without hemorrhage and vitritis.

The ability of ganciclovir and foscarnet to suppress retinitis does not distinguish them from each other. Instead, the choice is based on their ability to affect life expectancy and their toxicity profiles. In the only controlled study involving both medications, each increased the median life expectancy compared with untreated patients with CMV retinitis. Ganciclovir patients lived 9 months after diagnosis, and foscarnet patients lived 13 months.

In spite of their clinical efficacy, these are toxic medications associated with many complications. Ganciclovir's primary toxicity is to the immune system and often results in neutropenia, an important problem in patients with compromised immunity. Because it gen-

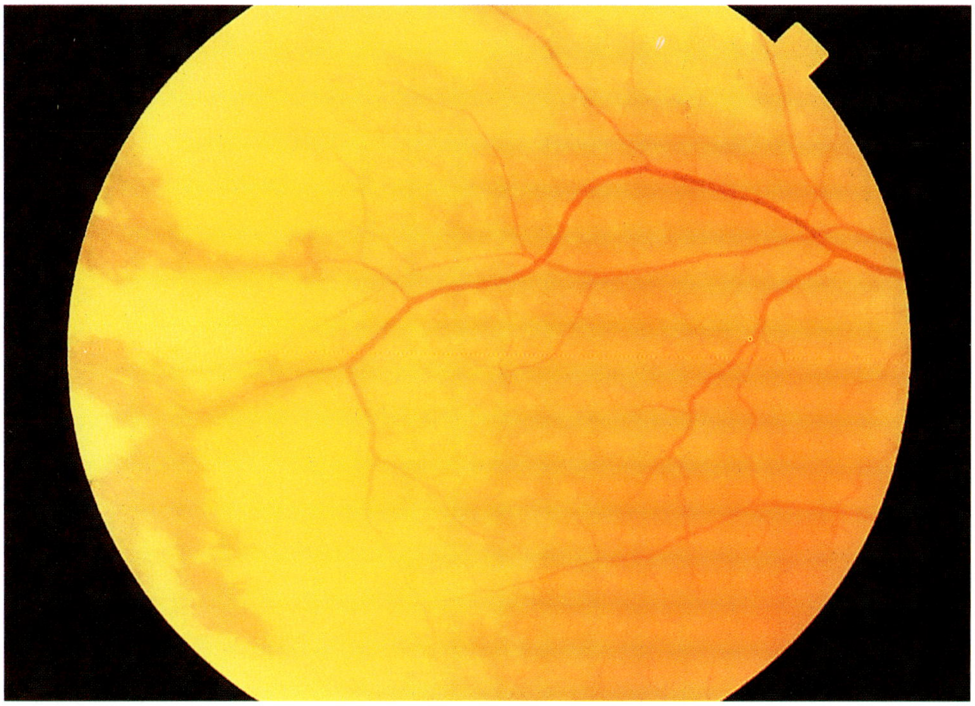

FIGURE 23.3. Ophthalmoscopic appearance of toxoplasmosis retinitis in a patient with human immunodeficiency virus.

erally supresses the blood cell–producing systems of the body, ganciclovir usually cannot be used concurrently with zidovudine (AZT), which suppresses bone marrow. Although foscarnet may be used with AZT, its primary complication is renal failure, a serious problem because AIDS patients are often on multiple medications and require excellent renal function to eliminate waste.

After a diagnosis of CMV retinitis, the patient is hospitalized for induction therapy with either ganciclovir or foscarnet, typically administered and monitored by an infectious disease specialist. The decision of which antiviral to use is often forced since many patients cannot tolerate the neutropenia of ganciclovir, whereas others with renal problems cannot take foscarnet. After 2 weeks of high-dose induction therapy, patients have an indwelling subclavian catheter placed to administer intravenous maintenance therapy at home. Maintenance therapy is continued as long as it can be tolerated. The retina should be monitored periodically for breakthrough retinitis, an observation that dictates increased dosage or alternate medical therapy.

TOXOPLASMOSIS

Toxoplasmosis retinochoroiditis is a less common manifestation of AIDS. It is typically a simple diagnosis in patients with normal immunity. There are characteristic white fluffy lesions, often accompanied by a scar, with surrounding edema and overlying vitritis (Figure 23.3). The ophthalmoscopic picture in immune-suppressed patients is similar, with some important differences. The lesion is frequently larger, indicating the immune system is less able to contain the infection. The lesion is often not accompanied by a scar, indicating an acquired infection, not a reactivation. There is less vitritis in AIDS patients, because there are fewer white blood cells available. Finally, AIDS patients with toxoplasmosis retinochoroiditis commonly have toxoplasmosis encephalitis, and a neurologic consult must be considered. The antimicrobial agents of choice are sulfadiazine or clindamycin combined with pyrimethamine. The response to therapy is diminished in immune-suppressed patients, and these medications are frequently toxic.

SYPHILIS

Syphilis, known as the great imitator, must be considered in the differential diagnosis of any infectious retinitis. This is particularly true in an AIDS patient, as coinfection with HIV and syphilis is common, though retinal infection is in fact rare. Syphilis can manifest as pigmentary retinitis, hemorrhagic retinitis, periphlebitis, or neuroretinitis. AIDS patients with ocular syphilis commonly have coinfection of the central nervous system. When ocular syphilis is suspected, the most sensitive laboratory test is the fluorescent treponema antibody absorption test. Other tests can yield false-negative results when a patient has been treated for primary syphilis and has seroconverted, but still has ocular or neurologic infection. Treatment with aqueous penicillin is required to cross the blood–brain barrier and effectively treat the ocular and neurologic infection.

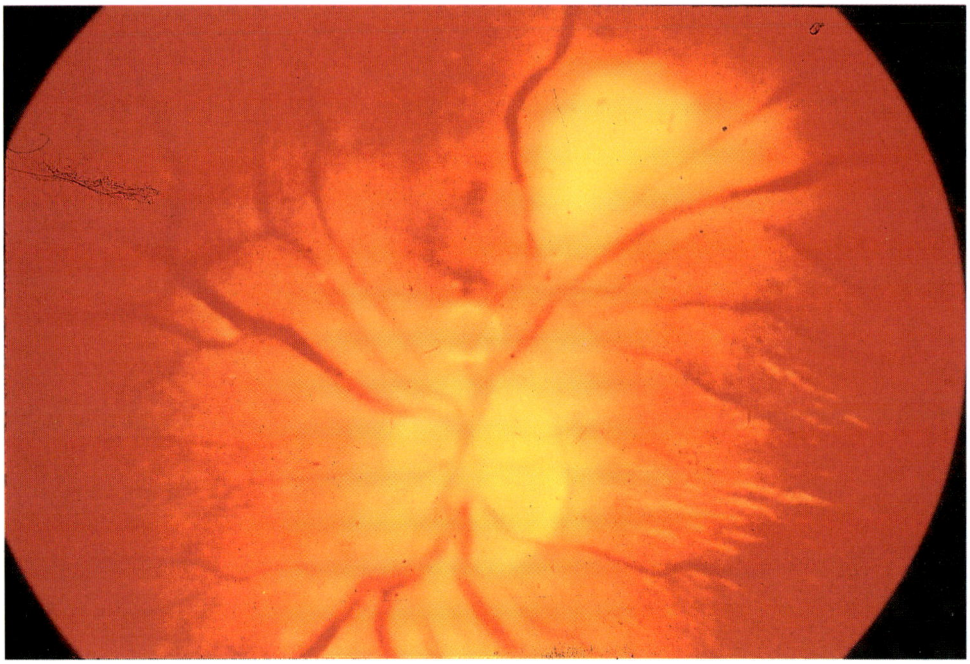

FIGURE 23.4. An example of herpes simplex retinitis.

TUBERCULOSIS

Tuberculosis (TB) is the second most common opportunistic infection in AIDS. AIDS patients with TB have extrapulmonary or nonpulmonary infection 50% of the time, although ocular involvement is rare. In the eye, TB may be seen as anterior uveitis, choroiditis, retinal periphlebitis, and hemorrhagic retinitis. Diagnosis is supported by skin test and chest radiography. Although there are increasing cases of drug resistance, most AIDS patients do respond to multidrug antituberculosis therapy. The mainstays of treatment are isoniazid and rifampin.

HERPES VIRUSES

Herpes simplex and herpes zoster rarely infect the retina in AIDS resulting in retinal necrosis and vasculitis (Figure 23.4). While the macula is frequently spared, it is at risk from complications of macular pucker or from rhegmatogenous retinal detachment. Treatment is with acyclovir, frequently at dosages high enough to require intravenous therapy.

NONINFECTIOUS RETINOPATHY

The most common (although least threatening) retinal findings are not infectious but are vascular in nature. CWS, microaneurysms, and hemorrhages (indications of microvasculopathy) are seen in over half of AIDS patients (Figure 23.5). The appearance is similar to diabetic retinopathy, but the cause is still debated. Possibilities include damage to endothelial cells of the retinal vessels by HIV infection, deposition of immune complexes, or altered blood flow.

The macula is rarely involved, so vision is usually not affected. Though macular edema can develop, it is not yet known whether laser photocoagulation is helpful.

CWS must be differentiated from early CMV retinitis. This can be done by following the patient for retinal changes. CWS do not progress in size and often disappear, whereas CMV rapidly progresses. A useful strategy in following CWS is to examine the patient frequently when the lesions are first noted; if they appear stable, gradually increase the follow-up interval. (For example, once CWSs are observed, see the patient 1 week later; if stable, see the patient 2 weeks later; if still stable, see the patient 1 month later, eventually settling on a 3- or 6-month follow-up schedule.) If rapid progression is observed, then infectious retinopathy should be suspected.

SUMMARY

Patients with AIDS represent a particularly challenging dilemma for the primary care clinician. The diverse response on the part of the retina and the potential for macular involvement require early diagnosis and treatment to reduce the risk of significant visual loss. The side effects and the inevitable toxic response of therapeutic agents also pose an important clinical challenge since patients must be monitored for progression of the disease as well as for tolerance of medication and the development of side effects. Exact etiologic diagnosis in AIDS

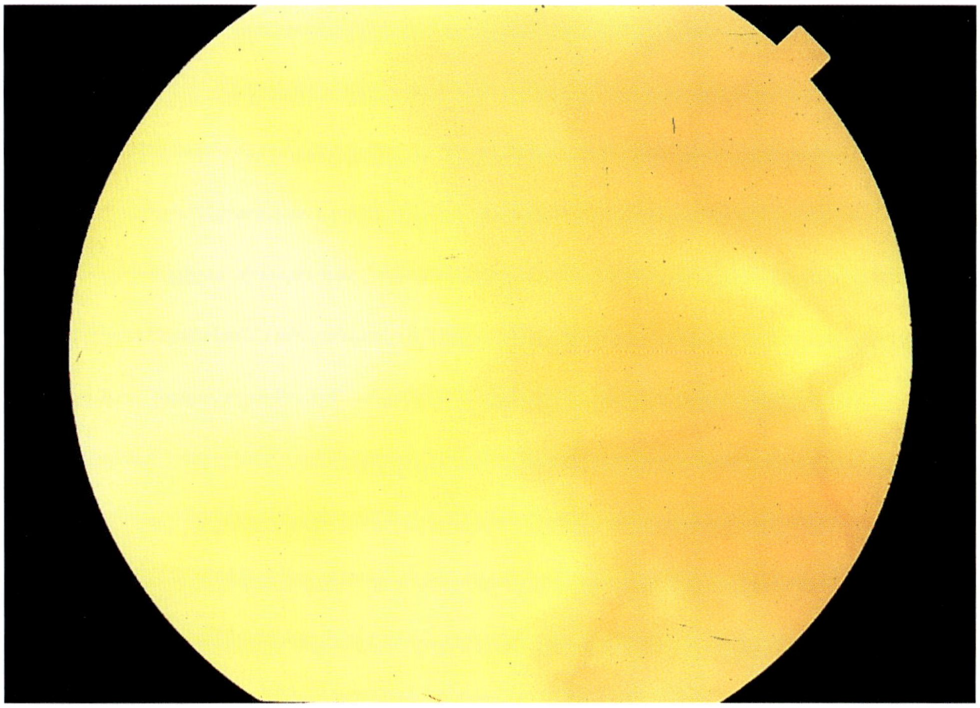

FIGURE 23.5. Cotton wool spots seen in a patient with human immunodeficiency virus in the absence of any additional fundus findings.

cases is imperative, and other unrelated causes of macular disease must always be considered in the differential diagnostic scheme.

SUGGESTED READING

Acheson JF, Shah SM, Spalton DJ, et al. Treatment of CMV retinitis in an AIDS patient. Br J Ophthalmol 1987;71:810–816.

AIDS Research Group, AIDS Clinical Trial Group. Mortality in patients with AIDS treated with either foscarnet or ganciclovir for CMV retinitis. N Engl J Med 1992;326:213–220.

Bach MC, Hedstrom PS. CMV retinitis treated with ganciclovir in AIDS. Ann Ophthalmol 1987;19:369–375.

Cochereau-Massin I, LeHoang P, Lautier-Frau M, et al. Ocular toxoplasmosis in HIV infected patients. Am J Ophthalmol 1992;114:130–135.

Culbertson WW. Infections of the retina in AIDS. Int Ophthalmol Clin 1989;29:108–118.

Drew WL, Buhles W, Erlich AH, et al. Herpes Virus Infections. In MA Sande, PA Volberding (eds), The Medical Management of AIDS. Philadelphia: Saunders, 1988;271–288.

Freeman WR, Lerner CW, Mines JA, et al. Prospective study of the ophthalmologic findings in AIDS. Am J Ophthalmol 1984;97:133–142.

Friedman AH. The retinal lesions of AIDS. Trans Am Ophthalmol Soc 1984;82:447–491.

Harkins T. CMV retinitis complicated by optic neuropathy. J Am Optom Assoc 1992;63:21–27.

Harkins T, Herriott KB. Medical management of AIDS: A review. J Am Optom Assoc 1992;63:35–42.

Heath PH, Hodges GR. Administration of ganciclovir. J Intrav Nurs 1988;11:176–177.

Henderley DE, Freeman WR, Smith RE, et al. CMV retinitis and response to therapy with ganciclovir. Ophthalmology 1987;94:425–434.

Henderley DE, Freeman WR, Smith RE, et al. CMV retinitis as the initial manifestation of AIDS. Am J Ophthalmol 1987;103:316–320.

Hennis HL, Scott AA, Apple DJ. CMV retinitis. Surv Ophthalmol 1989;34:193–203.

Holland GN. Acquired immune deficiency syndrome and ophthalmology. Am J Ophthalmol 1992;114:86–95.

Holland GN, Buhles WC, Mastre B, et al. The UCLA CMV retinopathy study group. Arch Ophthalmol 1989;107:1759–1766.

Holland GN, Sison RF, Jatulis DE, et al. Survey of patients with AIDS after development of CMV retinopathy. Ophthalmology 1990;97:204–211.

Jabs DA. Treatment of CMV retinitis—1992. Arch Ophthalmol 1992;110:185–187.

Jabs DA, Enger C, Bartlett JG, et al. CMV in AIDS. Arch Ophthalmol 1989;107:75–80.

Jabs DA, Newman C, DeBustros S, et al. Treatment of CMV retinitis with ganciclovir. Ophthalmology 1987;94:824–830.

Khadem M, Kalish SB, Goldsmith J, et al. Ophthalmic findings in AIDS. Arch Ophthalmol 1984;102:201–206.

McLeish WM, Pulido JS, Holland S, et al. The ocular manifestations of syphilis in the HIV infected host. Ophthalmology 1990;97:196–203.

Newsome DA. Noninfectious ocular complications of AIDS. Int Ophthalmol Clin 1989;29:95–97.

Pepose JS. Acute Retinal Necrosis Syndrome. In SJ Ryan (ed), Retina. St. Louis: Mosby, 1989;617–623.

Pepose JS, Holland GN, Nestor NS, et al. Acquired immune deficiency syndrome—Pathogenic mechanisms of ocular disease. Ophthalmology 1985;92:472–484.

Polis MA. Foscarnet and ganciclovir in the treatment of CMV retinitis. J AIDS 1992;5:S3–S10.

Resta S, Wolitz R, Merigan TC. CMV retinitis in the AIDS patient. AIDS Updates 1990;3:1–12.

Schuman JS, Orellana J, Friedman AH, et al. Acquired immune deficiency syndrome. Surv Ophthalmol 1987;31:384–410.

Smith RE. Toxoplasmic retinochoroiditis as an emerging problem in AIDS patients. Am J Ophthalmol 1988;106:738–739.

Teich SA, Castle J, Friedman AH, et al. Active CMV particles in eyes of an AIDS patient being treated with ganciclovir. Br J Ophthalmol 1988;72:293–298.

Teich SA, Cheung TW, Friedman AH. Systemic antiviral drugs used in ophthalmology. Surv Ophthalmol 1992;37:19–53.

Wilson RJ. CMV retinitis in AIDS. J Am Optom Assoc 1992;63:49–58.

PART

VI

Retinal Vascular Disease

CHAPTER

24

Diabetic Macular Edema

Jerry D. Cavallerano

The visual threat of proliferative diabetic retinopathy (PDR) is usually recognized, but diabetic macular edema (DME) is sometimes overlooked as a common cause of visual loss from diabetes mellitus. DME, however, is a frequent ocular complication of diabetes.

An estimated 14–15 million Americans have diabetes mellitus, all of whom are at risk of developing ocular complications of diabetes. Studies indicate that approximately 500,000 Americans have DME, and 325,000 of these have clinically significant macular edema (CSME) and are at risk of moderate visual loss (MVL), i.e., a doubling of the visual angle. The annual incidence of new cases of DME and clinically significant DME is estimated at 75,000 and 50,000, respectively.

The value of therapeutic laser photocoagulation surgery for DME was addressed in the Early Treatment Diabetic Retinopathy Study (ETDRS). Study results indicate that appropriate focal laser photocoagulation surgery can reduce the 5-year risk of MVL from macular edema by at least 50%; consequently, proper diagnosis of macular edema and referral to a retinologist for evaluation and consideration of focal laser surgery are crucial.

There is no known means of curing or preventing diabetic retinopathy or DME, but laser surgery significantly reduces the risk of visual loss from both proliferative diabetic retinopathy and DME. Since these conditions may be present and pose a significant visual threat without causing any visual symptoms, and since the conditions are frequently most amenable to treatment before symptoms develop, regular examination and screening for all diabetic persons is valuable, and referral for evaluation and laser surgery can preserve vision for many diabetic patients. Clinical management and guidelines for treatment of diabetic retinopathy and DME have been established by the ETDRS and the Diabetic Retinopathy Study.

DIABETIC EFFECTS ON MACULAR STRUCTURE AND FUNCTION

Diabetic macular disease may be present at any level of diabetic retinopathy and afflicts persons with insulin-dependent diabetes mellitus and noninsulin-dependent diabetes mellitus alike. Diabetes can alter the structure of the macula in any of the following ways, significantly affecting its function:

- Macular edema—a collection of intraretinal fluid in the macula, with or without lipid exudates and with or without cystoid changes
- Nonperfusion of parafoveal capillaries, with or without intraretinal fluid
- Traction on the macula by fibrous tissue proliferation, causing dragging of the retinal tissue, surface wrinkling, or detachment of the macula
- Intraretinal or preretinal hemorrhage in the macula
- Lamellar or full-thickness retinal hole formation
- Combinations of the processes listed previously

CLINICAL PRESENTATION

A person with DME may have no ocular or visual symptoms, and visual acuity may be 20/20 or better. In advanced cases, or when edema threatens or involves the center of the macula, a patient may complain of blurred vision, distorted vision, or warping of straight lines. Some patients complain that bathroom tile patterns, or similar patterns, appear distorted.

Different tests of visual function are useful in evaluating and monitoring progression of macular edema and educating patients about macular disease (Table

TABLE 24.1. Tests of Macular Function

Test	*Comment*
Visual acuity	May be 20/20 or better
	May be reduced
Contrast sensitivity	May be normal
	May be reduced, particularly in high-frequency range
Color vision	May be normal
(D-15, Munsell 100 Hue tests)	Tritan/blue-yellow defect
Amsler grid	May be normal
	Central or paracentral metamorphopsia or loss of contrast

24.1). Warping or distortion on Amsler grid testing is not infrequent, particularly when macular edema involves the center of the macula. Contrast sensitivity testing may show a reduction in sensitivity, especially in the high- and mid-frequency pattern range. Color vision testing on Desaturated D-15 Panel or Farnsworth-Munsell 100 Hue tests may show decreased blue-yellow sensitivity because of disruption of macular cones. However, Amsler grid testing, contrast sensitivity acuity, and color vision can all be normal in the presence of CSME.

Clinical Description and Diagnosis

Proper evaluation for DME requires stereoscopic evaluation of the macula through dilated pupils with either stereoscopic fundus photography or fundus biomicroscopy. *No* test of visual function, including visual acuity, Amsler grid testing, contrast sensitivity testing, or color vision testing, can replace proper stereoscopic evaluation of the macula, although such ancillary tests are helpful in educating patients concerning the effects of macular disease, monitoring the status of macular disease, and evaluating the response to laser photocoagulation. Fluorescein angiography (FA) is usually necessary in determining treatable lesions for focal laser surgery for macular edema, but FA is usually not necessary for diagnosing macular edema. Indeed, there may be areas of leakage in the macular area on FA, but if there is not an accumulation of fluid or thickening in the macular area, macular edema is not present (Figure 24.1).

Macular edema is not always easy to identify, and its presence may be questionable. On examination, macular edema may show as a dull or gray area, or there may be other subtle changes in retinal color or loss of retinal transparency in the macula.

In stereoscopic macular examination, the pit of the fovea in a healthy eye appears to lie on the retinal pigment epithelium, without any apparent thickness. This image is most clearly appreciated with stereoscopic fundus photography. The retinal thickness of the area of the posterior pole, approximately 0.5–1.0 disc diameters (DD) from the center of the macular, corresponding to the hill of Clivus,

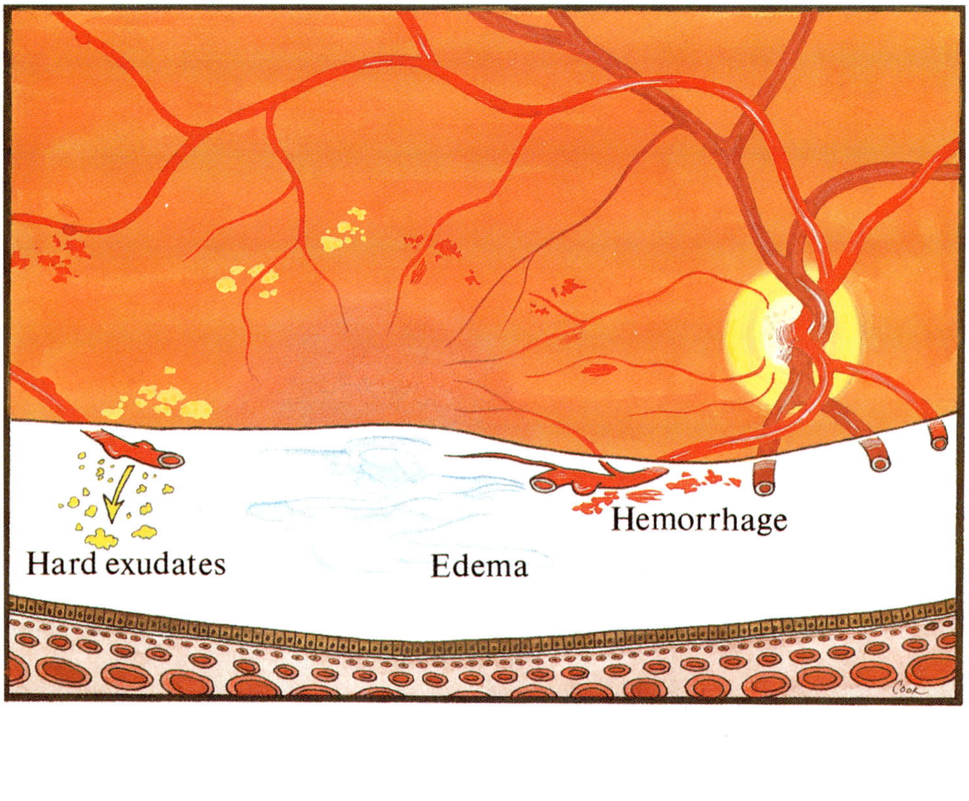

FIGURE 24.1. Schematic depiction of diabetic macular edema. Leakage of fluid and protein into the sensory retina results in retinal thickening. While hard exudates may be easily discerned with a direct ophthalmoscope, retinal thickening is much more subtle and requires stereoscopic evaluation with a fundus lens and biomicroscope. Patients with suspicion of retinal edema, hard exudates, and hemorrhages or microaneurysms in the macular area or decreased vision of unknown or questionable cause should be referred to a retinal specialist for evaluation.

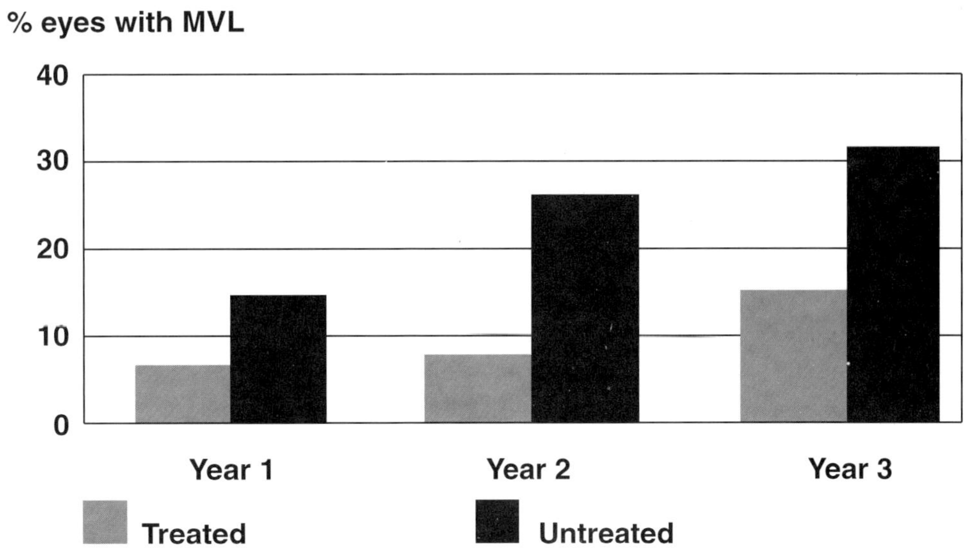

FIGURE 24.2. Bar graph based on Early Treatment Diabetic Retinopathy Study results illustrating the benefit of focal laser photocoagulation in preventing moderate visual loss for eyes with mild-to-moderate nonproliferative diabetic retinopathy and edema involving or threatening the center of the macula. (MVL = moderate visual loss.)

appears approximately twice the diameter of a normal retinal vein at the disc margin. This area is assumed to be the thickest area of the retina in a healthy eye and is a useful reference gauge for the presence or absence of retinal thickening. The diameter of the optic nerve head, which is approximately 1,500 μ, is a useful reference gauge to evaluate the position of retinal thickening or hard exudates in relation to the center of the macula.

The presence in the macula of hard exudates, intraretinal microvascular anomalies, hemorrhages, or microaneurysms is a strong indicator that macular edema may be present. Hard exudates are comparatively easy to identify. They are shiny white or yellowish-white deposits, usually with sharp borders, within the outer layers of the retina. When retinal edema is present, the waxy exudates may be more superficial in the retinal layers. The exudates may be isolated, individual spots, confluent patches, or full or partial rings. These rings of exudates frequently surround areas of retinal edema or areas of leaking microaneurysms, from which the exudates emanate. The exudates are composed of fluids, lipids, and small molecules and are a sign of a leaky capillary bed. Hard exudates may or may not be accompanied by retinal thickening.

Hard exudates are not to be confused with "soft" exudates or cotton wool spots. Soft exudates are more superficial in the retina and represent focal areas of swelling of the nerve fiber layer resulting from ischemia within this layer. The edges of the soft exudates are usually more feathery than the discrete borders of hard exudates.

Clinically, macular edema is retinal thickening within 2 DD of the center of the macula (*not* fluorescein leakage without thickening). Retinal thickening or hard exudates with adjacent retinal thickening that threaten or involve the center of the macula is considered to be CSME. To summarize, CSME exists when any one of the following conditions is present:

- Thickening of the retina located less than or equal to 500 μ from the center of the macula
- Hard exudates with thickening of the adjacent retina located less than or equal to 500 μ from the center of the macula
- A zone or zones of retinal thickening, 1 DD or larger in size, located less than or equal to 1 DD from the center of the macula

MANAGEMENT

The ETDRS has shown conclusively that focal laser photocoagulation reduces the risk of MVL (a doubling of the visual angle, e.g., 20/30 reduced to 20/60) by 50% or more for eyes with CSME (Figure 24.2). In the ETDRS, focal treatment for DME reduced the risk of MVL, was more likely to improve the level of visual acuity, reduced the amount of retinal thickening, and had no adverse side effects on central visual fields and color vision compared with eyes assigned to treatment deferral.

Although focal laser photocoagulation is the only proven method of reducing the risk of visual loss from DME, various strategies have been attempted to control or cure it. Pharmacologic methods have been used to decrease total serum lipids, but this therapy has not proven effective. Diet modification, with a reduction of fats and cholesterol levels, seems to have some positive impact in reducing hard exudates. Carbonic anhydrase inhibitors and other intraocular pressure-lowering agents have also been attempted and may have some efficacy.

TABLE 24.2. Primary Care Management of Diabetic Macular Edema[a]

Clinical finding	*Management*
Reduced visual acuity	Prompt referral[b]
Distortion on Amsler grid testing	Referral
Acquired blue-yellow color defect	Referral
Clinically significant macular edema	Prompt referral
Macular edema, not clinically significant macular edema	Referral
Hemorrhages or microaneurysms in macular area, with or without retinal thickening	Referral

[a]The presence of proliferative retinopathy or eyes with diabetic macular edema and severe or worse nonproliferative diabetic retinopathy warrants prompt referral; the presence of diabetic macular edema with symptoms or conditions such as nephropathy, hypertension, and hyperlipidemia also warrants prompt referral.
[b]Referral is to a retinologist skilled in the management of diabetic eye disease.

Patients who have or are suspected of having macular edema should be evaluated by a retinal specialist (Table 24.2). The ETDRS recognized specific macular lesions that pose a significant threat of MVL. The presence of any one of these lesions signifies CSME (Figures 24.3 and 24.4).

Patients with CSME should normally undergo focal laser photocoagulation. In some cases, macular edema that has not reached the level of CSME may be treated with focal photocoagulation. For example, scatter (panretinal) laser photocoagulation may cause or increase preexisting macular edema; eyes that seem to be progressing toward high-risk proliferative retinopathy may be treated with focal photocoagulation even if the edema is not at the CSME stage. Coincident medical conditions, such as renal disease and hypertension, also may be an indication for focal laser photocoagulation, even if an eye is not at the CSME stage. These treatment decisions are best made by a retinologist skilled in the management of diabetic eye disease.

Focal laser treatment for DME involves either *direct* focal treatment to discrete areas of leaking thought

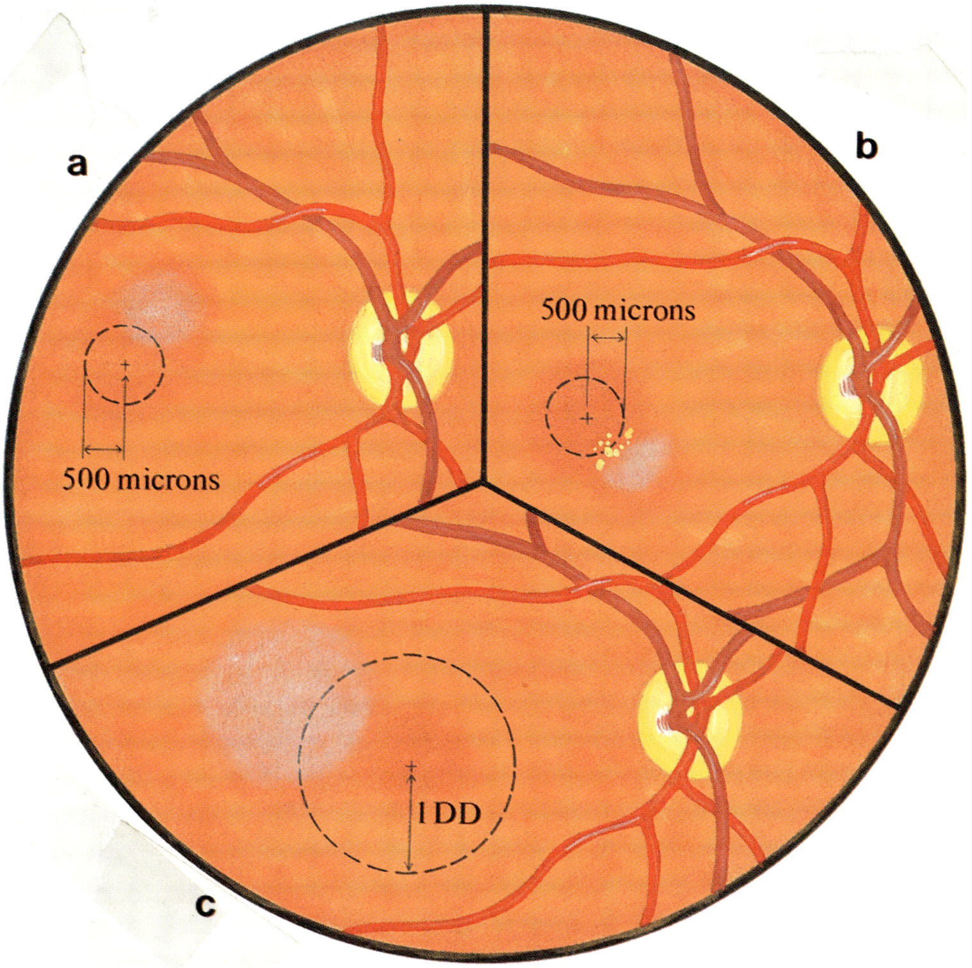

FIGURE 24.3. Composite schematic showing the various lesions of clinically significant macular edema. Macular edema or macular thickening may only be seen by stereoscopic evaluation of the macula with fundus lens and stereobiomicroscope or by stereofundus photography. The presence or absence of macular edema is frequently difficult to detect, even for experienced examiners. The presence of macular edema, the suspicion of its presence, or unexplained visual loss warrants referral. Tests such as Amsler grid testing, contrast sensitivity testing, and color vision testing, while important adjunct tests of visual function, cannot replace appropriate macular examination. a. Thickening of the retina less than 500 μ from the center of the macula. b. Hard exudates less than or equal to 500 μ from the center of the macula accompanied with retinal thickening. c. Retinal thickening greater than or equal to 1 DD in size with a portion of the thickening less than 1 DD from the center of the macula.

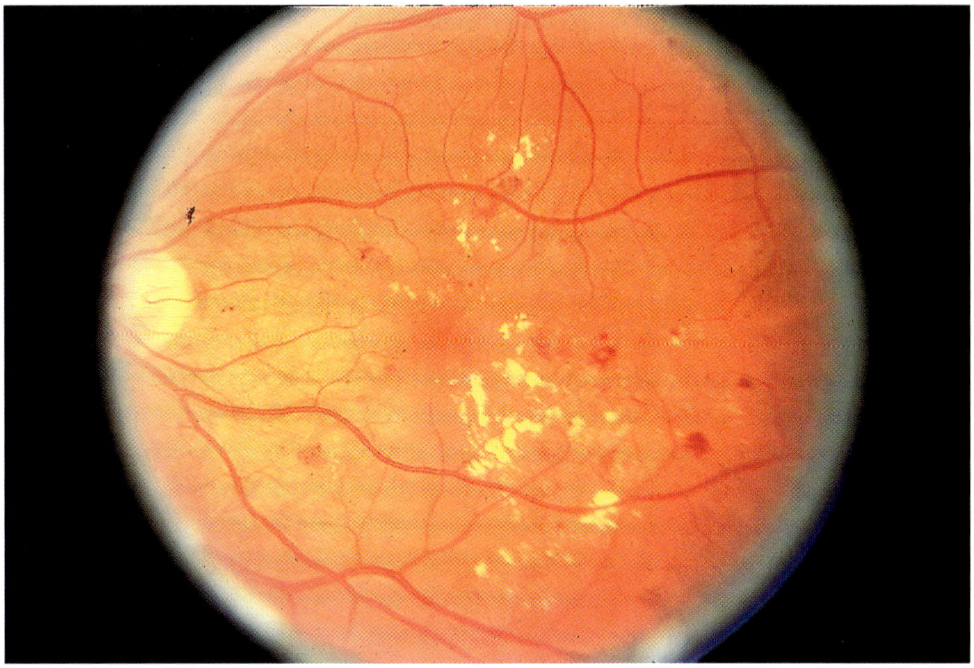

FIGURE 24.4. Clinical appearance of hard exudates less than 500 μ from the center of the macula. There is thickening of the adjacent retina not appreciated without stereoscopic observation. Visual acuity is 20/20.

to be contributing to retinal thickening identified on FA, *grid* focal treatment to areas of diffuse leakage or areas on nonperfused retina that is thickened, or combinations of grid and direct focal treatment. FA is used to identify these "treatable lesions" (Table 24.3). In managing CSME, there are particular retinal lesions identified on FA by the ETDRS that are amenable to treatment. These "treatable lesions" associated with macular edema include those shown in the following list:

- Focal leaks greater than 500 μ from the center of the macula thought to be causing retinal thickening or hard exudates (Figure 24.5)
- Focal leaks 300–500 μ from the center of the macula thought to be causing retinal thickening or hard exudates if it appears that treatment is likely to destroy the remaining perifoveal capillary network and visual acuity is 20/40 or worse
- Areas of diffuse leakage (Figure 24.6) from extensive numbers of microaneurysms or from many intraretinal microvascular anomalies
- Avascular zones, other than the normal foveal avascular zone, not previously treated (Figure 24.7)

Table 24.3 summarizes the management recommendations for CSME at the various retinopathy levels.

The 3-year risk of MVL from macular edema in the ETDRS without focal laser treatment was 30%. Focal laser surgery for CSME reduced this risk to 15%, reducing the risk of MVL by approximately 50%. Focal treatment also increased the chance of improvement in visual acuity of one line or more. On the other hand, scatter (panretinal) laser surgery was not effective in managing DME and, in some cases, may have had a deleterious effect on the progression of macular edema.

The timing of focal laser photocoagulation for DME requires the judgment of an experienced examiner guided by the findings of the ETDRS. Eyes with CSME and retinopathy that are approaching high-risk PDR are best treated first with focal photocoagulation for the macular edema 6–8 weeks before initiating scatter (panretinal) laser surgery. Eyes with mild or moderate nonproliferative diabetic retinopathy and CSME respond best to prompt focal photocoagulation with scatter treatment delayed, unless very severe nonproliferative diabetic retinopathy or high-risk PDR occurs.

Delaying scatter photocoagulation while focal treatment is being completed is unlikely to increase the risk of severe visual loss, provided the retinopathy is not progressing rapidly and careful follow-up can be maintained. Delaying scatter photocoagulation while focal treatment is completed in eyes with high-risk PDR usually is not advisable.

Focal treatment was not attended by adverse effects on central visual field or color vision compared with eyes assigned to deferral of focal treatment in the ETDRS. Any harmful effects of early photocoagulation reflected by constriction of the peripheral visual fields seem to be due mostly to scatter photocoagulation. Because the principal goal of treatment is to prevent a further decrease in visual acuity, focal laser surgery should be considered in

TABLE 24.3. General Management Recommendations

	Natural course (rate of progression to)		*Evaluation*		*Treatment strategies*		
Level of retinopathy	*PDR, 1 year*	*High-risk characteristics, 5 years*	*Color fundus photography*	*Fluorescein angiography*	*Panretinal photocoagulation*	*Focal*	*Follow-up (months)*
Mild NPDR	5%	15%					
No macular edema			No	No	No	No	12
Macular edema			Yes	Occasionally	No	No	4–6
CSME			Yes	Yes	No	Yes	2–4
Moderate NPDR	12–27%	33%					
No macular edema			Yes	No	No	No	6–8
Macular edema (not CSME)			Yes	Occasionally	No	No	4–6
CSME			Yes	Yes	No	Yes	2–4
Severe NPDR	52%	60%					
No macular edema			Yes	No	Rarely	No	3–4
Macular edema (not CSME)			Yes	Occasionally	Occasionally after focal	Occasionally	2–3
CSME			Yes	Yes	Occasionally after focal	Yes	2–3
Very severe NPDR	75%	75%					
No macular edema			Yes	No	Occasionally	No	2–3
Macular edema			Yes	Occasionally	Occasionally after focal	Occasionally	2–3
CSME			Yes	Yes	Occasionally after focal	Yes	2–3
Non–high-risk PDR	—	75%					
No macular edema			Yes	No	Occasionally	No	2–3
Macular edema			Yes	Occasionally	Occasionally after focal	Occasionally	2–3
CSME			Yes	Yes	Occasionally after focal	Yes	2–3
High-risk PDR	—	—					
No macular edema			Yes	No	Yes	No	2–3
Macular edema			Yes	Yes	Yes	Usually	1–2
CSME			Yes	Yes	Yes	Yes	1–2

PDR = proliferative diabetic retinopathy; NPDR = nonproliferative diabetic retinopathy; CSME = clinically significant macular edema.

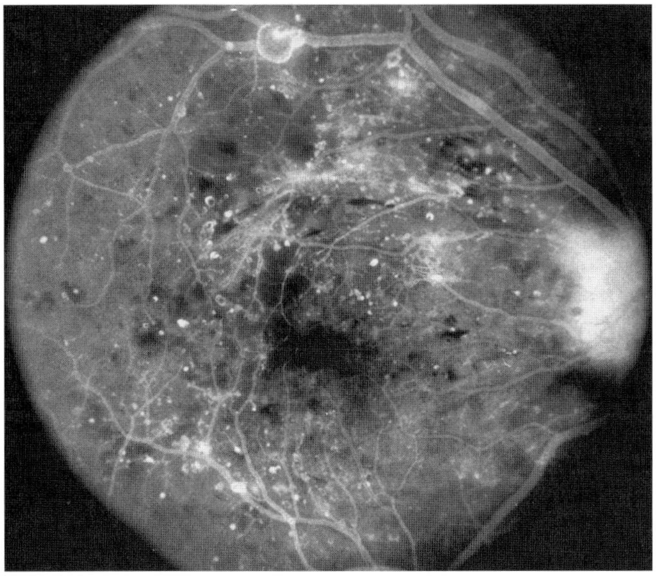

FIGURE 24.5. Fluorescein angiogram showing focal leaks from microaneurysms greater than 500 μ from the center of the macula. There is decreased perfusion in the macular area. Visual acuity is 20/20.

all eyes with CSME, especially if the center of the macula is threatened or involved, even if normal visual acuity is present.

SUMMARY

Timely and appropriate focal laser photocoagulation can significantly reduce the risk of MVL from DME. Since macular edema frequently is most amenable to treatment before there is any loss of visual acuity or other visual symptoms, regular eye examinations by a skilled examiner are important in reducing the risk of visual loss from this condition (Table 24.4). All patients should be encouraged to have an annual eye examination, and patients who have or are suspected of having macular edema, even if it has not reached the clinically significant level, should be referred to a retinal specialist for treatment consideration. Proper management and treatment can significantly reduce the risk of visual loss.

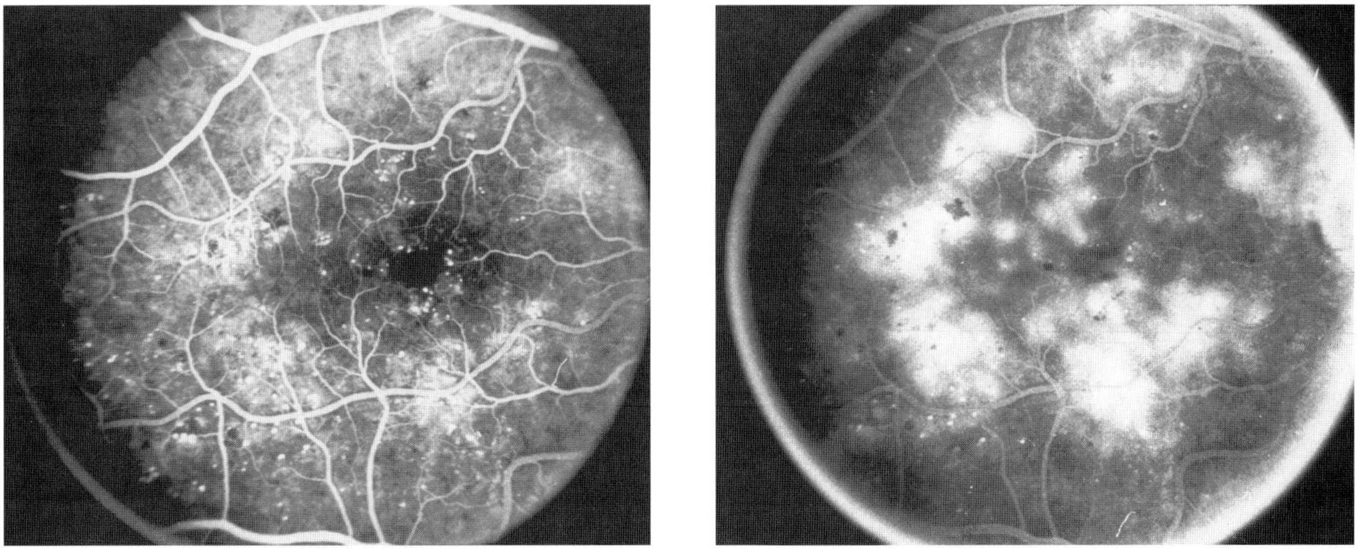

A B

FIGURE 24.6. Areas of diffuse leakage from extensive numbers of microaneurysms. A. There is poor perfusion centrally in the macular area. There are also areas of focal leakage at 500 μ from the center of the macula. Farther out from the center of the macula are multiple microaneurysms with hyperfluorescence. B. In the late phase of the angiogram, diffuse leakage results in staining and accumulation of fluid within the macular area.

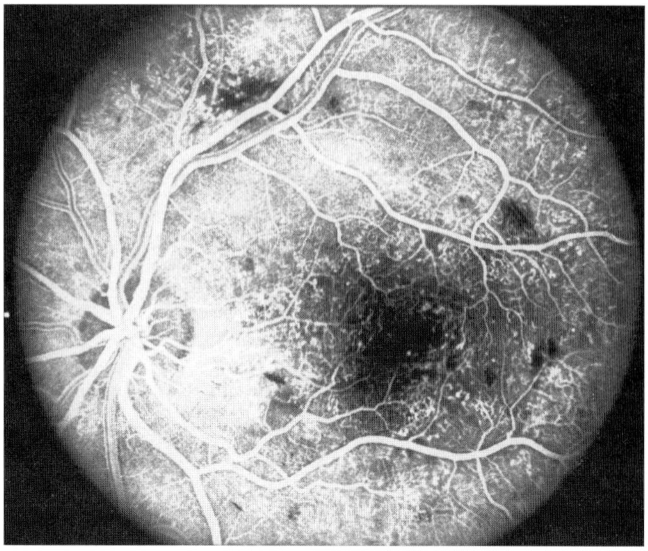

FIGURE 24.7. Avascular zone evident on fluorescein angiography showing poor perfusion within the macular area.

TABLE 24.4. Eye Examination Schedule

Type of diabetes mellitus	*Recommended time of first examination*	*Routine minimum follow-up**
Type I insulin-dependent diabetes mellitus	5 years after onset or during puberty	Yearly
Type II non–insulin-dependent diabetes mellitus	At time of diagnosis	Yearly
During pregnancy	Prior to pregnancy for counseling Early in first trimester Each trimester or more frequently as indicated 3–6 months postpartum	

*Abnormal findings dictate more frequent follow-up examinations (see Table 24.3).

SUGGESTED READING

Diabetic Retinopathy Study report number 10: Factors influencing the development of visual loss in advanced diabetic retinopathy. Invest Ophthalmol 1985;26:983–991.

Diabetic Retinopathy Study report number 11: Intraocular pressure following panretinal photocoagulation for diabetic retinopathy. Arch Ophthalmol 1987;105:807–809.

Diabetic Retinopathy Study report number 12: Macular edema in Diabetic Retinopathy Study patients. Ophthalmology 1987;94:754–760.

Diabetic Retinopathy Study report number 13: Factors associated with visual outcome after photocoagulation for diabetic retinopathy. Invest Ophthalmol 1989;30:23–28.

Diabetic Retinopathy Study report number 14: Indications for photocoagulation treatment of diabetic retinopathy. Int Ophthalmol Clin 1987;27:239–253.

Early Treatment Diabetic Retinopathy Study report number 1: Photocoagulation for diabetic macular edema. Arch Ophthalmol 1985;103:1796–1806.

Early Treatment Diabetic Retinopathy Study report number 2: Treatment techniques and clinical guidelines for photocoagulation of diabetic macular edema. Ophthalmology 1987;94:761–774.

Early Treatment Diabetic Retinopathy Study report number 3: Techniques for scatter and local photocoagulation treatment of diabetic retinopathy. Int Ophthalmol Clin 1987;27:254–264.

Early Treatment Diabetic Retinopathy Study report number 4: Photocoagulation for diabetic macular edema. Int Ophthalmol Clin 1987;27:265–272.

Early Treatment Diabetic Retinopathy Study case report numbers 3 and 4: Case reports to accompany Early Treatment Diabetic Retinopathy Study report numbers 3 and 4. Int Ophthalmol Clin 1987;27:273–333.

Early Treatment Diabetic Retinopathy Study report number 5: Detection of diabetic macular edema. Ophthalmoscopy versus photography. Ophthalmology 1989;96:746–751.

Early Treatment Diabetic Retinopathy Study report number 7: Early Treatment Diabetic Retinopathy Study design and baseline patient characteristics. Ophthalmology 1991;98:741–756.

Early Treatment Diabetic Retinopathy Study report number 8: Effects of aspirin treatment on diabetic retinopathy. Ophthalmology 1991;98:757–765.

Early Treatment Diabetic Retinopathy Study report number 9: Early photocoagulation for diabetic retinopathy. Ophthalmology 1991;98:766–785.

Early Treatment Diabetic Retinopathy Study report number 10: Grading diabetic retinopathy from stereoscopic color fundus photographs—An extension of the modified Airlie House Classification. Ophthalmology 1991;98:786–806.

Early Treatment Diabetic Retinopathy Study report number 11: Classification of diabetic retinopathy from fluorescein angiograms. Ophthalmology 1991;98:807–822.

Early Treatment Diabetic Retinopathy Study report number 12: Fundus photographic risk factors for progression of diabetic retinopathy. Ophthalmology 1991;98:823, 833.

Early Treatment Diabetic Retinopathy Study report number 13: Fluorescein angiographic risk factors for progression of diabetic retinopathy. Ophthalmology 1991;98:834–840.

ETDRS Study Group. Early Treatment Diabetic Retinopathy Study Manual of Operations. Baltimore: ETDRS Coordinating Center, University of Maryland, 1985;4:15;18:18–38.

Klein R, Klein BEK, Moss SE, et al. The Wisconsin Epidemiologic Study of Diabetic Retinopathy. II. Prevalence and risk of diabetic retinopathy when age at diagnosis is less than 30 years. Arch Ophthalmol 1984;102:520–526.

Klein R, Klein BEK, Moss SE, et al. The Wisconsin Epidemiologic Study of Diabetic Retinopathy. III. Prevalence and risk of diabetic retinopathy when age at diagnosis is 30 or more years. Arch Ophthalmol 1984;102:527–532.

CHAPTER

25 The Macula in Retinal Vascular Disease

Leland W. Carr

The retinal blood vessels mirror the state of the body's vascular system and can provide the clinician with important information regarding the patient's general health. Changes in the retinal vessels reflect abnormalities of the blood, blood-forming organs, and the cardiovascular system, and are directly related to changes that occur in the general circulatory system. Although devoid of retinal vessels, the macula can react in a number of ways to various retinal vascular disease states and, because of its unique architecture, responds in a very specific fashion.

The retinal blood vessels can react to insult in several ways. The blood vessel walls may thicken, the lumen may narrow, the vessels may become compressed, an embolus may become lodged within the vessel, or turbulent blood flow at a stricture point may lead to thrombosis with occlusion. The retinal blood flow volume and velocity may vary depending on numerous factors. Retinal vascular perfusion is autoregulated by a combination of factors, including intraocular pressure (IOP) and intrinsic blood oxygen level. The integrity of retinal blood vessel walls can become compromised, resulting in increased permeability and leakage, or in some instances, vascular outpouchings in the form of microaneurysms or macroaneurysms may develop. New retinal vessels can develop if the oxygen level within the retina is sufficiently diminished, and shunt or collateral vessels may form to improve venous outflow.

Retinal vascular disease may significantly impair retinal and subsequently macular function. The extent and location of the vascular compromise will determine the effect on vision and is determined by the degree of dyschromatopsia, dysmorphopsia, and loss of visual function.

Retinal hemorrhages, edema, and exudates may collect at various levels within the retina, leading to photoreceptor and retinal pigment epithelial (RPE) dysfunction. Diseased retinal vessels may cause edema, which can alter the macular thickness and transparency. Blood or fluid accumulation between the sensory retina and the RPE or beneath the RPE may lead to separation of either or both of these layers.

RETINAL VASCULAR OCCLUSIVE DISEASE

Retinal vascular occlusive disease represents an important clinical consideration in the etiopathogenesis of certain macular disease states. Vascular occlusive disease includes branch and central retinal artery and vein occlusion, each occurring with varying degrees of frequency. Branch retinal vein occlusion (BRVO) is more prevalent, whereas arterial occlusive disease is relatively rare but yields a poorer prognosis. The symptoms of vascular occlusive disease vary depending on the site of occlusion and the extent of retinal damage. Typically, the patient reports a sudden, painless, unilateral, partial-to-complete loss of vision. The visual loss may go unnoticed if the patient fails to separate visual function of each eye or if the macula is spared. The significance of retinal vascular occlusion rests with the high probability that systemic disease is present and inadequately controlled.

Following retinal vascular occlusion, the prognosis for visual recovery is dependent on the overall status of the patient's vascular system. The faster blood flow is reestablished, the less likely there will be long-term retinal tissue damage. This phenomenon is particularly important in arterial occlusive disease, where rapid vasodilation and improved perfusion pressure may restore retinal blood flow by dislodging a thrombus or embolus. Should this occur, vision loss will be transient, a condition referred to as *amaurosis fugax* or *fleeting monocular vision loss*. Similarly, an undamaged venous and capillary system can recover from central retinal vein occlusion (CRVO) or BRVO and recanalization may occur around a blockage point. Collateral or shunt venous channels may develop from preexisting, smaller caliber veins and capillaries that become distended in order to resume the normal vascular drainage of the occluded vessel.

Systemic disease is an important consideration in retinal vascular disease. Important systemic vascular disease states include arteriosclerosis, hypertension, diabetes, and carotid artery and coronary artery disease. Arteriosclerosis disposes patients to all four types of retinal vascular occlusion. An evaluation for underlying systemic vascular disease should be aggressively pursued in patients with vascular occlusion. Systemic hypertension, diabetes mellitus, carotid artery disease, and coronary artery disease must be considered, along with clotting disorders causing thrombus and embolus formation. These conditions include cardiac valve disease, cardiac arrhythmia, systemic lupus erythematosus, syphilis, temporal arteritis, sickle cell disease, and the primary dysproteinemias. Ocular ischemic syndrome and primary open-angle glaucoma should also be considered.

MACULAR EDEMA

The extent of macular damage resulting from a retinal vascular occlusive event depends on two factors: the amount and duration of edema in the fovea, and the degree of infarction and necrosis of the papillomacular pathway linking the fovea and the optic nerve.

The extent, distribution, and consistency of macular edema determines the amount of permanent damage. Macular edema can lead to RPE and photoreceptor disruption and permanent loss of central visual function. The integrity of the capillary network will influence the formation as well as the drainage of fluid from the macula. Diffuse or cystoid macular edema (CME) frequently accompanies venous occlusive disease but is rarely a factor in arterial occlusion. Chronic CME can lead to epiretinal membrane formation and possibly to macular hole formation.

ARTERIAL OCCLUSIVE DISEASE

Branch and central retinal arterial occlusions represent the same disease process and have similar etiologies. Arterial occlusive disease occurs more frequently at or beyond the sixth decade and is slightly more prevalent in men. There is an acute onset of vision loss that may cause total loss of visual function. The visual field loss may manifest as a small paracentral scotoma, a hemianopsia, or total loss of the visual field resulting in no light perception. The extent of visual field loss depends on the site of obstruction and the area of retina compromised by the occlusion.

Clinical Features of Central Retinal Artery Occlusion

- Sixth decade
- Positive afferent pupillary defect
- Threadlike, segmented arterial column during acute phase
- Grayish-white, thickened retina with obscured view of underlying choroidal detail
- Foveal cherry-red spot
- Subtle optic nerve head pallor
- Slight arteriolar caliber narrowing
- Arteriolar wall sheathing
- Optic atrophy

Clinical Features of Branch Retinal Artery Occlusion

- Narrowed arteriolar blood column
- Relucent retina surrounding involved area
- Arteriolar wall sclerosis

Arterial blockage typically occurs in an elderly patient with a well-established history of atherosclerosis and may be caused by thrombus formation at a narrow portion of the artery or an embolic event. Occasionally younger patients are encountered who are prone to clotting disorders resulting from inflammatory vasculitis, as seen in systemic lupus erythematosus, syphilis, or polyarteritis nodosa.

Systemic Conditions Frequently Associated with Retinal Arterial Occlusive Disease

- Arteriosclerosis
- Systemic hypertension
- Carotid artery disease
- Diabetes mellitus
- Cardiac valve disease
- Collagen vascular disease
- Hypercoagulation states
- Giant cell arteritis

Immediately after an occlusion occurs, the arterial blood column distal to the point of blockage becomes threadlike and segmented. Some degree of blood flow is almost immediately reestablished, and only a subtle reduction in the caliber of the flow column remains. Within minutes following occlusion of the central retinal artery, the retinal nerve fiber layer is compromised, and the patient acquires a relative afferent pupillary defect.

If retinal circulation is not adequately restored within 1–2 hours, oxygen deprivation leads to infarction

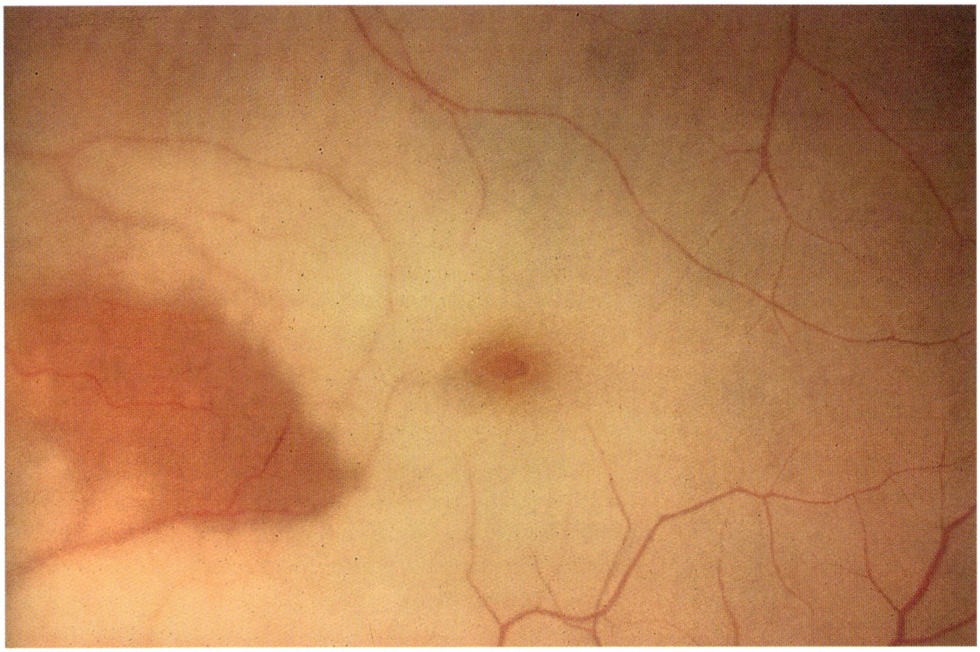

A

FIGURE 25.1. A. Central retinal artery occlusion depicting opaque, edematous, necrotic retina with the foveal red spot and healthy retina nasal to the fovea served by the cilioretinal artery. (Courtesy of J. Cavallerano.) B. Branch retinal artery occlusion in a patient with anterior ischemic optic neuropathy demonstrating hemorrhage and edema of the optic disc.

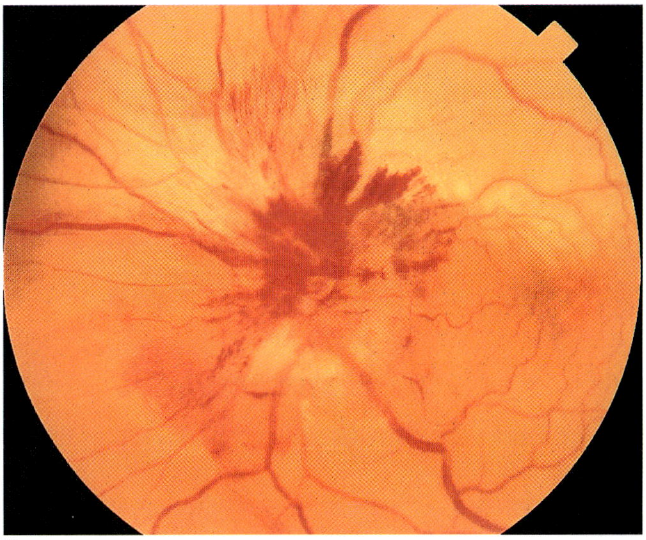

B

and permanent retinal tissue damage. Ischemic damage to the ganglion cell and nerve fiber layers of the papillomacular bundle interrupts foveal communication with the visual pathway. Ischemia also causes severe damage to the inner sensory retina due to the high metabolic demand of the axons within the papillomacular bundle.

The site of arterial obstruction dictates the appearance of the retina. A gray, hazy appearance is observed in mild cases, and if severe, the retina may become totally opaque (Figure 25.1). Optic nerve head edema often accompanies intracellular edema and necrosis. The absence of inner retinal layers at the fovea, combined with the columnar arrangement and dense subfoveal RPE cells and the density of the underlying choriocapillaris, cause the fovea to appear brownish-red in comparison to the adjacent retina. This explains the appearance of the characteristic cherry-red spot observed in arterial occlusive disease. Intraretinal hemorrhage is extremely rare with arterial occlusive disease and should increase the index of suspicion for an accompanying venous stasis retinopathy.

Inner retinal tissue necrosis occurs so rapidly in arterial occlusive disease that angiogenesis and release of vasoproliferative factors does not occur, and retinal neovascularization, neovascularization of the iris (NVI), and subsequent neovascular glaucoma rarely occur.

Approximately one out of five eyes contains one or more cilioretinal arteries that originate from the choroidal vascular system. These vessels pass through the temporal optic nerve head and along the papillomacular pathway, sometimes reaching the fovea. Cilioretinal arteries are independent from the retinal circulation and remain patent following central retinal artery occlusion. A segment of viable retina will be maintained, and the patient describes a central sparing of visual function. Conversely, the cilioretinal artery may occlude as an isolated event, leading to significant loss of vision to the corresponding area of the retina served by the artery.

Management of Arterial Occlusive Disease

Vision loss associated with retinal arterial occlusive disease is typically profound and permanent. The prognosis for preservation of visual function can be improved if treatment is instituted immediately. Management typically involves a rapid lowering of the IOP while elevating the blood perfusion pressure to the eye by inducing arterial dilation. The goal is to dislodge the embolus and promote distal movement along the arterial pathway. Paracentesis is performed to reduce IOP rapidly, and a retrobulbar injection of lidocaine without epinephrine may help to stimulate dilation of the central retinal artery. Alternatively, inhalation of 5% carbon dioxide with 95% oxygen (Carbogen) or breathing into a bag may be used to induce vasodilation. Oral carbonic anhydrase inhibitors and topical beta-blockers are often added to help maintain a low IOP.

Treatment for Acute (<24-Hour Old) Retinal Arterial Occlusive Disease

- Reduce IOP immediately
- Induce arterial vasodilation
- Increase blood flow to the eye

Failure to reverse the ischemic process within 24 hours results in permanent vision loss and at this point emphasis should be directed to identifying the underlying systemic disease. The patient should be monitored regularly for neovascular changes of the posterior and anterior segments.

Prognosis Following Acute Retinal Artery Occlusion

- Less than 35% recover to 20/100 or better
- Eighteen percent suffer stroke within 6 years
- Thirty-four percent die within 6 years (myocardial infarction, most common cause)
- Ocular neovascularization occurs in less than 5% of cases

VENOUS OCCLUSIVE DISEASE

Retinal venous occlusive disease is classified according to the site of obstruction. BRVO, in which the peripheral or tributary portion of the system is blocked, is more common than CRVO. In CRVO, venous outflow is obstructed by occlusion or compression of the retinal vein at the disc. Ischemic and nonischemic venous occlusions are also classified according to the degree and extent of remaining capillary perfusion.

Retinal venous occlusion is commonly associated with systemic hypertension or arteriosclerosis. Other conditions such as inflammatory phlebitis or diabetes promote occlusion by reducing blood flow through increased blood viscosity. Optic nerve head anatomy may dispose the patient to retinal vein occlusion. Deep glaucomatous cupping and acute coursing and kinking of the vessels as they pass over the edge of the optic disc may also lead to occlusion. Acute or progressive elevation of IOP may provide the small additional force needed to trigger an occlusion in one of the veins along the disc. IOP measurements should be obtained in both eyes, and prophylactic pressure reduction should be considered by use of topical agents.

Conditions Frequently Associated with Occlusive Retinal Venous Disease

- Arteriosclerosis
- Systemic hypertension
- Diabetes mellitus
- Open-angle glaucoma
- Hyperlipidemia, hyperviscosity, cryofibrinogenemia
- Platelet-coagulation abnormalities
- Carotid artery disease

CRVO often involves compression of the soft, pliable venous wall by the rigid arteriosclerotic central retinal artery. This usually occurs within the optic nerve at the level of the lamina cribrosa. At this location, the artery and vein are held together by a common sheath of fascial connective tissue, with the central retinal vein being physiologically narrowed as it passes through its scleral canal. Additionally, the laminar edge may provide a stiff scaffold against which the vein can be compressed, constricting the vein and reducing blood flow. As the vein becomes progressively flattened, its lumen narrows, leading to turbulent flow and predisposing to thrombus formation and occlusion.

NONISCHEMIC VENOUS OCCLUSIVE RETINOPATHY

CRVO may develop slowly over time, often as the result of insidious compression of the retinal veins. This leads to progressive slowing of venous outflow from the retina, which translates directly into increased levels of venous backpressure and vessel distension. This is sometimes referred to as *venous stasis retinopathy*, and impaired retinal drainage produces microvascular damage throughout the affected vascular watershed. Capillaries are distended, tortuous, and dotted with microaneurysms. Small-to-moderate flame-shaped hemorrhages and edematous retina develop as vessel wall integrity becomes compromised. Cotton wool spots (CWS), if present, are generally few and small. Severe retinal ischemia and widespread capillary nonperfusion are not typical features of nonischemic venous occlusion. Instead, capillary dilatation and fluid leakage into the macula area may compromise vision through the production of cystoid and other forms of edema. CME is characterized by increased fluid in the spaces of the macula and a diffuse loss of transparency accompanied by thickened tissue (Figure 25.2).

Clinical Presentation of Nonischemic Central Retinal Vein Occlusion

- Sixth decade
- Visual acuity often 20/50 or better

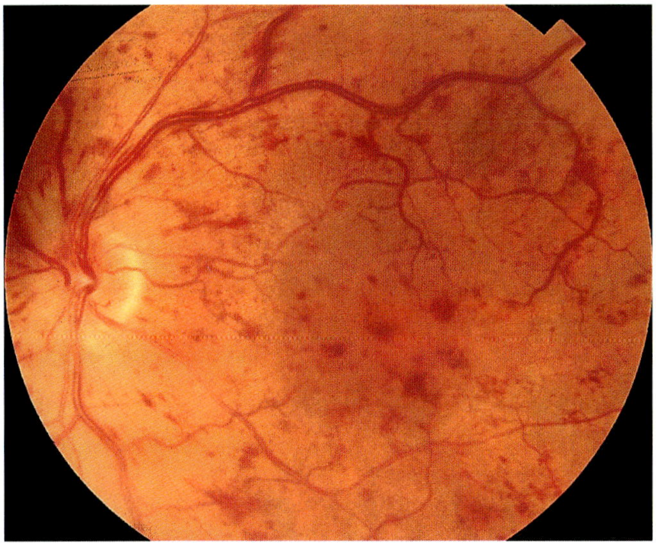

A

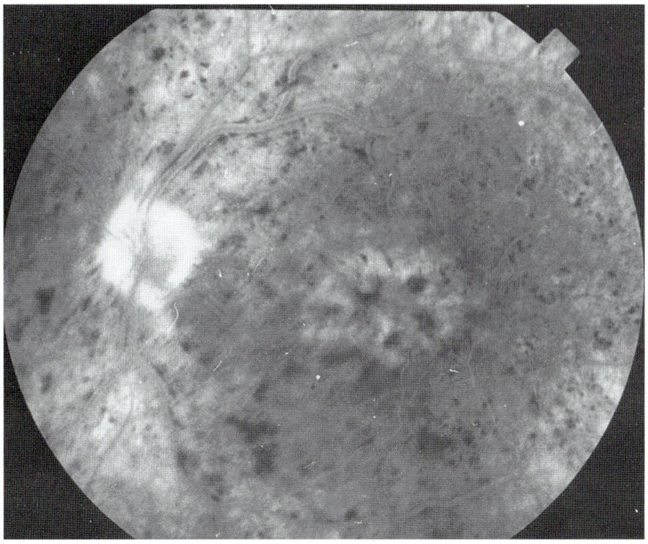

B

FIGURE 25.2. Clinical photograph (A) and the late phase of a fluorescein angiogram (B) revealing the petalloid pattern of hyperfluorescence in the left eye of a patient with cystoid macular edema from central retinal vein occlusion.

- Thirty percent show positive afferent pupillary defect
- Distended retinal veins
- Irregular venous caliber
- Intraretinal hemorrhages following the venous distribution
- Macular hemorrhages and edema
- Intraretinal collateral venous-to-venous shunt vessels
- Opticociliary collateral network on optic nerve head
- Neovascularization of retina, optic disc, and iris possible

With nonischemic CRVO, the retinal vascular system can remain functional through alternative means. Preexisting capillary channels become dilated and form collateral circulation, while opticociliary shunt vessels develop at the disc to create a new pathway for retinal drainage. Here, venous blood is shunted into the underlying choroidal system for drainage through the vortex veins, thus bypassing the occluded central retinal vein. Venous-to-venous collateral networks may also develop adjacent to areas of poor venous outflow in the retina.

Prognosis for Nonischemic Central Retinal Vein Occlusion

- Visual acuity often 20/40 or better
- Occasionally persistent macular edema and pigment degeneration
- Retinal neovascularization rare
- Neovascular glaucoma in less than 1% of cases

Management of Nonischemic Venous Occlusive Retinopathy

Treatment of nonischemic venous occlusion is directed at addressing the tendency for clot formation. Treatment or improved control of hypertension along with anticoagulation therapy, initially in the form of low-dose aspirin, should be considered. Neovascularization is not a common sequela but may develop, and patients should be monitored at routine intervals for complications of neovascularization including neovascularization of the disc and neovascularization elsewhere. A small percentage of nonischemic CRVO convert to the ischemic form.

NVI typically starts within the collarette zone, adjacent to the pupil, but may rarely begin within the anterior chamber angle. Careful examination of the iris prior to dilation and gonioscopy is advisable.

Fluorescein angiography (FA) may be indicated to identify areas of capillary nonperfusion. If substantial areas of retinal ischemia are detected, scatter laser photocoagulation may be considered to prevent the release of vasoproliferative factors that may induce subsequent neovascularization.

ISCHEMIC VENOUS OCCLUSIVE DISEASE

Ischemic venous occlusive disease can be more devastating to the patient than the nonischemic form because of the attendant complications. When venous occlusion is sudden and complete, as with acute thrombosis at a point of arteriovenous compression, retinal ischemia may develop. This form of occlusion produces hemorrhagic retinopathy, and the retinal veins are engorged, irregular

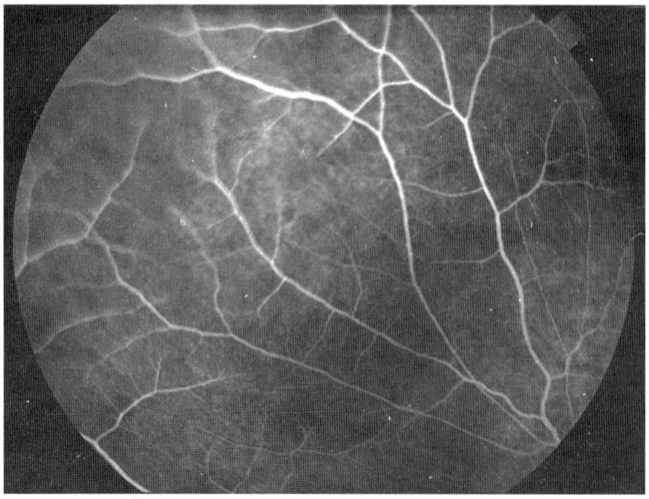

FIGURE 25.3. Fluorescein angiogram in ischemic venous occlusion with dark areas indicating capillary nonperfusion and retinal ischemia.

in caliber, and tortuous. Large, flame-shaped hemorrhages, numerous CWS, and diffuse retinal edema are evident. Extensive areas of capillary nonperfusion can also be present in hemorrhagic retinopathy, putting the patient at risk for neovascularization of the disc, neovascularization elsewhere, and NVI (Figure 25.3). Neovascularization is usually evident during the first 2–4 months following the occlusion. An effective collateral drainage network may develop if enough capillary channels remain patent.

Clinical Presentation of Ischemic Central Retinal Vein Occlusion

- Sixth decade
- Vision 20/400 or worse
- Positive afferent pupillary defect
- Blurred or obscured disc margins
- Grossly irregular retinal veins
- Numerous large, flame-shaped retinal hemorrhages and CWS
- Numerous intraretinal hemorrhages
- Occasional preretinal and vitreous hemorrhages
- Intraretinal venous-to-venous collateral shunts
- Opticociliary network on optic nerve head
- Neovascularization of retina, optic disc, and iris

Prognosis of Ischemic Central Retinal Vein Occlusion

- Visual recovery rare
- Persistent macular edema, hemorrhage, exudate, and cysts
- Perifoveal capillary nonperfusion
- Macular holes
- Ocular neovascularization
- Neovascular glaucoma in 50% of cases

Management should include careful monitoring for NVI, neovascular glaucoma, neovascularization of the disc, and neovascularization elsewhere during the first 6 months, and control of systemic hypertension and anticoagulant therapy should be considered.

BRANCH RETINAL VEIN OCCLUSION

BRVO usually occurs in the temporal retina at a point of compression created by an arteriovenous crossing. Typically, the arterial wall thickens and becomes rigid as a result of arteriosclerosis. A shared fascial sheath allows the nonpliable arterial vessel to flatten the unprotected, nonmuscular venule. This creates distortion of the venous lumen, leading to restricted and turbulent flow, thus disposing it to clot formation. As the occlusion develops, venous pressure extends away from the constriction point, back toward the capillary bed, thus reducing the overall net flow velocity.

Clinical Presentation of Branch Retinal Vein Occlusion

- Fifth decade
- Often asymptomatic
- Visual acuity variable depending on extent of macular involvement
- May be preceded by splinter hemorrhage at site of arteriovenous crossing compression (Bonnet's sign)
- Affected venules are dilated and tortuous
- Intraretinal hemorrhages in involved area
- CWS with capillary nonperfusion
- Collateral vascularization
- CME and other edema
- Ocular neovascularization

Branch venous occlusion often goes unnoticed by the patient because the macula is not always involved. However, capillary nonperfusion, vascular leakage, intraretinal hemorrhage, and the accumulation of cystic or non-CME may affect vision. Branch vein occlusions affecting the superior arcades are more likely to involve the macula simply due to gravitational influence. If the perifoveal capillary bed remains undamaged, central visual function often returns after the hemorrhage and edema resolve. This process typically requires anywhere from 3 to 6 months following the occlusive event.

The ischemic event can cause generalized changes in the larger, nonoccluded veins and arteries as they course through the nonperfused section of retina. Although these vessels remain patent, their outer walls

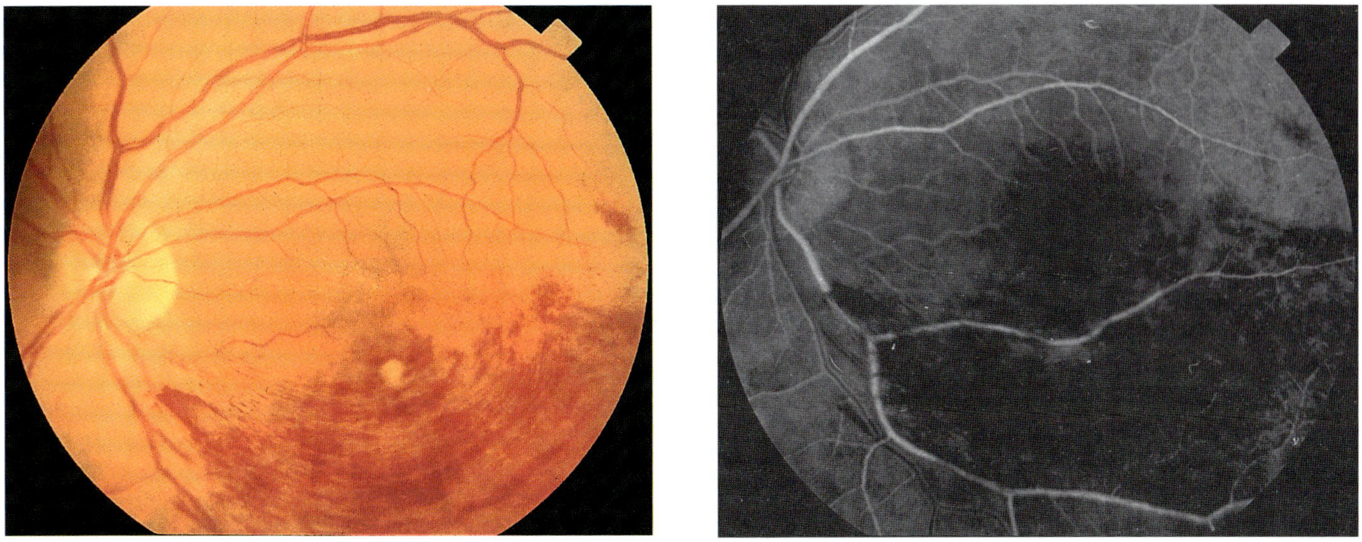

A B

FIGURE 25.4. A. Inferior branch retinal vein occlusion with loss of transparency of the retina in the macular area due to macular edema. B. Substantial areas of capillary nonperfusion are apparent in the macula in the arteriovenous phase of the fluorescein angiogram. Treatment by laser photocoagulation may prevent further vision loss due to macular edema and helps to militate against retinal neovascularization. (Reprinted with permission from A Cavallerano. Cystoid macular edema. Clin Eye Vis Care 1992;4:87–91.)

suffer damage from ischemia, taking on the thickened, white, opaque appearance of vessel sheathing. Although vessel sheathing occurs, giving the illusion of possible obstruction, FA demonstrates that these vessels remain fully patent.

Chronic capillary compromise may lead to permanent impairment of vision. Chronic CME and other edema, secondary epiretinal gliosis, or ischemia can render the affected retina nonfunctional. Focal or grid-pattern macular photocoagulation may have value in reducing chronic macular edema associated with BRVO. Controversy exists as to whether photocoagulation is most effective early on or when the macular edema is long-standing.

Hard exudates in the macula often accompany venous occlusive disease when perifoveal capillary network nonperfusion is present. The remaining viable capillaries become dilated, distended, and engorged, responding to the need for collateral drainage. This results in loss of vessel wall integrity, increased permeability, and exudative leakage into the macular area. This creates a clinically distinctive pattern, observed ophthalmoscopically, of stellate configuration of exudative material in the macular area.

Obstruction of a major retinal vein often leads to extensive capillary nonperfusion. As venous pressure increases, the capillary flow stops, and the clot within the precapillary arteriolar area leads to severe, widespread, retinal ischemia. Numerous CWS and retinal hemorrhage are observed at all levels of the retina, and FA confirms the presence of extensive nonperfusion.

Macular Branch Vein Occlusion

A subclassification of BRVO deserving special consideration involves macular branch vein occlusion. Small venous channels are located between the superior and inferior vascular arcades and are vital for macular drainage. When occluded, the patient almost always experiences blurred vision due to edema. Fundus biomicroscopy reveals foveal thickening and CME. Small aneurysms are typically seen under high magnification, and tiny collateral channels may be observed. Diagnostic confirmation is made through FA. Treatment of macular edema includes focal and grid-pattern laser photocoagulation. Neovascular complications are extremely rare (Figure 25.4).

Management of Branch Retinal Vein Occlusion

Following a BRVO, the eye suffering from severe ischemia may respond by releasing a vasoproliferative factor, and neovascularization may occur. NVI is an uncommon sequela of BRVO and occurs in only 1–3% of cases. A greater threat is posed by retinal neovascularization, which occurs in approximately 20% of all cases of BRVO, most commonly within the retinal area

TABLE 25.1. Incidence of Ocular Neovascularization with Venous Occlusion

	Central retinal vein occlusion (%)	*Branch retinal vein occlusion (%)*
Neovascularization of the disc	11	11
Neovascularization elsewhere	2	21
Neovascularization of the iris	15	2
Neovascular glaucoma	8–25	1

served by the occluded vessel (Table 25.1). Vitreous hemorrhage may also occur. When neovascularization occurs, scatter laser photocoagulation may be effective in eliminating or reducing retinal neovascularization, and early scatter treatment of large ischemic patches may be warranted as a prophylactic measure. Management of BRVO should also include identification and treatment of underlying systemic disease.

OVERVIEW OF PHOTOCOAGULATION STUDIES: BRANCH VEIN OCCLUSION STUDY GROUP (1984 AND 1986) AND CENTRAL RETINAL VEIN OCCLUSION STUDY GROUP (1988 TO PRESENT)

Disagreement regarding the benefit of photocoagulation in the management of retinal venous occlusive disease has led to several multicenter clinical trials designed to evaluate the role of early laser treatment. The Branch Vein Occlusion Study Group findings, commissioned in 1984 and 1986, may be summarized as follows:

A. In patients with macular edema and visual acuity reduction to 20/40 or worse:
   1. Delay FA and photocoagulation until significant clearing of retinal hemorrhages has occurred. However, the following should be considered:
      a. Foveal hemorrhage may be partly responsible for visual acuity reduction.
      b. The FA is difficult to evaluate through the massive intraretinal hemorrhage.
      c. Retinal hemorrhage makes photocoagulation extremely difficult.

B. In patients with vision reduction to 20/40 or worse, perform FA only after sufficient clearing of retinal hemorrhage has occurred.
   1. If macular edema is present, argon green laser photocoagulation should be applied to individual areas of macular leakage.
   2. Photocoagulation is contraindicated in BRVO with vision reduction resulting from macular ischemia (capillary nonperfusion) or from disruption and atrophy of the macular RPE.
   3. Krypton red photocoagulation may be indicated in cases involving vitreous hemorrhage, intraretinal hemorrhages, or advanced lenticular opacification.
   4. Additional treatment is indicated if visual function remains reduced and macular edema persists at a 4-month follow-up evaluation.

C. Patients with BRVO who develop ocular neovascularization (disc, peripheral vessels, or iris) should be treated with scatter laser photocoagulation across all zones of retinal capillary nonperfusion. The following protocol is adhered to:
   1. Argon green is the preferred wavelength.
   2. Krypton red may be indicated in cases involving vitreous hemorrhage, intraretinal hemorrhage, or advanced lenticular opacification.
   3. Neovascularization that persists at the 4-month follow-up visit after laser treatment is considered an indication for additional scatter photocoagulation.

The Central Retinal Vein Occlusion Study (CVOS), a nine-center, controlled clinical trial sponsored by the National Eye Institute, was designed to provide additional insight regarding the natural course of CRVO and the effect of argon green grid-pattern photocoagulation on macular edema resulting from CRVO. Additional insight has been obtained regarding the impact of prophylactic scatter photocoagulation on ischemic forms of CRVO.

Patients were recruited from 1988 through 1991 and were randomly assigned to treatment versus observation groups. Each patient was followed for at least 2 years subsequent to entering the study, and all patients were followed closely for the development of NVI. Any patient who developed 2 or more clock hours of NVI or any patient who developed neovascularization within the anterior chamber angle was immediately assigned to undergo initial (or additional) scatter laser treatment.

Results of the CVOS showed that laser photocoagulation did not improve visual acuity in patients with macular edema secondary to CRVO. The CVOS also demonstrated that for eyes with ischemic CRVO with 10

DD of nonperfusion, there was no benefit in performing panretinal photocoagulation before the development of NVI or anterior chamber angle.

SUMMARY

The macula is affected by retinal vascular anomalies in a variety of ways. Cystoid and other forms of macular edema are a frequent manifestation of venous occlusive disease and a common cause of reduced central vision. The clinician should also be aware of the likelihood for retinal ischemia and its sequelae, namely neovascularization of the retina and NVI with secondary glaucoma. There should be a consistent strategy for patient follow-up to monitor for each of these conditions, and a complete medical evaluation is indicated to rule out any systemic causes for the vascular occlusion.

Arterial occlusive disease requires an immediate referral for a medical evaluation to rule out carotid, cardiac, and cardiac valvular disease. The retinal response is one of necrosis, and the prognosis for retention of usable vision is extremely poor. If detected extremely early in the course of the arterial occlusion, immediate intervention should include the administration of Carbogen, or carbon dioxide by other means, or paracentesis. Digital massage and immediate reduction of the IOP by other means may help to retain some useful vision. Any patient with arterial occlusion should be monitored closely to preserve the integrity of the fellow eye.

SUGGESTED READING

Appen RE, Wray SH, Cogan DG. Central retinal artery occlusion. Am J Ophthalmol 1975;79:374–381.

Brown GC, Magargal LE. Central retinal artery obstruction and visual acuity. Ophthalmology 1982;89:14–19.

Ellenberg G, Freedman J. Retinal vein occlusion and ocular hypertension. Ann Ophthalmol 1982;14:920–922.

Gass JDM. Stereoscopic Atlas of Macular Diseases. St. Louis: Mosby, 1987;422–434.

Gutman FA. Evaluation of a patient with central retinal vein occlusion. Ophthalmology 1983;90:481.

Hayreh SS, Rojas P, Podhajsky P, et al. Ocular neovascularization with retinal vascular occlusion. III. Incidence of neovascularization with retinal vein occlusion. Ophthalmology 1983;90:488–506.

Hayreh SS, van Heuven WAJ, Hayreh MS. Experimental retinal vascular occlusion: I. Pathogenesis of central retinal vein occlusion. Arch Ophthalmol 1978;96:311–323.

McGrath MA, Wechsler F, Hunyor ABL, et al. Systemic factors contributing to retinal vein occlusion. Arch Intern Med 1978;138:216–220.

Morse PH. Vitreoretinal Disease (2nd ed). Chicago: Year Book, 1989.

Sanborn GE, Magargal LE. Arterial Obstructive Disease of the Eye. In W Tasman, EA Jaeger (eds), Duane's Clinical Ophthalmology (Vol 3). Philadelphia: Lippincott, 1992;1–29.

Sanborn GE, Magargal LE, Jaeger EA. Venous Occlusive Disease of the Retina. In W Tasman, EA Jaeger (eds), Duane's Clinical Ophthalmology (Vol 3). Philadelphia: Lippincott, 1992.

Savino PJ, Glaser JF, Cassady J. Retinal stroke: Is the patient at risk? Arch Ophthalmol 1977;95:1185–1189.

Wesley RE, Johnston DT, Gutow GS. Central retinal artery occlusion. Ophthalmic Surg 1987;18:123–125.

CHAPTER

26 Cotton Wool Spots

Rodney K. Gutner

Cotton wool spots (CWS), or cytoid bodies, are retinal abnormalities manifested by localized areas of retinal edema. The lesions were first described by Heymann in 1856 and were thought to be areas of degenerated, axonal ganglion cells. Found predominantly in the posterior pole, these lesions are often associated with vascular abnormalities of the retina or elsewhere. Although diabetes mellitus is the most common systemic disease associated with this abnormality, other maladies have been implicated.

CWS are the most common ocular lesions found in patients with acquired immunodeficiency syndrome (AIDS) and have reportedly been observed in disease states as diverse as hypertension, collagen disease, blood dyscrasias, and toxemic retinopathy of pregnancy. The observation of one CWS in an otherwise normal retina demands a careful and extensive medical evaluation. CWS are always a manifestation of an underlying retinal vascular or systemic disorder that warrants careful evaluation.

CWS are focal areas of retinal edema that probably represent areas of microinfarct in the nerve fiber layer of the retina. The dense, white appearance and feathered edge is distinctive, and the lesion may sometimes appear to extend into the vitreous. There is a collection of cytoid material within the lesions, probably representing an accumulation of axoplasmic debris. These lesions are generally referred to as soft exudates, to distinguish them from the hard exudates seen in other retinal vascular disease (Figure 26.1).

When encountered in the diabetic patient, the lesions are thought to be due to the primary precapillary infarction of the arteriole resulting in ischemia. In fact, CWS can be encountered prior to the onset of other retinal manifestations of diabetic retinopathy, including microaneurysms.

When seen as a manifestation of AIDS, the lesions are thought to be caused by vaso-occlusion. In other instances, the exact cause is unclear, but vascular compromise seems to be a requirement for the pathogenesis of these lesions (Figure 26.1B).

The clinical presentation of these retinal lesions is highly distinctive. A white to yellowish lesion with blended edges is seen within the posterior pole, with a predilection for the temporal quadrant. The lesions are often observed between the arteriole and venule, and the typical lesion rarely exceeds 1/4 DD in size. Visual acuity can be temporarily affected depending on the location of the lesion and the amount of concomitant retinal disease. Patients who are good observers and historians may also report the presence of an isolated scotoma, which can be documented by perimetric examination.

Patients with CWS should be evaluated for the presence of underlying systemic diseases. There are many systemic conditions of consequence that can cause CWS, and it is essential for the practitioner to communicate the ophthalmoscopic findings to the patient's primary care physician.

DIFFERENTIAL DIAGNOSIS OF UNDERLYING CAUSES OF COTTON WOOL SPOTS

- Diabetes
- Collagen disease
  - Scleroderma
  - Disseminated lupus erythematosus
  - Rheumatoid arthritis
  - Polyarteritis nodosa
- Blood diseases
  - Aplastic anemia
  - Leukemia

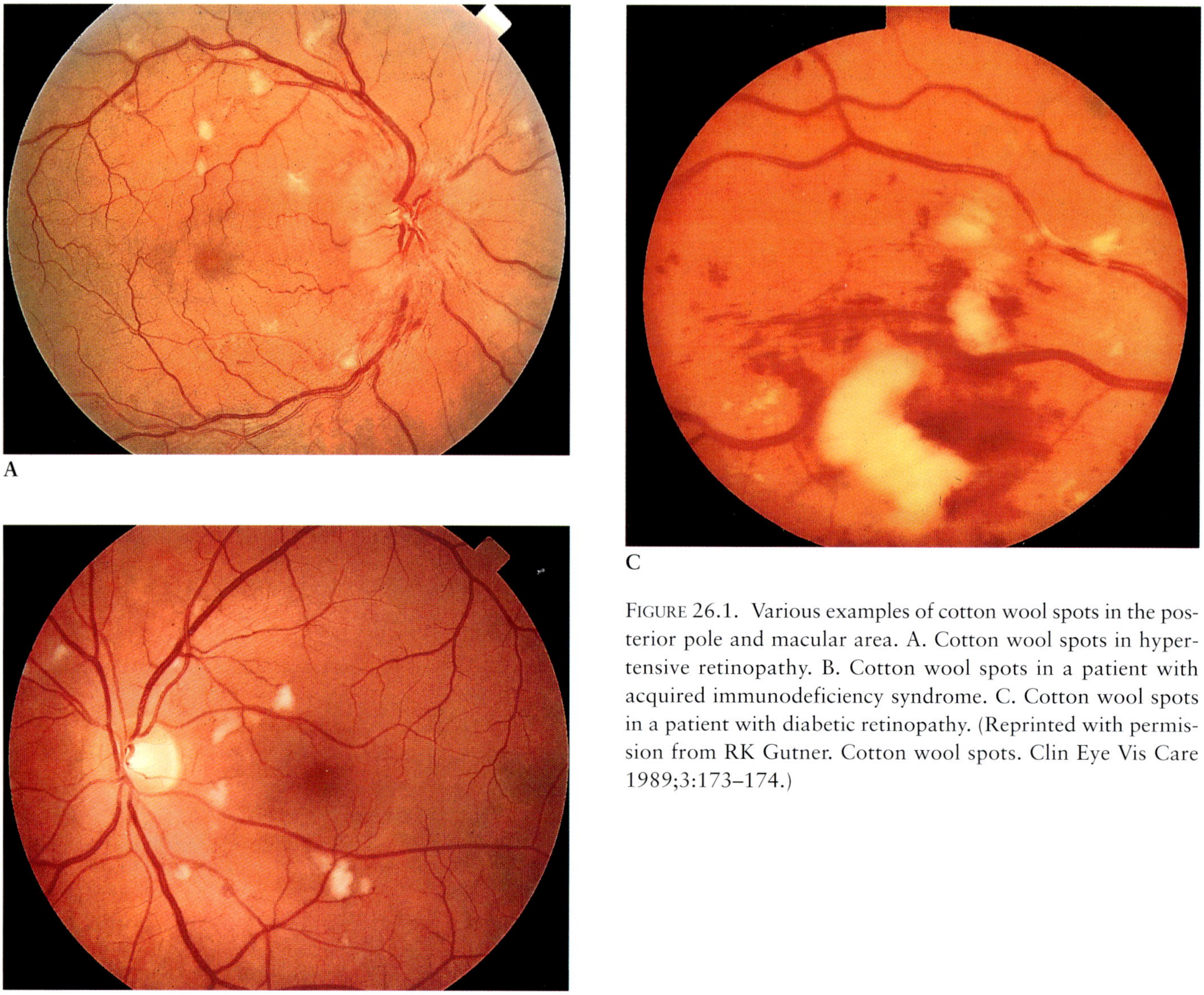

A

B

C

FIGURE 26.1. Various examples of cotton wool spots in the posterior pole and macular area. A. Cotton wool spots in hypertensive retinopathy. B. Cotton wool spots in a patient with acquired immunodeficiency syndrome. C. Cotton wool spots in a patient with diabetic retinopathy. (Reprinted with permission from RK Gutner. Cotton wool spots. Clin Eye Vis Care 1989;3:173–174.)

- Pernicious anemia
- Multiple myeloma

Hodgkin's disease

Infectious conditions

- AIDS
- Pneumonia
- Rheumatic fever
- Rocky Mountain spotted fever
- Subacute bacterial endocarditis

Untreated malignant hypertension

Renal disease

Toxemic retinopathy of pregnancy

SUGGESTED READING

Brown GC, Brown MM, Hiller T, et al. Cotton-wool spots. Retina 1985;5:206–214.

Mansour AM, Jampol LM, Logani S, et al. Cotton-wool spots in acquired immunodeficiency syndrome compared with diabetes mellitus, systemic hypertension, and central retinal vein occlusion. Arch Ophthalmol 1988;106:1074–1077.

McLeod D. Reappraisal of the retinal cotton-wool spot: A discussion paper. J R Soc Med 1981;74:682–686.

Roy FH. Ocular Differential Diagnosis. Philadelphia: Lea & Febiger, 1989;522–524.

Roy MS, Rick ME, Higgins KE, et al. Retinal cotton-wool spots: An early finding in diabetic retinopathy? Br J Ophthalmol 1986;70:772–778.

Tanenbaum M, Russell S, Richmond P, et al. Calcified cytoid bodies in acquired immunodeficiency syndrome. Retina 1987;7:84–88.

CHAPTER

27

White-Centered Retinal Hemorrhage

Rodney K. Gutner

White-centered retinal hemorrhage (WCRH) was initially described by Moritz Roth in the early 1870s, and the association of the phenomenon with subacute bacterial endocarditis was made by Litten almost a decade later. Roth's name was then associated with these retinal lesions, and the condition was mistakenly ascribed to the appearance of retinal hemorrhages seen in leukemia, a phenomenon now referred to as *pseudo-Roth spot.* Today it is known that WCRH is associated with numerous clinical entities and represents a local clinical sign of an underlying systemic vascular disease process.

Little epidemiologic information is available concerning WCRH since it is seen in conjunction with a multitude of systemic disorders. However, a distinction has been made between the lesions occurring in subacute bacterial endocarditis, where the white center has been ascribed to infectious emboli, and those appearing in leukemia, where the white center is due to an aggregate of inflammatory white cells.

Contrary to earlier clinical observations, the singularly unique appearance of the white center to the retinal hemorrhage arises from local and systemic conditions other than subacute bacterial endocarditis and leukemia. The circumstances causing WCRH are varied and include certain retinal hemorrhagic disorders, such as hypertension and diabetes, carcinoma of the lung, difficult labor and delivery in mothers, battered child syndrome, and ischemia associated with increased venous pressure.

A suitable pathophysiologic explanation for the white center of these hemorrhages is arrived at from an understanding of the common features associated with some of the systemic disorders. The distinctive white center is the result of either aggregates of leukocytes and debris (leukemia), a septic emboli (bacterial endocarditis), or an accumulation of fibrinous platelet material.

Any anoxic phenomenon resulting in a sudden increase in venous pressure will alter the permeability of the endothelium of the retinal capillaries. This, in turn, will allow the passage of whole blood through the capillary wall and finally initiate a reparative coagulation process, resulting in an aggregation of fibrinous material that produces a white center. In this process, the white center appears to be a manifestation of the healing process.

WCRH produces no symptoms unless there is macular involvement. The characteristic fundoscopic appearance is distinctive and reveals a retinal hemorrhage of any shape with a homogeneous white center (Figure 27.1). Several other retinal disease manifestations can mimic WCRH, including a hemorrhage with an overlying nerve fiber layer infarct (cotton wool spot), intraretinal microvascular anomalies, or a resolving center of a homogeneous hemorrhage. Fluorescein angiography may be useful in distinguishing the previously mentioned conditions from one another. There are many important systemic conditions that can cause WCRH, and it is essential for the practitioner to communicate the ophthalmoscopic findings to the patient's primary care physician. WCRH is ideally suited to comanagement with a primary care physician, either an internist, a family practitoner, or a hematologist.

DIFFERENTIAL DIAGNOSIS OF UNDERLYING CAUSES OF WHITE-CENTERED RETINAL HEMORRHAGE

Infectious processes
- Sepsis
- Endocarditis
- Syphilitic aortitis
- Viral pneumonia

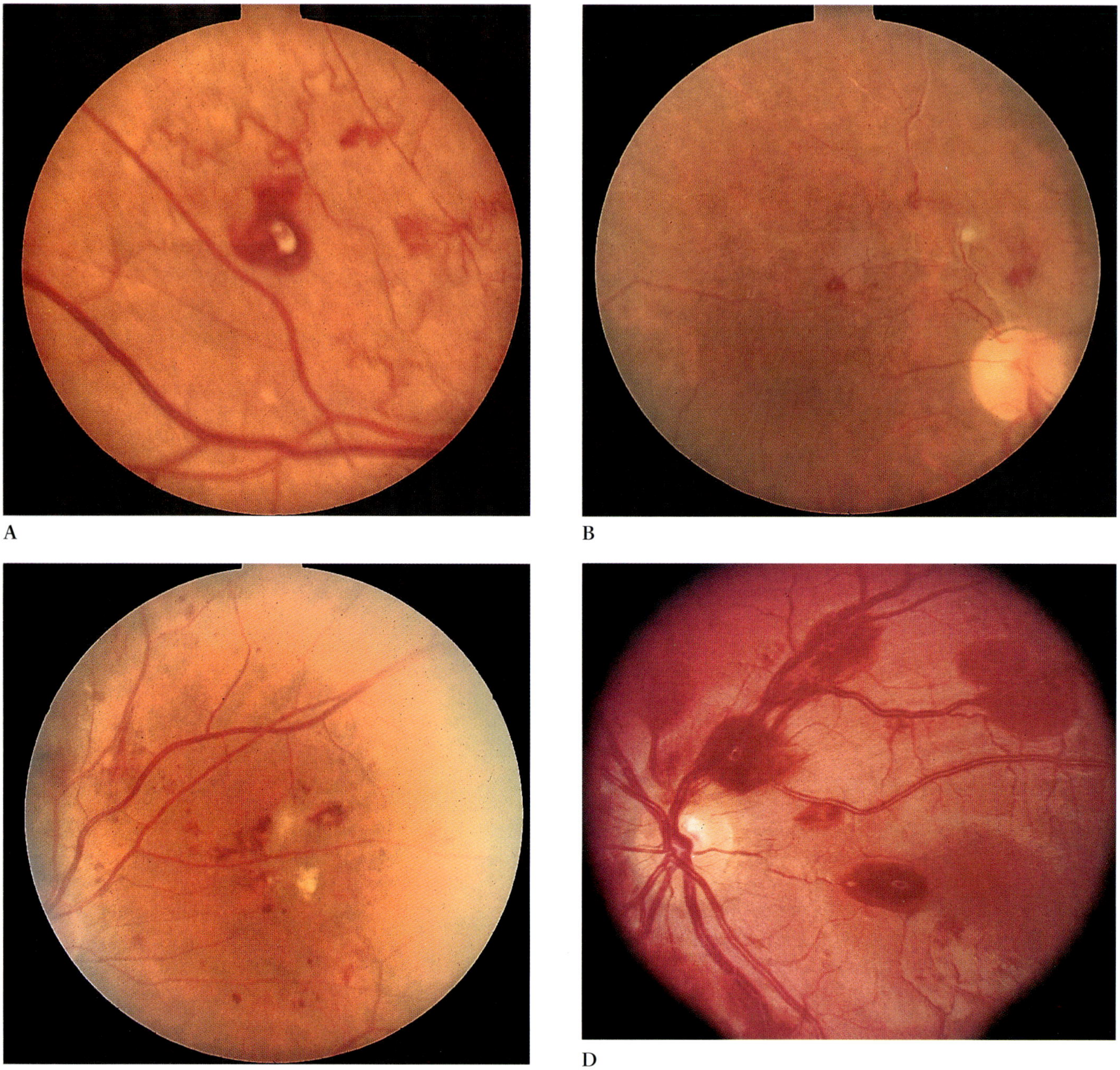

A B C D

FIGURE 27.1. Various expressions of white-centered retinal hemorrhages. A, B. White-centered hemorrhage in two patients with branch retinal vein occlusion. C. White-centered retinal hemorrhage in a patient with nonproliferative diabetic retinopathy. D. White-centered retinal hemorrhage in a patient with Valsalva's retinopathy involving the macula.

  - Rocky Mountain spotted fever
  - Arteritis
- Collagen vascular diseases
  - Systemic lupus erythematosus
  - Rheumatic heart disease
- Blood disorders
  - Leukemia
  - Hemorrhagic shock
  - Pernicious anemia
- Capillary fragility
  - Hypertension
  - Diabetes
- Anoxia
  - Carbon monoxide poisoning
  - Anemia
- Carcinoma of the lung

Intracranial hemorrhage
Increased venous pressure

SUGGESTED READING

Catalano D, Tannenbaum HL, Majerovics A, et al. White-centered retinal hemorrhages in diabetic retinopathy. Ophthalmology 1987;94:388–392.

Clarkson JG, Green WR. Endogenous Fungal Endophthalmitis. In TD Duane (ed), Clinical Ophthalmology (Vol 3). New York: Harper & Row, 1982;11.

Duane TD, Osher RH, Green WR. White-centered retinal hemorrhages: Their significance. Ophthalmology 1980;87:66–69.

Kincaid MC, Green WR. Ocular and orbital involvement in leukemia. Surv Ophthalmol 1983;27:211–232.

Roy FH. Ocular Differential Diagnosis. Philadelphia: Lea & Febiger, 1989;510–511.

Spencer WH (ed). Ophthalmic Pathology. Philadelphia: Saunders, 1985.

Van Uitert RL, Solomon GE. White-centered retinal hemorrhages: A sign of intracranial hemorrhage. Neurology 1979;29:236–239.

Walsh JB. Cardiovascular Disorders. In TD Duane (ed), Clinical Ophthalmology (Vol 5). New York: Harper & Row, 1982;22.

PART

VII

Traumatic Retinopathy

CHAPTER

28

Traumatic Maculopathy

Anthony A. Cavallerano

Direct or indirect trauma to the posterior segment often affects the macula. Blunt trauma, penetrating intraocular foreign bodies, surgical trauma, and photic injuries can cause tissue damage in the macular area with resultant decreased visual function in some cases (Figure 28.1). The following list summarizes the posterior segment manifestations of posterior ocular trauma:

- Vitreous hemorrhage (Terson's syndrome)
- Macular hole
- Traumatic retinal pigment epitheliopathy
- Retinal dialysis (peripheral involvement)
- Retinal breaks and detachment
- Commotio retina
- Subretinal and intraretinal hemorrhage
- Purtscher's retinopathy
- Choroidal rupture
- Evulsed optic nerve
- Ruptured globe

PHOTIC INJURY

The direct and cumulative effects of light are not completely understood, but there is a growing body of evidence to suggest that harmful effects can occur if the macula is unprotected. Damage can occur through photochemical, photocoagulative, or mechanical effects of visible light.

Photochemical damage occurs when visible light causes tissue damage without significantly raising the temperature. Photochemical damage to the retina occurs chiefly with shorter wavelengths.

Photocoagulative damage occurs when the tissue temperature is increased by 10–20°C above the body temperature. The temperature elevation causes disruption of tissue proteins with resultant injury.

Ocular protective mechanisms exist that shield the retina from the harmful effects of light rays. The cornea protects against ultraviolet (UV) light below 300 μ but is transparent between 300 and 400 μ. It is this range that is potentially harmful to the posterior segment of the eye. UVB, between 280 and 315 μ, and UVA, between 315 and 400 μ, fall within this range. The crystalline lens absorbs wavelengths between 300 and 400 μ and does so with increasing efficiency as nuclear sclerosis and yellowing of the lens develop with age.

The retina also has some protective features to safeguard against the deleterious effects of visible light, including the carotenoid pigment, especially xanthophyll. This latter pigment, which serves as a chromophore, is located in the inner and outer plexiform layers of the retina, and has its densest concentration in the foveal region. In addition to diminishing light exposure levels of the retinal tissue, especially the macular region, it also reduces chromatic aberration.

The outer segments of the photoreceptors also offer protection by shedding photopigment-containing disks. By removing these structures, which might be damaged, the retinal pigment epithelium (RPE) maintains an environment that is protected against the phototoxic and photochemical effects of light. Other protective agents include melanin, which is densest in the foveal area, and antioxidants, including vitamin E.

Lipofuscin safeguards against the damaging effects of light. Lipofuscin increases in concentration with age, and the ratio of melanin to lipofuscin reverses during the aging process. The greatest increase occurs between the

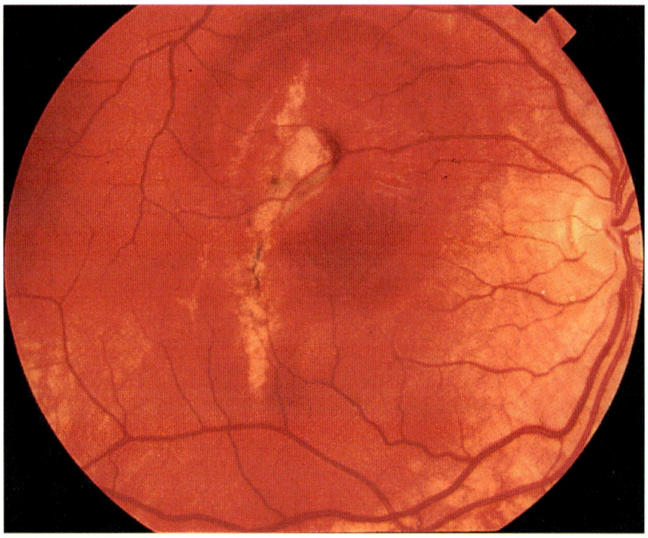

A

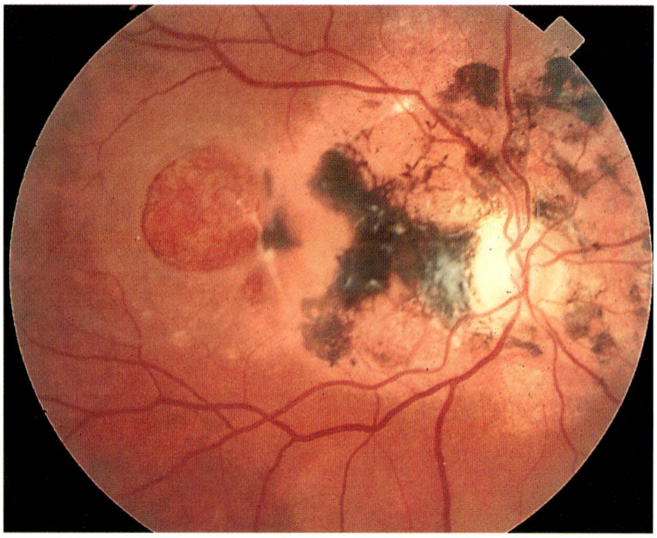

B

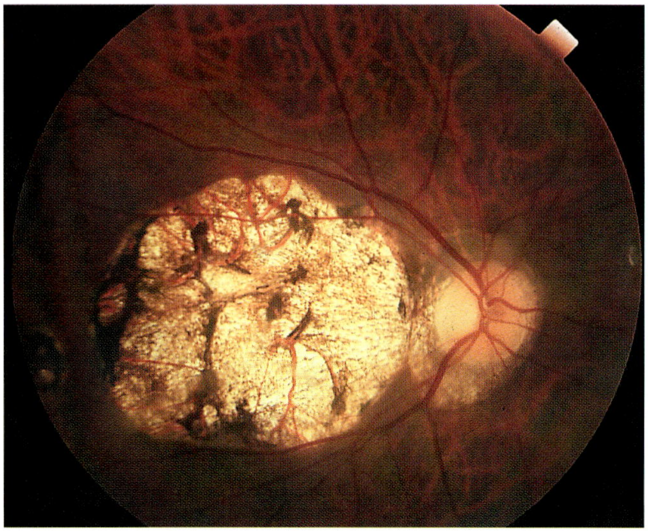

C

FIGURE 28.1. Various manifestations of posterior segment ocular trauma. A. Choroidal rupture. B. Traumatic macular hole. C. Commotio retina.

first and second decade of life, when there is a corresponding decrease in melanin.

SOLAR MACULOPATHY

Photochemical damage to the macula results from exposure to sunlight. The most likely cause is a photochemical response, and the blue wavelengths of light are probably responsible. There is a greater potential for harm with younger patients because of their clear media.

Solar retinopathy can also occur following eclipse viewing, and the condition is often bilateral. Longer wavelengths are responsible for the damage to the retinal tissue, which usually occurs directly in the center of the fovea. A local edematous response is observed during the first few days following exposure, and a cuff of edema surrounds the involved area. Vision is decreased during the acute stage but will often return almost to normal in many cases. The patient will also report a central scotoma or after-image in the center of their field for days following the photic injury.

BLUNT OCULAR TRAUMA

Blunt ocular trauma can result in retinal damage and, depending on the extent of macular involvement, may have no effect on vision if the peripheral retina is involved or may significantly alter visual function if the macula is injured. Both direct and indirect contussive trauma can result in retinal injury. Commotio retina, macular holes, traumatic optic neuropathy, including evulsed optic nerves, retinal dialysis, and choroidal tears, are posterior segment signs of direct or indirect blunt trauma.

Commotio Retina

Commotio retina results in what appears to be retinal edema and subsequent changes in the RPE. However, it has been demonstrated that the blood–retinal barrier is intact, and the opalescent appearance of the retina is due to a loss of integrity of the outer photoreceptor segments. The opaque appearance of the affected retina eventually resolves over time. Pigment migration has been shown to occur, and full-thickness macular holes can develop; there is also liquefaction of the overlying vitreous (Figure 28.1C). Treatment should include protection of the involved eye with a Fox shield or safety glasses and surveillance until the retinal edema resolves.

Choroidal Rupture

Choroidal rupture can be caused by blunt ocular trauma, and tears of the choroid and RPE have been noted. Direct or coup injuries result in crescent tears parallel to the ora serrata, and contracoup injuries result in crescent-shaped lesions concentric to the optic disc. Subretinal and sometimes sub-RPE hemorrhages are reported in conjunction with this type of injury. In many cases, choroidal neovascularization is present during the healing stage of the process, and the patient is at risk for choroidal neovascularization development with attendant visual complications throughout the rest of his or her life. A direct alteration of vision takes place if the lesion is located in the macular area. Management should include surveillance, and the patient should be monitored regularly for choroidal neovascularization (Figure 28.1A).

Macular Holes

Traumatic retinal holes can occur following blunt trauma and are rarely associated with peripheral retinal breaks and detachment. Macular holes following injury may be relatively large and may have regular or irregular borders. They may also be associated with subretinal hemorrhage and choroidal ruptures (Figure 28.1B).

SUMMARY

Patients with a recent or remote history of blunt ocular trauma often manifest posterior segment changes with macular involvement. The clinician should monitor the patient at least annually for complete examination, even if visual function is intact. The primary care clinician should educate the patient as to the signs and symptoms of visual loss following trauma, and the patient should be advised to return for evaluation with new onset of decreased vision or dysmorphopsia. Eye protection in the form of safety glasses and industrial or athletic eye wear should be routinely recommended, especially in monocular patients.

SUGGESTED READING

Cooling RJ. Traumatic retinal detachment: Mechanisms and management. Trans Ophthalmol Soc UK 1986;105:575–579.

Mansour AM, Green WR. Histopathology of commotio retinae. Retina 1992;12:24–28.

Parver LM. Eye trauma: The neglected disorder. Arch Ophthalmol 1986;104:1452–1453.

Pulido JS, Blair NP. The blood-retinal barrier in Berlin's edema. Retina 1987;7:233–236.

Vinger PF. Eye injury resulting from violence: Research and prevention. Arch Ophthalmol 1992;110:765–766.

PART

VIII

Hereditary Macular Disorders

CHAPTER

29

Hereditary Macular Disorders

Susan A. Primo

Categorization of the macular dystrophies may be based on the primary retinal layer of involvement. Six of the most common disorders that are described here are central areolar choroidal dystrophy (CACD), Stargardt's disease, Best's disease, pattern dystrophy, cone dystrophy, and juvenile X-linked retinoschisis (JXR). These dystrophies are all characterized by bilaterality (with relative symmetry), progression to varying degrees, and lack of systemic or laboratory findings. Genetic patterns of inheritance as well as fluorescein angiography (FA) and electrodiagnostic testing (electroretinography [ERG] and electro-oculography [EOG]) play an integral role in the differentiation and subsequent identification of these conditions. It is important for the clinician to follow a step-by-step process in diagnosing a specific dystrophy:

1. Identify the general color of the macular area (and background), i.e., white, black, or yellow (Figure 29.1).
2. Attempt to determine the genetic pattern from the patient's family ocular history. The value of examining other family members to establish a diagnosis cannot be overemphasized.
3. Perform or order appropriate ancillary tests such as electrodiagnosis, color vision, FA, and visual fields (routine screening or threshfield).

Completion of these three steps identifies the hereditary macular disorder. In all likelihood, it will be one of the six described in this chapter. Others do exist, but they are very rare. Consultation with a retinal specialist is indicated to ensure the proper diagnosis if it seems unclear.

Macular Dystrophies and Associated Primary Anatomic Fundus Layer

Choriocapillaris
- CACD

Retinal pigment epithelium
- Stargardt's disease
- Best's disease
- Pattern dystrophy

Sensory retina
- Cone dystrophy
- JXR

Genetic Patterns

Dominant patterns
- CACD
- Best's disease
- Pattern dystrophy (except Sjögren's dystrophy)
- Cone dystrophy
- Some cases of Stargardt's disease

Recessive transmission
- Stargardt's disease
- Sjögren's reticular dystrophy

X-linked transmission
- JXR

Electrodiagnostic Findings

Reduced ERG
- Cone dystrophy (photopic)
- JXR (b-wave only)
- Late stages of Stargardt's disease

Reduced EOG
- Best's disease

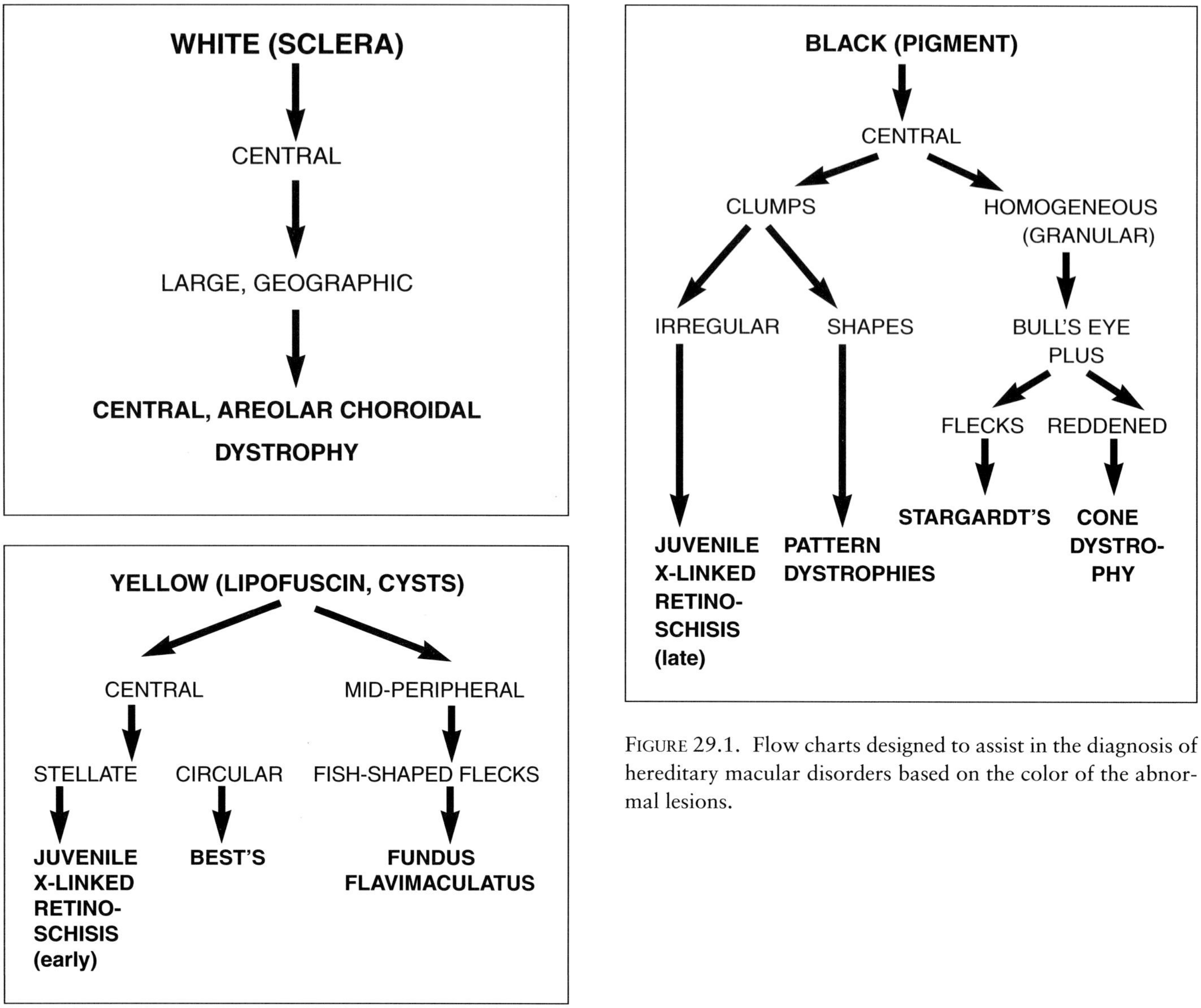

FIGURE 29.1. Flow charts designed to assist in the diagnosis of hereditary macular disorders based on the color of the abnormal lesions.

Pattern dystrophy
Late stages of Stargardt's disease

THE DYSTROPHIES

Central Areolar Choroidal Dystrophy

CACD is the only macular disorder that primarily affects the choriocapillaris. As a result, the white central background (bared sclera) represents a regional, geographic area of choroidal as well as retinal pigment epithelial (RPE) atrophy (Figure 29.2). Coursing through the lesion may be large, yellowish-white or orange-red, thickened, choroidal "sclerotic" vessels. FA demonstrates patterns consistent with the well-circumscribed area of atrophy. Visual acuity loss begins during the third to fourth decade of life and is generally moderate to severe (culminating around 20/200). The genetic pattern of inheritance is autosomal dominant. Electrodiagnostic findings in CACD are usually normal to subnormal depending on the stage of atrophy.

Stargardt's Disease

Stargardt's disease is perhaps the most common macular dystrophy that is encountered. The classic appearance is a bull's-eye pigment pattern or beaten-bronze metallic sheen to the macular area (Figure 29.3). The lesion is approximately 1 disc diameter (DD) in size. Decreased visual acuity usually begins in the first or second decade of life and eventually decreases to the point of legal blindness by the third or fourth decade. Stargardt's disease patients report no photophobia and have normal color vision until late in the disease's pro-

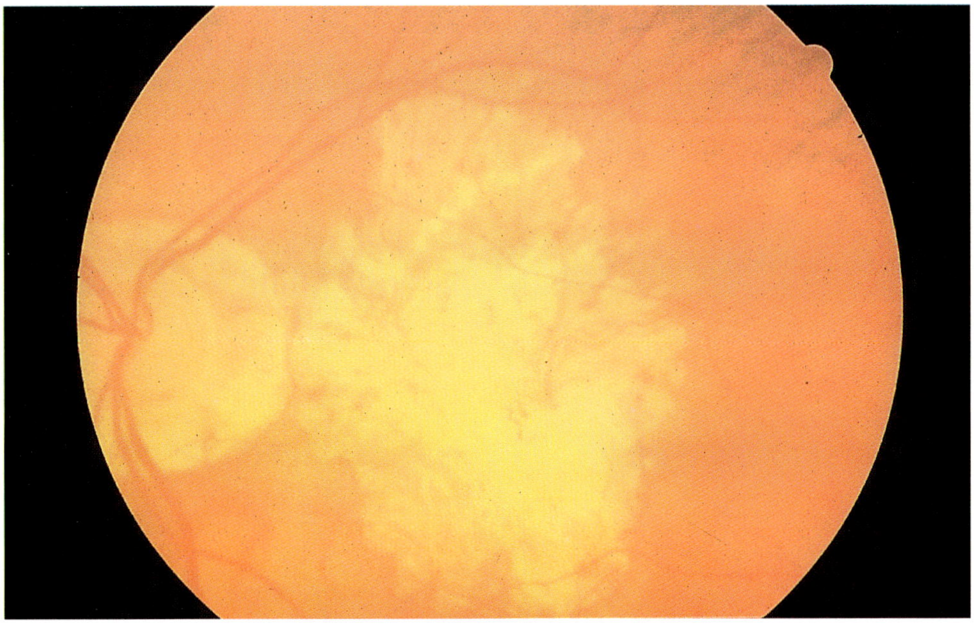

FIGURE 29.2. Central areolar choroidal dystrophy. Note regional area of choroidal atrophy revealing sclera tissue. Visual acuity is 20/400.

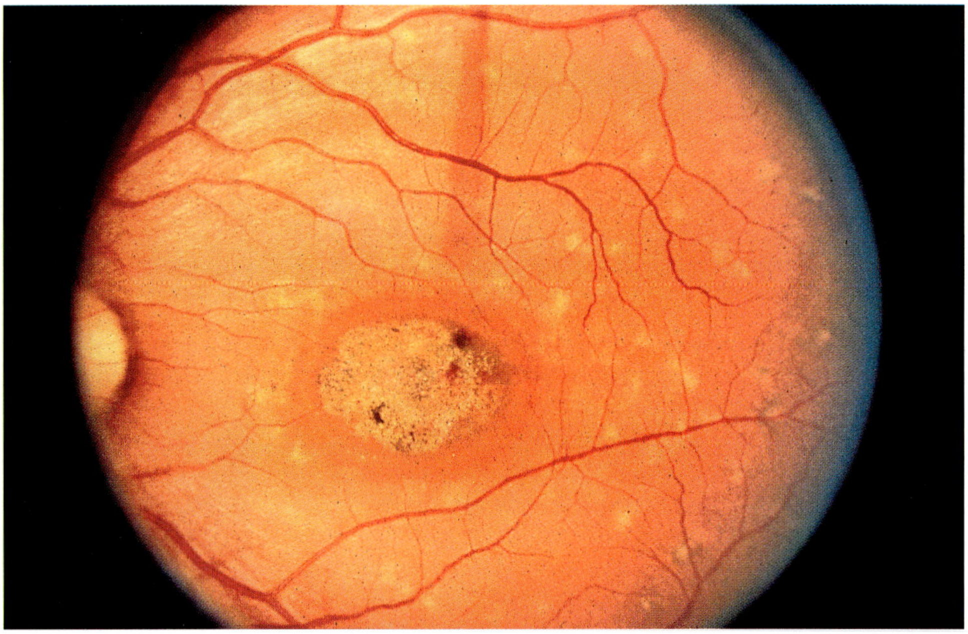

FIGURE 29.3. Stargardt's disease. Note bull's-eye maculopathy and presence of midperipheral flecks (fundus flavimaculatus). Visual acuity is 20/120.

gression. The disorder is typically an autosomal recessive inheritance, but autosomal dominant inheritance has been reported in some pedigrees.

Fundus Flavimaculatus

Fundus flavimaculatus, thought to be the same entity as Stargardt's disease, is characterized by round, oval, linear, or fishtail-shaped flecks that are localized deep in the retina. The yellowish flecks, found in the posterior pole and midperipheral regions, may or may not accompany the macular lesion of Stargardt's disease. Perhaps the most distinctive feature of Stargardt's disease or fundus flavimaculatus is the classic "dark choroid" (of the background) demonstrated on FA (Figure 29.4). This finding is present in 85% of patients with both macular changes and flecks, and its cause is essentially unknown. Other fluorescein patterns show scattered areas of hyperfluorescence in and around the macular area and reflect the RPE disturbance (Figure 29.4). Electrodiagnosis plays an

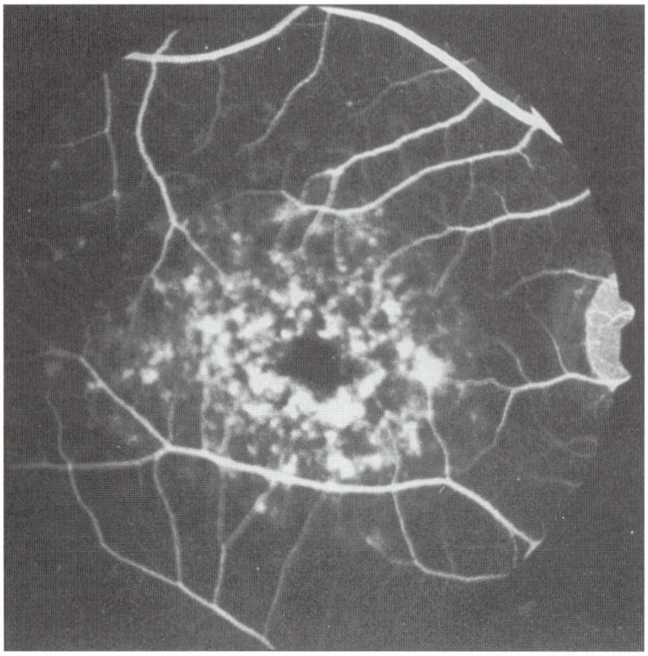

FIGURE 29.4. Fluorescein angiogram of dark choroid (absence of choroidal flush) in Stargardt's disease. Note hyperfluorescent areas in and around the macula.

important part in establishing the diagnosis and differentiating it from cone dystrophy; the ERG and EOG are normal until late in the course of the disorder.

Best's Disease

Best's disease characteristically presents as a small, yellow, egg yolk–like lesion in the macular area. This vitelliform lesion is thought to be a homogeneous viscous material, probably secreted by the RPE and outer segments of the photoreceptors. Unlike the other dystrophies, Best's disease has distinct stages with corresponding visual acuity reduction. Stages 0 and I (beginning in the first to second decade of life) present with subtle RPE granularity and mild macular hypoplasia. Approximately 80% of patients have visual acuity of 20/20 and remain at this level for several years. The typical vitelliform lesion occurs in stage II, when visual acuity starts to decrease to around 20/30 (Figure 29.5). The later part of this stage is characterized by rupture of the cyst ("scrambled egg" phase). Fluorescein patterns at this point show central hypofluorescence (corresponding to the yellowish material) and then irregular transmission when the cyst ruptures. Fluid development within the vitelliform cyst, the pseudohypopyon phase, represents stage III (Figure 29.6); approximately one-third of patients progress to this stage, with visual acuity between 20/60 and 20/80. Stage IV, the final stage, is distinguished by the appearance of an atrophic or fibrous scar (occurring in patients older than 55 years of age), and visual acuity drops to 20/200. Most patients with Best's disease ultimately remain in stage II or III and maintain vision at around 20/40.

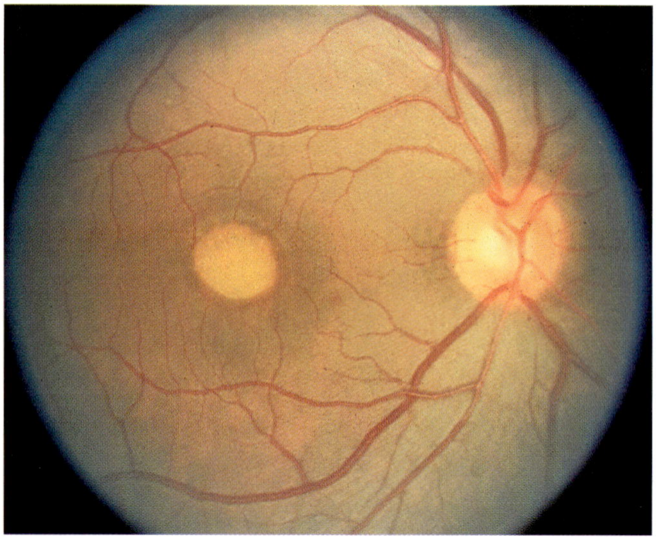

FIGURE 29.5. Best's disease (stage II). Note yellowish, egg yolk–like lesion. Visual acuity is 20/30.

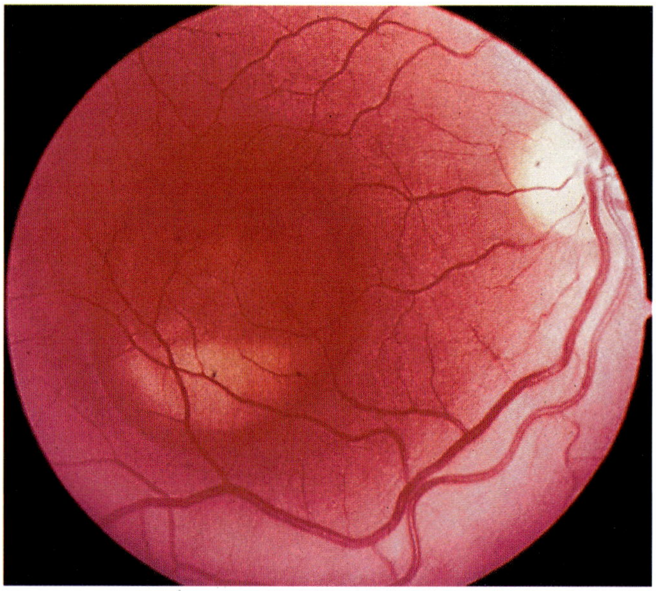

FIGURE 29.6. Pseudohypopyon phase of Best's disease, stage III. Note fluid level within the vitelliform cyst. Visual acuity is 20/80.

Since the defect arises in the RPE, the EOG is the most appropriate electrodiagnostic test. Results yield a reduced Arden ratio in the range of 1.35 or less (normal value is 1.8 and greater). In addition, patients with normal maculae who are descended from individuals with

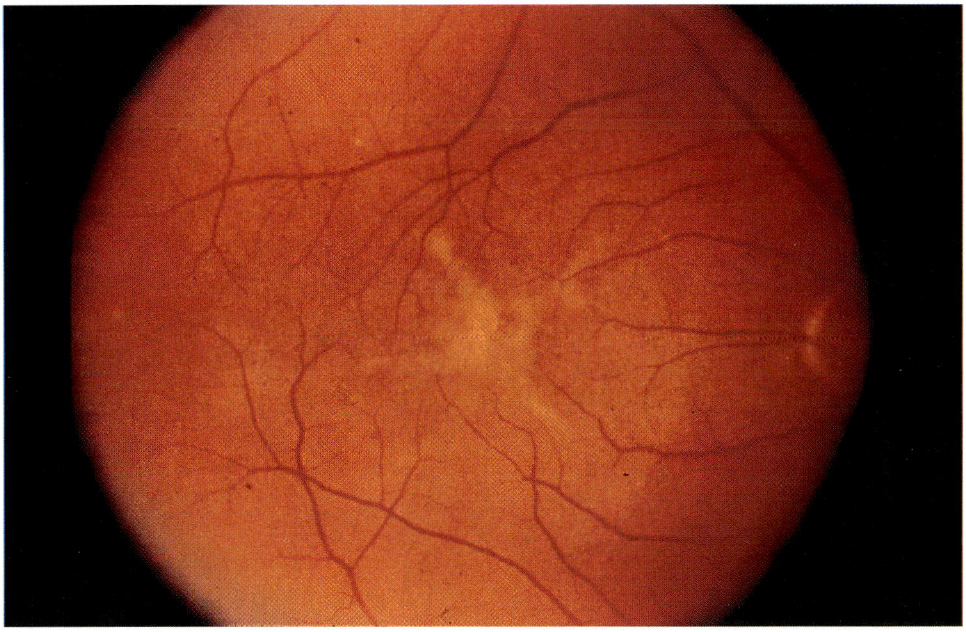

FIGURE 29.7. Butterfly pattern dystrophy. Note butterfly-shaped retinal pigment disturbance in the macula. Visual acuity is 20/30. (Courtesy of John Weiter, M.D.)

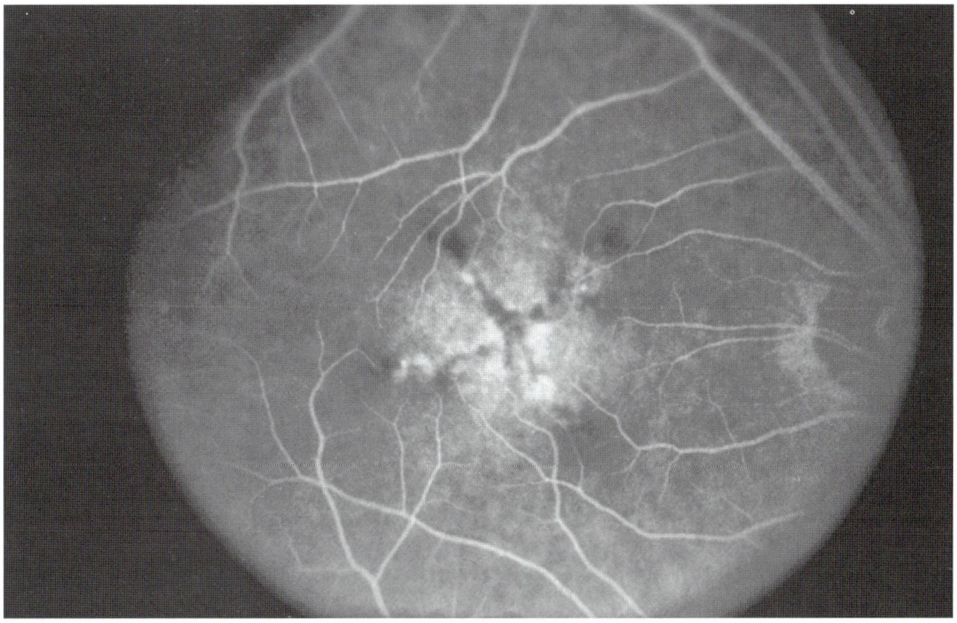

FIGURE 29.8. Fluorescein angiography of butterfly dystrophy. Note that hypofluorescence closely corresponds to funduscopic appearance. (Courtesy of John Weiter, M.D.)

known Best's disease (with abnormal EOGs) also have abnormal EOGs despite their normal fundus appearance.

Pattern Dystrophies

Pattern dystrophies of the RPE consist of five main types: butterfly, Sjögren's reticular, macroreticular, grouped pigmentary, and fundus pulverulentis. The three types that are described here are butterfly, Sjögren's, and macroreticular dystrophies. Most of the pattern dystrophies follow an autosomal dominant mode of inheritance, except for Sjögren's reticular (autosomal recessive) dystrophy. In general, vision is mildly reduced, and the disorder becomes evident during the first to third decade of life.

Butterfly dystrophy is so named because its reticular pigment pattern closely resembles the shape of a butterfly (Figure 29.7). The most striking demonstration of this shape becomes evident on FA in which the reticular hypofluorescent pattern corresponds to areas of hyperpigmentation (Figure 29.8). The dystrophy usually presents during the second to fifth decade of life, and visual acuity is mildly affected.

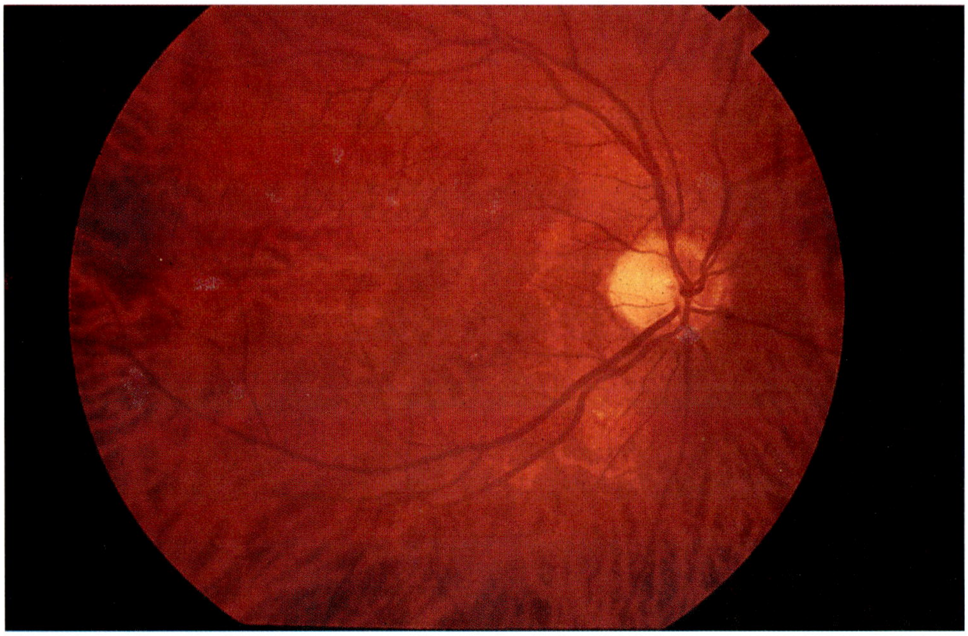

FIGURE 29.9. Macroreticular pattern dystrophy. Note subtle pigment pattern disturbance in the macula. Visual acuity is 20/20. (Courtesy of John Weiter, M.D.)

FIGURE 29.10. Fluorescein angiogram of macroreticular dystrophy. Note that hypofluorescence corresponds to and emphasizes areas of pigment accumulation. (Courtesy of John Weiter, M.D.)

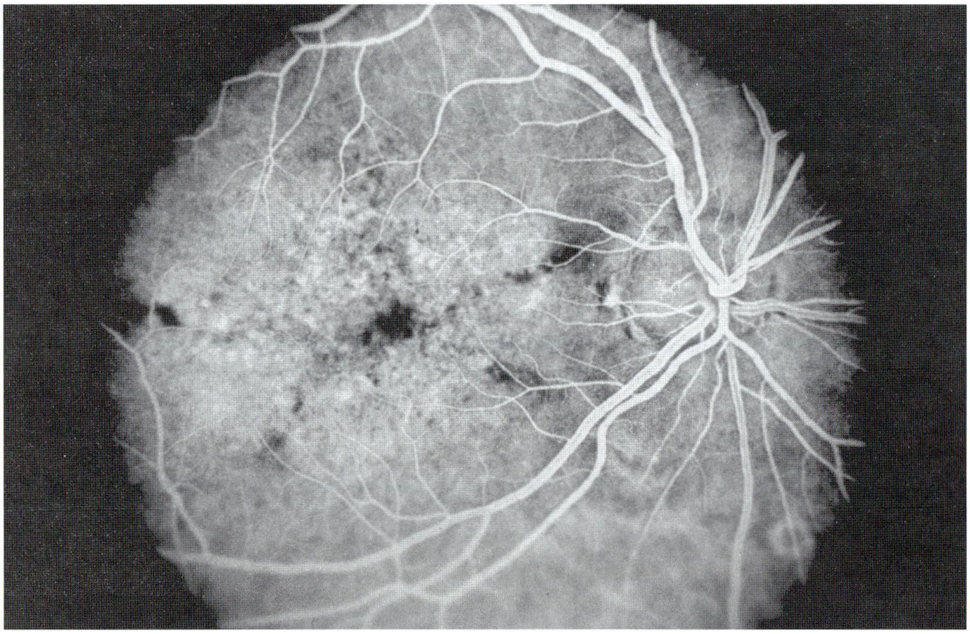

Sjögren's reticular dystrophy, although relatively rare, is unique in that it is the only one of the pattern dystrophies that follows an autosomal recessive mode of inheritance. This dystrophy occurs during the first decade of life, and visual acuity may be normal to mildly reduced with minimal progression, except perhaps later in life. A hyperpigmented network forms around a central dark pigment spot approximately 1 DD in size. Over time, the network gradually extends toward the midperiphery and becomes confluent and irregular in appearance. As with the other types, this pattern becomes strikingly obvious with FA.

Macroreticular dystrophy, which closely resembles Sjögren's reticular dystrophy, presents much later in life, around the fifth decade, and visual acuity is mildly to moderately affected. The inheritance pattern is autosomal dominant. Bands of hyperpigmentation (which become evident with FA) are arranged in reticular, propeller-like, or cross-hatched designs in the central macular area (Figures 29.9 and 29.10). As with Best's dystrophy, the EOG will be reduced in the range of 1.65 or less. The ERG findings in all patients with pattern dystrophies are normal.

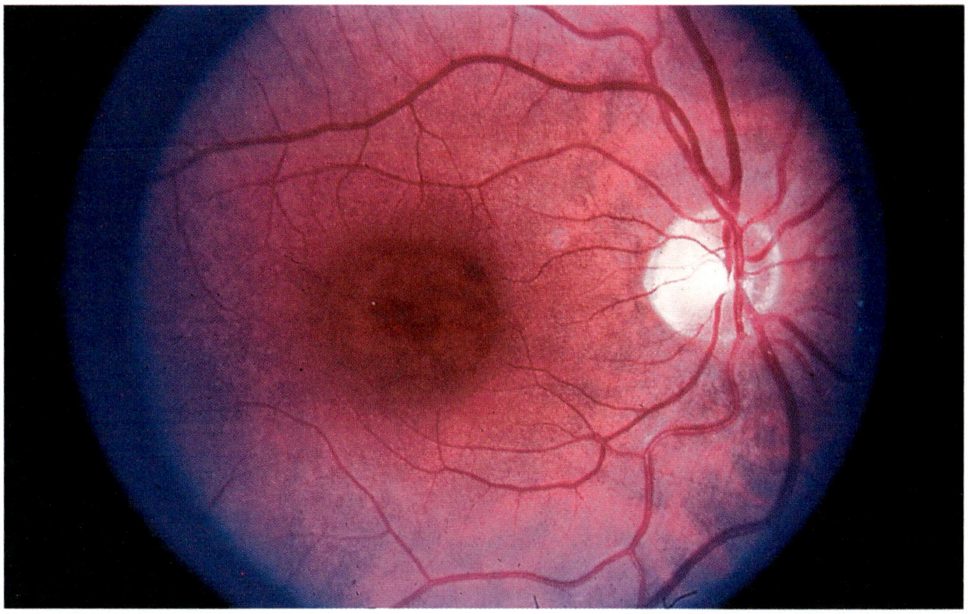

FIGURE 29.11. Cone dystrophy. Note homogeneous, reddened bull's eye area of macular involvement. Visual acuity is 20/300.

Cone Dystrophy

Cone (or cone-rod) dystrophy presents with a bull's-eye macular pattern similar to Stargardt's disease. The classic appearance is a central zone, typically a deep red, homogeneous area, which is surrounded by regions of depigmentation (Figure 29.11). The sharply demarcated zones of involved and uninvolved retina are most easily recognized with fluorescein studies, in which the surrounding area of depigmentation is seen as an early doughnut-shaped area of hyperfluorescence. The central zone is hypofluorescent corresponding to uninvolved RPE. The outer regions may enlarge and demonstrate hypofluorescence outside the doughnut-shaped area.

The second and less common presentation of cone dystrophy is diffuse spotty pigment clumping. Its appearance is one of fine pigment clumping interspersed with small atrophic spots throughout the macular area. With time, the clumps may enlarge and extend outward. This form of the dystrophy tends to show a more rapid progression and deterioration of visual function.

Cone dystrophy generally presents during the first or second decade of life, progressing to severe vision reduction (20/300 and worse). Since the appearance is similar to Stargardt's disease, it is important to differentiate the two because cone dystrophy implies a much more devastating course in terms of visual acuity loss, and it has an autosomal dominant pattern of inheritance. Most patients with cone dystrophy complain of poor color vision and photoaversion, often before significant acuity reduction. As mentioned previously, patients with Stargardt's disease generally have good color vision until late in the disease and no photophobia. Other features that help to differentiate the two are FA and electrodiagnostic testing. In Stargardt's disease, the majority of patients demonstrate the dark choroid finding and also normal ERG results (until very late). In cone dystrophy, the ERG is significantly reduced, particularly under photopic conditions. Therefore, if the clinician is referring the patient for electrodiagnostic studies, the suspected diagnosis of cone dystrophy must be relayed to the consultant performing the test so that appropriate recording techniques may be used to isolate cone and rod function selectively.

Juvenile X-Linked Retinoschisis

JXR is most unique in that not only is the inheritance X-linked (therefore, occurring in male subjects only), but it is also the only macular dystrophy that is actually vitreoretinal in nature, i.e., most of the retinal findings are directly related to vitreous changes. Its primary clinical feature is a bilateral, stellate-shaped maculopathy in 100% of affected boys and men. A peripheral retinoschisis is present 50% of the time. The pathognomonic macular feature is the result of the formation of yellowish cysts in a radial pattern (Figure 29.12). These cysts form between the nerve fiber layer and the rest of the retina where the dialysis has occurred. With time, the cysts coalesce secondary to a breakdown of the radial septa. The central cyst then collapses, leaving RPE disturbance resembling atrophic age-related macular degeneration (Figure 29.13).

The peripheral retinoschisis, almost always located inferotemporally in each eye, is also the result of a congenital cyst (Figure 29.14). This "vitreous veil" has its anterior edge stopping just posterior to the ora serrata, and its posterior edge may extend right up to the optic

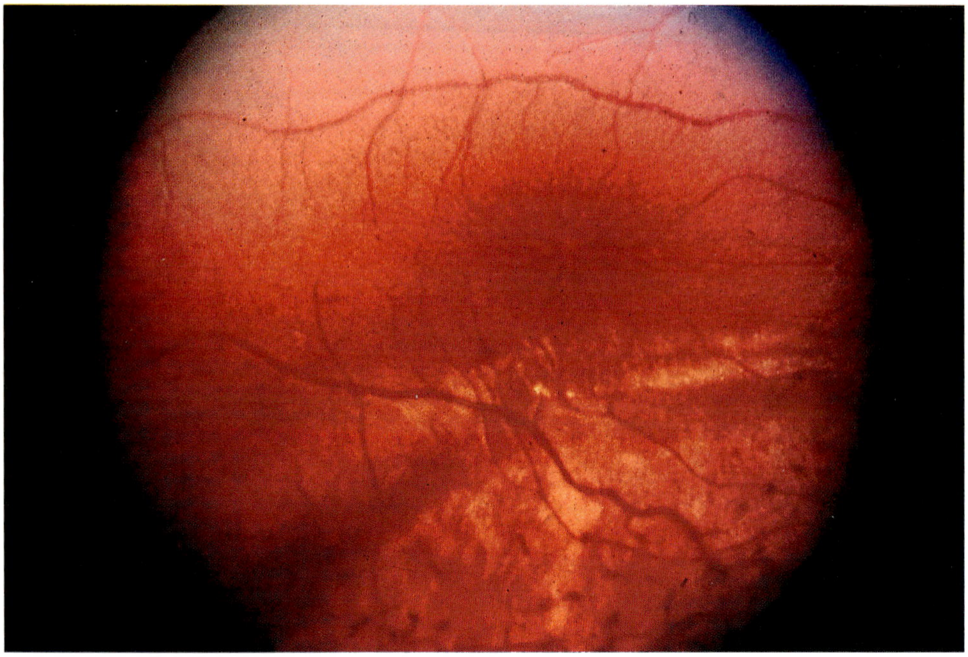

FIGURE 29.12. Juvenile X-linked retinoschisis (early). Note stellate maculopathy and posterior edge of peripheral retinoschisis inferotemporally. Visual acuity is 20/60. (Courtesy of John Loewenstein, M.D.)

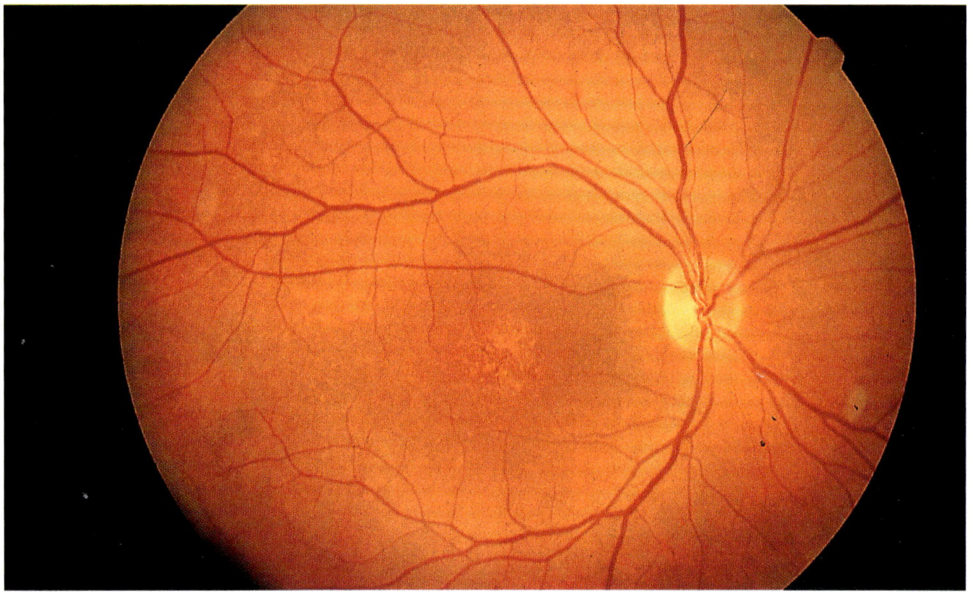

FIGURE 29.13. Juvenile X-linked retinoschisis (late). Note retinal pigment epithelial disturbance resembling age-related macular degeneration. Visual acuity is 20/120.

nerve head. Over time, the retinoschisis ultimately collapses as the vitreous undergoes degenerative changes, and large strands or floaters may be observed. Since the retinal dialysis in JXR occurs at the nerve fiber layer (versus the outer plexiform layer seen in acquired retinoschisis), the inner layer of the retinoschisis is very thin and thus prone to large holes or dehiscences (Figures 29.14 and 29.15). These large holes represent breaks in the inner layer. In addition, the fragile blood vessels that course through the thin inner layer may rupture, leading to vitreous hemorrhage. Outer layer breaks are less common but may also occur, potentially allowing fluid to seep under the RPE, causing a larger break and subsequent retinal detachment. Other peripheral fundus findings observed in the area of the retinoschisis are sheathed and dendritic opacified vessels and chorioretinal disturbance.

Visual acuity loss in JXR begins during the first or second decade of life and ranges from moderate to severe, with all patients approaching legal blindness by the fifth or sixth decade. Other common associated findings contributing to decreased acuity include strabismus, hyperopic astigmatism, and posterior subcapsular cataract. If the cataract is advanced enough, extraction generally provides a subjective increase in the patient's visual func-

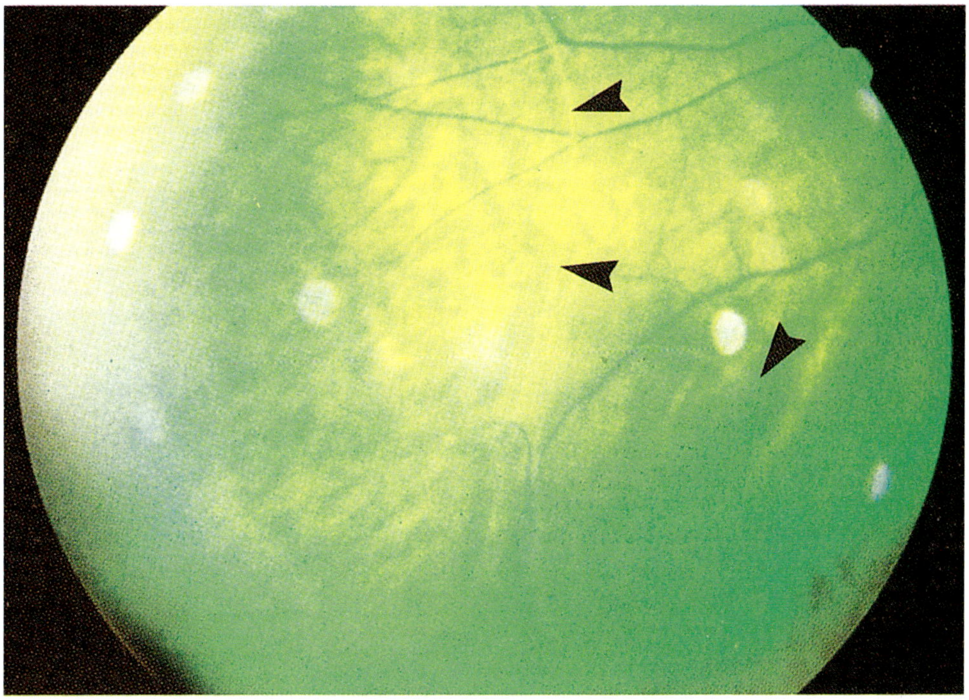

FIGURE 29.14. Peripheral retinoschisis in juvenile X-linked retinoschisis. Note large dehiscences (holes) in the inner layer (arrows).

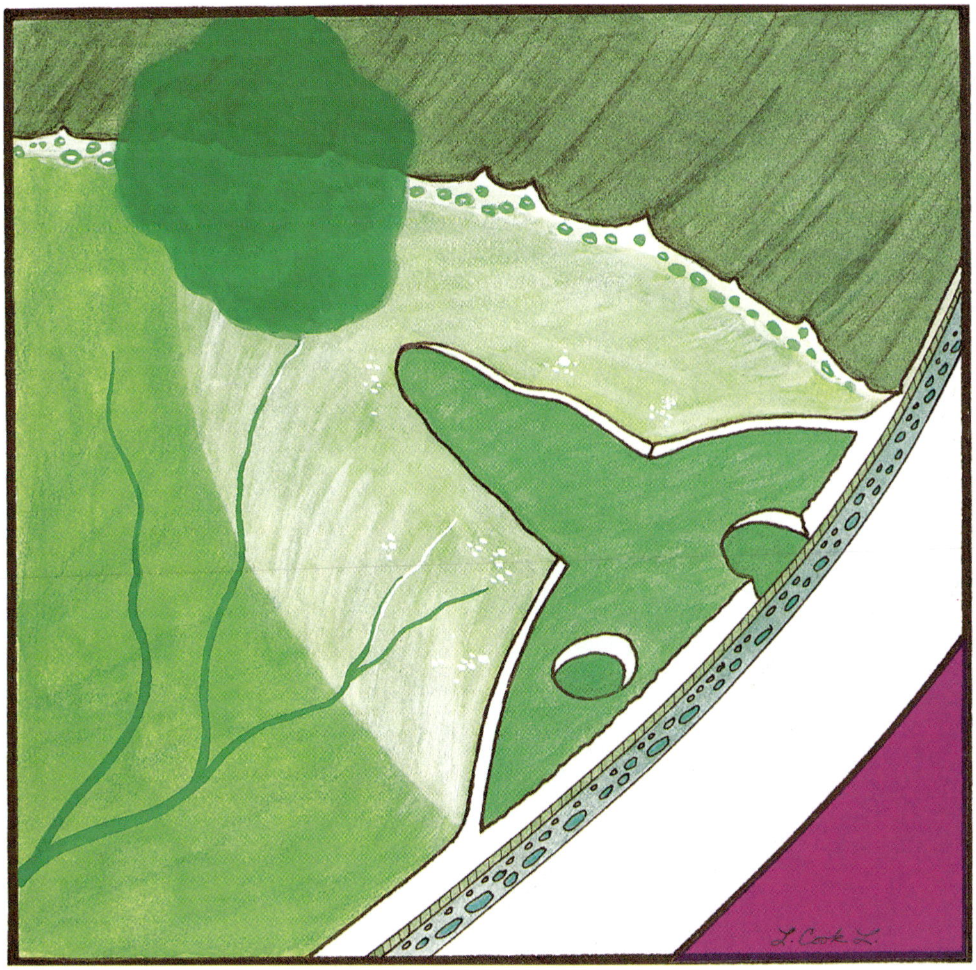

FIGURE 29.15. Congenital versus acquired peripheral retinoschisis. Note retinal splitting at the nerve fiber layer in congenital retinoschisis versus the outer plexiform layer in acquired schisis. Note also the thin inner layer in congenital retinoschisis, which is prone to large holes. Also, vitreous hemorrhage may occur secondary to rupture of fragile blood vessels.

tion. Surgical intervention should not be dismissed simply because objective visual acuity may not be improved. Another management strategy should include close observation of the peripheral retinoschises, if present, to avoid retinal detachment that might occur from outer layer breaks. If detachment ensues, immediate referral for surgery is indicated.

Electrodiagnostic studies reveal an interesting, characteristic decrease in the b-wave of the ERG. This finding corroborates the defective Müller's cell theory as the cause of congenital cysts in this dystrophy.

MANAGEMENT

Generally speaking, management of all of the macular dystrophies is directed toward visual rehabilitative measures since acuity loss is the major problem of most patients. Low vision devices as well as early intervention in school programs will allow for a child who has reduced acuity to function as well as possible. Adult patients may be managed appropriately depending on goal-specific needs. If the clinician feels that he or she cannot provide the appropriate low vision devices, etc., appropriate referral should not be delayed. In addition, genetic counseling for parents is indicated so that they may have a clear understanding of the potential effects on future offspring.

All of the dystrophies should be monitored yearly via dilated fundus evaluation. JXR suggests closer attention to possible retinal complications if peripheral retinoschises are present. See Table 29.1 for a summary of these conditions.

SUGGESTED READING

Bither PP, Berns LA. Dominant inheritance of Stargardt's disease. J Am Optom Assoc 1988;59:112–127.

Condon GP, Brownstein S, Wang N, et al. Congenital hereditary (juvenile X-linked) retinoschisis. Arch Ophthalmol 1986;104:576–583.

Deutman AF. Electro-oculography in families with vitelliform dystrophy of the fovea. Arch Ophthalmol 1969;81:305–316.

Deutman AF. Vitreoretinal Dystrophies. In AE Krill, AG Deutman (eds), Hereditary Retinal and Choroidal Diseases. Hagerstown, MD: Harper & Row, 1977;1053.

Deutman AG, van Blommestein JD, Henkes HE, et al. Butterfly-shaped pigment dystrophy of the fovea. Arch Ophthalmol 1970;83:558–569.

Ferry AP, Llovera I, Shafer DM. Central areolar choroidal dystrophy. Arch Ophthalmol 1972;88:39–43.

Gelisken O, De Laey JJ. A clinical review of Stargardt's disease and/or fundus flavimaculatus with follow-up. Int Ophthalmol Clin 1985;8:225–235.

Krill AE. Cone Degenerations. In AE Krill, AG Deutman (eds), Hereditary Retinal and Choroidal Diseases. Hagerstown, MD: Harper & Row, 1977;441.

Mohler CW, Fine SL. Long-term evaluation of patients with Best's vitelliform dystrophy. Ophthalmology 1981;88:688–692.

Watke RC, Folk JC, Lang RM. Pattern dystrophy of the retinal pigment epithelium. Ophthalmology 1982;89:1400–1406.

Yanoff M, Rahn EK, Zimmerman LE. Histopathology of juvenile retinoschisis. Arch Ophthalmol 1968;79:49–53.

TABLE 29.1. Summary of Hereditary Macular Disorders

Location/ dystrophy	*Heredity*	*Decade of onset*	*Acuity loss*	*Color vision*	*Posterior segment findings*	*Fluorescein angiography*	*Electrodiagnosis*	*Histopathology*
Choriocapillaris								
Central areolar choroidal	AD	3rd–5th	Moderate to severe	R-G late	RPE and choriocapillaris atrophy; begins nonspecific, then well circumscribed	Window defects; then large areas of atrophy	Normal to subnormal	—
RPE								
Stargardt's/fundus flavimaculatus	AR, AD	1st–2nd	Moderate to severe	R-G, B-Y late	Beaten bronze/bull's-eye ± fish-shaped flecks in posterior pole	Irregular RPE transmission; dark choroid	Normal to subnormal	—
Best's disease	AD (variable penetrance)	1st	Mild to severe	R-G, B-Y late	Mild RPE defects early; yellow circular lesion to atrophic or fibrous scar late	Window defects; hypofluorescence	Reduced EOG; normal ERG	Deposition of yellow, homogeneous material secreted by RPE
Butterfly	AD	2nd–5th	Mild	Normal	Butterfly-shaped pattern of pigmentation	Window defects; more obvious butterfly shape	Subnormal EOG; normal ERG	Abnormal lipofuscin material
Sjögren's reticular	AR	1st	None to mild	Normal	Irregular patch of pigmentation	Window defects	Normal to subnormal EOG; normal ERG	Abnormal lipofuscin
Macroreticular	AD (variable penetrance)	5th	Mild to moderate	Normal	Pigmented band in various patterns, e.g., propeller-like	Window defects	Normal to subnormal EOG; normal ERG	Abnormal lipofuscin
Sensory retina								
Cone	AD, AR(?)	1st–2nd	Moderate to severe; photoaversion	Severe loss	Bull's-eye; pigment clumping	Doughnut-shaped area of hyperfluorescence	Reduced to flat, photopic ERG; normal to subnormal EOG	—
Juvenile X-linked retinoschisis	X-linked	1st–2nd	Moderate to severe	B-Y, R-G late	Foveal schisis—100%; peripheral schisis—50%	Window defects late; defects if chorioretinal atrophy or breaks	Reduced b-wave of ERG; normal EOG	Splitting of retina at nerve fiber layer

RPE = retinal pigment epithelium; AD = autosomal dominant; AR = autosomal recessive; R-G = red-green; B-Y = blue-yellow; EOG = electro-oculography; ERG = electroretinography.

PART

IX

Treatment, Management, and Prevention

CHAPTER 30

Prevention and Medical Management of Age-Related Macular Degeneration

Stuart P. Richer

Animal research and epidemiologic studies, as well as single-blind European and U.S. human clinical supplementation trials, have enhanced our understanding of the pathophysiologic relationships and risk factors linking age-related macular degeneration (AMD) to cardiovascular disease, nutritional status, and chronic ultraviolet blue (UVB) visible light exposure. Human twin studies demonstrate that genetic factors also appear to play a factor, although most likely a limited one compared with environmental stress. Thus, in anticipation of the results of ongoing and future double-blind intervention studies, recent efforts to prevent and treat AMD have been directed toward nutrition and UVB visible light protection, as the potential benefits far outweigh the risks and the "baby boom" population is fast approaching the age when prevention now could make a significant difference later. Furthermore, experts project that the life span for Americans born at the beginning of the next century will exceed 85 years.

AMD is not a hopeless disease. Specifically, basic science research is directed at determining those nutrients, especially antioxidants and trace metals for antioxidant enzymes, that lessen the damage to the metabolically active Bruch's membrane–retinal pigment epithelium (RPE) complex, which is subjected to chronic, high levels of stress from long-term exposure to oxygen free radicals and radiation. Clinical science has yet to catch up with important, compelling basic science discoveries and animal data. Many of the data are consistent with the broad-based "free radical" paradigm of aging, health, and disease.

FREE RADICALS AND ANTIOXIDANTS

There is growing evidence that the pathologic mechanism for atrophic or dry AMD, sometimes a precursor for neovascular (wet) AMD, is related to acute or chronic photoreceptor–RPE exposure to high-energy, short-wavelength radiation with or without the action of photosensitizers. The photoreceptors are unique in containing highly polyunsaturated fatty acids, especially in their outer segment membranes, which are readily oxidized in chain lipid peroxidative reactions. In the metabolically active, oxygen-rich environment of the retina, UVB visible radiation initiates the production of active, more damaging forms of oxygen known as *hydroxyl* and *superoxide free radicals.* These forms of biochemically destructive oxygen are known as *oxygen free radicals.* However, *vitamin-derived free radicals,* from the major soluble antioxidant vitamin ascorbic acid (ascorbyl radical) or from the major lipid membrane–soluble vitamin tocopherol or vitamin E (tochpheroxyl radical), also exist when vitamin recycling is incomplete. Thus, antioxidants can alternately act as oxidants dependent on the physiologic environment.

The age-related lipid/protein by-products of free radical oxidative damage to photoreceptors are known as *lipofuscin* and visualized as drusen. The material accumulates over time as a result of the aforementioned oxidative processes. Mechanisms for removing this material exist but are compromised with aging. In addition to vitamins A, C , E, and xanthophylls, the RPE complex employs gene-derived antioxidant enzymatic systems to protect itself against unquenched forms of reactive oxygen and vitamin-derived free radicals while providing the functions of phagocytosis, digestion, recycling, and metabolism. These endogenous antioxidant enzymes use one of the body's 12 trace metals. For example, copper and zinc are cofactors for the enzyme superoxide dismutase. The eye is also exposed to oxidants of hydrogen peroxide and derivative oxidants, namely aldehydes of polyunsaturated fatty acids generated during detoxification. Table 30.1 summarizes the type, location, and nutritional requirements of major putative ocular antioxidants and antioxidant enzymes that neutralize free radicals.

TABLE 30.1. Type, Location, and Nutritional Requirements of Major Putative Ocular Antioxidants and Antioxidant Enzymes That Neutralize Free Radicals in Age-Related Macular Degeneration

Enzymes	*Type*	*Location*	*Nutritional requirements*
Superoxide dismutase	Gene-derived	Photoreceptor outer segments	Zinc, copper, iron, manganese
Glutathione peroxidase	Gene-derived	Retina, RPE	Selenium, zinc, copper, iron
Glutathione reductase	Gene-derived	Retina	Riboflavin
Catalase	Gene-derived	RPE	Zinc, copper, iron
Retinal reductase	Gene-derived	Retina	Zinc
Vitamin E + vitamin C (work in concert)	Nutrient	Retina	Oral vitamin C and oral vitamin E
Vitamin A	Nutrient	Retina	Oral vitamin A
Metallothionein	Gene-derived	RPE	Zinc

RPE = retinal pigment epithelium.

Free radicals sometimes serve useful purposes in the body. They are produced as a normal consequence of cellular mitochondrial respiration, glucose oxidation, nucleic acid breakdown, production of prostaglandins, and macrophage attack. However, errant free radicals, if left unchecked, can impair or destroy lipids (in membranes and liposomes) and proteins, including enzymes involved in intermediary cellular metabolism (glycolysis and the Kreb cycle), and disturb both electrolyte balance and antioxidant protective systems themselves. The body has multiple layers of defense against free-radical damage, but these defenses can be overcome by environmental stress and aging.

ANIMAL STUDIES

Animal studies 15 years ago demonstrated that monkeys develop AMD in only 14 weeks when xanthophyll pigments (lutein and zeaxanthin) are withheld from the diet. Recent human clinical reports from the National Eye Institute (NEI) confirm the protective nature of these pigments found in dark green, leafy vegetables. The yellow (macula lutea) xanthophyll pigments found in primates protect retinal tissue from oxidizing sun damage in a similar way to that which occurs in the leaves and petals of plants and flowers. Monkeys or humans are not born with a yellow macula lutea, and it is a highly variable quantity because it is acquired from plant stuffs. In humans, the macula lutea is depleted more rapidly with cigarette smoking. Melanin (pigmentation) has also been found to be an important "radiation sink" against free radicals in animal studies.

In addition to the pigments (xanthophyll and melanin), numerous laboratory studies have confirmed that previous light exposure, duration and intensity of light, time in the diurnal cycle, as well as antioxidant capacity of the exposed animal retina or the animal diet itself (specifically vitamins C, E, and the carotenoid beta carotene) modulate the extent of sensory retinal-RPE oxidant damage in a predictable fashion.

Considerable data point to glutathione (GSH), a sulfur-containing tripeptide, and related enzymes—riboflavin-dependent GSH-reductase and selenium-dependent GSH-peroxidase—as protective against AMD. GSH, the cell's master antioxidant, works in conjunction with vitamins C and E and protects against cataractogenesis. GSH levels are dramatically boosted by the amino acid cysteine (or methionine and vitamin B_6, which convert to cysteine). Exposure to sunlight reduces GSH in the retina. Green, leafy vegetables, in addition to containing vitamins, minerals, and carotenoid pigments, are good sources of protein-bound and nonprotein-bound GSH.

Figure 30.1 summarizes the etiopathogenic factors in the development of AMD.

EPIDEMIOLOGY

Blue Visible and Ultraviolet Radiation Exposure Emerging as a Secondary Factor

It has been demonstrated that just 1 photon of UVB or 1 millionth of a watt can damage retinal cells. While the greatest amount of sun exposure occurs during youth, a younger retina has greater antioxidant protection than an aged retina. Results of two recent retrospective, large-scale clinical studies found no association in older individuals between long-term ocular exposure to ultraviolet (UV) light and AMD: the Chesapeake Bay Waterman Study found no association between individual exposure to ambient UVA, UVB, and AMD; and the Beaver Dam Eye Study found no association between ambient UVB exposure and AMD. Both study results are consistent

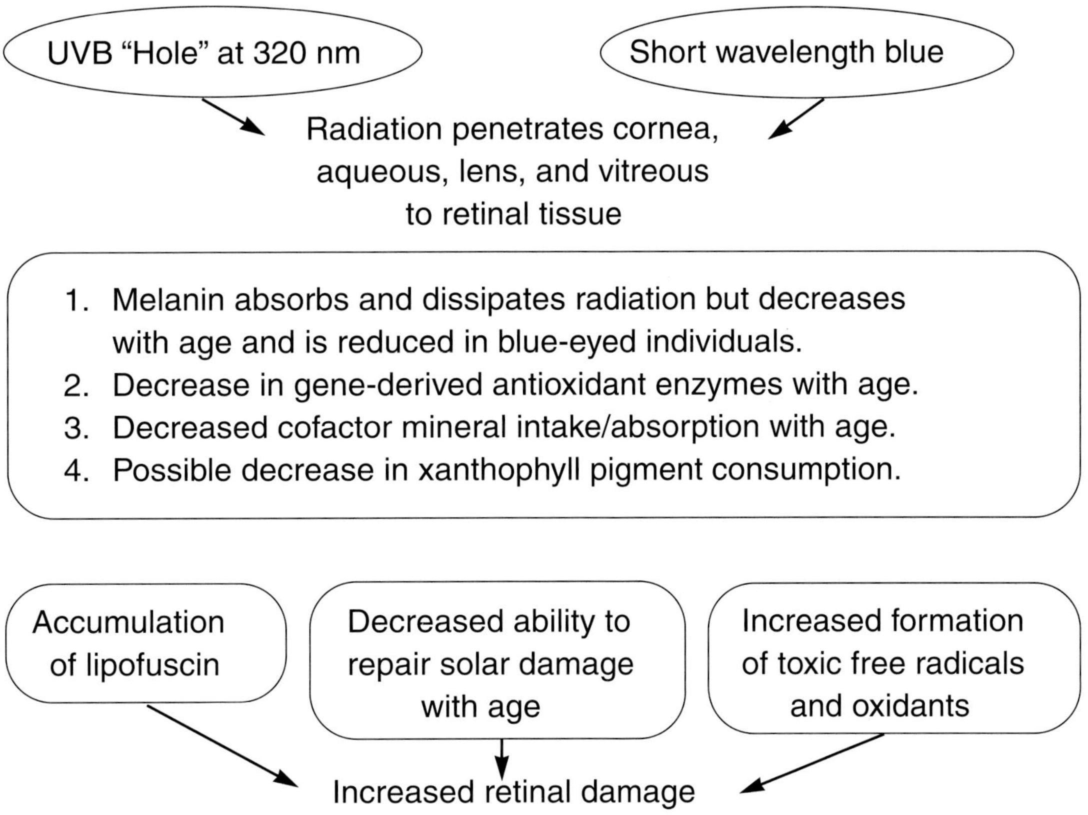

FIGURE 30.1. Summary of the etiopathogenic factors in the development of age-related macular degeneration. (UVB = ultraviolet/blue visible light.) (Adapted from LJ Alexander. Optometry clinics. Ocular Pharmacol Update 1992;2:1–34.)

with the conclusion that the protective role of lenticular chromophores prevents most UV radiation from reaching the retina. However, re-analysis of the Chesapeake Bay Waterman Study data revealed that more advanced cases of AMD were associated with greater exposure to blue visible light over the proceeding 20 years, consistent with animal studies. Furthermore, in the Beaver Dam Eye Study, the amount of time spent outdoors in the summer was associated with increased retinal pigment, while the use of eyeglasses, hats, and sunglasses was inversely associated with soft, indistinct drusen. The amount of leisure time spent outdoors in the summer was also significantly associated with exudative AMD.

Association with Atherosclerotic-Cardiovascular Disease and Nutrition

Most human epidemiologic studies now link chronic multifactorial diseases such as atherosclerosis-cardiovascular disease and their attendant risk factors to AMD. The multifactorial risk factors identified in AMD are summarized below. Note that many are identical to those for cardiovascular disease. Arteriosclerotic histopathologic changes in orbital arteries supplying the human eye are ubiquitous in persons over 70 years of age, and vascular insufficiency via correlative increased vascular resistance has been demonstrated in the short posterior ciliary arteries in humans. High intake of saturated fat and cholesterol was associated with higher risk of AMD in the Beaver Dam study.

Risk Factors for Age-Related Macular Degeneration Identified in Epidemiologic Studies

- Aging whites
- Postmenopausal women without estrogen replacement
- Cardiac disease
- Photosensitizing drug use
- Resident of southern United States
- Cigarette smokers
- Hyperopes
- Elevated alpha$_2$ globulin levels
- Elevated cholesterol levels
- Elevated systolic blood pressure

- Less education
- Scandinavian ancestry
- Pre-1984 pseudophakes
- Retinal drusen
- Diet without carotenoids
- Unprotected outdoor activity
- Small cup-disk ratio
- Higher body mass index
- Elevated fibrogen levels
- Elevated triglyceride levels
- Decreased physical activity

High serum values of vitamin E protect against AMD. Vitamin E, a lipid-soluble membrane antioxidant, protects low denisty lipoproteins from oxidation and is also a hypocholesterolemic agent. But vitamin E also benefits the cardiovascular system by decreasing blood viscosity via a decrease in platelet aggregation.

In 1988, a report showed that zinc slowed the progression of AMD, and this drew widespread attention in the news media, spawning over 20 different zinc-based dietary supplements. (Zinc deficiency is common in the elderly population.) An abundant trace element, zinc is required for RNA and DNA function and is plentiful in ocular tissue, acting as a cofactor for multiple cellular enzymatic retinal pathways. It is also necessary for the transport of vitamin A from the liver. Even a mild deficiency of zinc may result in impaired dark adaptation and contrast sensitivity, as well as decreased wound healing, taste, and smelling acuity. The protective effect of zinc against AMD has been demonstrated clinically.

The Veterans Affairs/Pacific University College of Optometry clinical study group found a low intake of cardioprotective nutrients (vitamin E and zinc but also magnesium, vitamin B_6, and folic acid) in veterans with AMD, compared with NHANES III (National Health and Nutrition Examination Survey) age-, sex-, and race-stratified data.

The NEI/Eye Disease Case Control group has learned that plant pigments (yellow xanthophyll carotenoids [lutein and zeaxanthin]), found, for example, in spinach and dark green vegetables, protect against the development of severe exudative AMD in agreement with earlier animal studies. Peak macula lutea pigment density, which passively protects the macula against actinic damage and actively protects the macula by quenching free radicals, has been shown to be reduced in smokers. Smokers are known to have 2.5 times the risk of developing macular degeneration during their lifetime.

The findings of additional risk factors for AMD, such as low magnesium and B vitamin intake, concur with a recent epidemiologic report that there are as yet unidentified risk factors for AMD. Low intake of magnesium is a risk factor for ischemic heart disease, acute myocardial infarction, hypertensive vascular disease, diabetic vascular disease, insulin resistance, atherosclerosis, and vasospasm. Magnesium is an important determinant of vascular tone, contractility, and reactivity. B vitamins assist in preventing atherosclerosis by retarding the buildup of homocysteine, an undesirable oxidant in the blood, and are also an independent risk factor for homocysteinuria and 15% of all cardiovascular diseases.

The basic science finding that melanin (as well as xanthophyll pigments) acts as a "radiation sink" against free radicals is supported by most epidemiologic studies, which show that patients with light-colored irises are at a higher risk of developing AMD.

PROSPECTIVE INTERVENTION STUDIES

In *Acta Ophthalmologica* in 1958, Vannas and Orma published the results of the first successful treatment of dry AMD, which they termed *arteriosclerotic retinopathy*. This was a placebo-controlled trial of patients receiving alternating intravenous heparin and vitamins A (30,000 U) and E (70 mg), both four times per day. Two-thirds of patients reported improved sight, including resolution of scotomas with Amsler grid testing.

At least five positive studies appeared in the German medical literature in the late 1970s and early 1980s, repeating the Helsinki studies but substituting a vasodilating drug, pentifylline, for heparin with similar results as confirmed by visual fields and fluorescein angiography. This is the current treatment for AMD in Germany.

In 1987, Crary, in the United States, reported treating 102 AMD patients for 7–12 years with a combination of vitamin C (500 mg/day), vitamin E (400 mg/day), beta carotene (9 mg/day), and selenium (250 µg/day). He found this treatment plan halted or improved degenerative macular changes in 60% of patients.

In 1988, Newsome et al. reported that high-dose zinc (200 mg) supplementation slowed the progression of dry AMD and incidentally resulted in fewer neovascular events. This study did not control for lens opacification. The positive effect may have been due to either zinc's ability to enhance transport of vitamin A from the liver to retina or zinc's melanin-binding properties, or both. Since that time, use of large doses of zinc (above 45 mg) are questioned because of possible stunting effects on the immune system. Newsome subsequently recommends "broad-spectrum" antioxidants with moderate amounts of zinc.

In 1991, Mamalis and Pomerance showed a 35% protective effect on contrast sensitivity of orally ingested, multiple-component, broad-spectrum antioxidants. This was a prospective, single-blinded, nonrandomized clinical trial studying 244 patients with dry AMD. Statistical analysis of the data suggested that antioxidant supplementation using LaHaye Labs I-Caps multivitamin, multimineral formulation twice daily could significantly decrease and in some cases reverse the progression rate of AMD. LaHaye Labs (Redmond, WA) initiated a prospective evaluation of 2,400 patients with eight clinical sites in 1991. Hoffman La Roche has a "React" clinical trial and is nearing completion of a 3-year study of 300 patients.

Currently, the NEI/National Insititutes of Health in collaboration with Storz Ophthalmics is in the midst of a large-scale (4,600 patient), 5-year, 11-center study on the treatment of AMD and cataracts using four different antioxidants and minerals (antioxidant enzyme cofactors) in different combinations. In 1993, the Eye Disease Case Control Study Group demonstrated that patients having the highest dietary intake of beta carotene or an "antioxidant index" composed of serum levels of antioxidants (vitamins C and E and selenium and carotenoids) had less risk of developing severe exudative AMD.

Today, more than 25 companies market antioxidant tablets or capsules to eye patients, yet a double-blind study evaluating any formulation has not been published to date.

CONSERVATIVE PREVENTION AND TREATMENT STRATEGY

Decreased intake of cardioprotective nutrients and sedentary lifestyles combined with age are of compelling significance as age itself brings additional degenerative changes in retinal tissues (over the age of 50), including gradual loss of melanin pigment and declines in gene-derived cellular antioxidant defenses (GSH peroxidase, superoxide dismutase, catalase, and metallothionine). With age, there is also decreased absorption of cofactor minerals ultimately used in antioxidant enzymatic reactions at the cellular level. Reduced antioxidant defense of the sensory retina–RPE complex combined with the cumulative effects of lifetime exposure to solar radiation places enormous stress on aging retina, especially the RPE.

In light of exhaustive animal, epidemiologic, and positive nonblinded but placebo-controlled U.S. and European clinical intervention supplement trial scientific data, the primary care clinician is in both a unique and vital position to develop a conservative prevention and treatment strategy:

1. Identify risk factors for AMD and seek internal medicine comanagement where necessary concerning cardiovascular disease, diet, and exercise.
2. Emphasize the importance of a well-balanced diet centered around plant foods to all patients. The basic science and clinical evidence of the benefit against cataractogenesis has been established. Proper well-balanced, plant-centered nutrition based on the U.S. Department of Agriculture Food Pyramid is especially important to patients with early signs of AMD or risk factors in the absence of visual loss.
3. Specifically recommend the intake of 5 ounces per day of fresh or frozen green, leafy vegetables five times per week. Spinach, for example, appears to be especially important to AMD patients as an excellent source of B vitamins, protective carotenoids (B carotene, zeaxanthin, and lutein), GSH, GSH precursors, and magnesium.
4. Since only 9% of the U.S. population follows the U.S. government recommendations concerning increased consumption of plant-based foods (five to nine portions of fruits and vegetables per day) and many westerners are largely inactive and consume high amounts of fat and cholesterol, it is appropriate and desirable for the primary care clinician to make specific recommendations concerning supplementation. Patients with added stress, i.e., smokers (who develop AMD 7 years before nonsmokers), as well as inner city patients who are not including any or minimal plant-derived food in their diet, are especially strong candidates for supplementation.
5. Prescribe a spectacle blue-blocking type tint or lens designed to protect the eye from UV exposure up to 430–450 nm in the visible spectrum. The current labeling standard for sunglasses developed by the Sunglass Association of America in conjunction with the U.S. Food and Drug Administration has been strongly criticized by researchers across the world for liberal standards on UVB radiation. Partially protective sunglasses may provide a false sense of security. The untoward effects of UVB radiation include cataractogenesis, pterygium, and other ocular diseases that may degrade vision. Blue-blocking type filters also improve vision by reduction of chromatic aberration and glare. Permitting unfiltered sun rays to enter the eyes while attempting to counter with nutritional intervention and exercise seems foolish. Those patients with blue or light-colored irides, all patients with aphakia, patients with pseudophakia who underwent cataract surgery prior to 1984 (when UV barriers were not incorporated into implants), those with silicon lens implants, and younger patients are all particularly vulnerable and would benefit from UVB radiation protection.

FURTHER CONSIDERATIONS IN PREVENTION AND TREATMENT

Although many functions, including visual acuity, color vision, and glare sensitivity, are compromised in AMD, prevention or treatment is problematic in that no clinical consensus exists to define or gauge subtle changes in visual function. Part of the explanation for this is the unique pathophysiology of the disease process itself.

Electron microscopy correlating the clinicomorphologic evolution of geographic RPE and rod photoreceptor atrophy has documented both primary RPE and photoreceptor atrophy and drusen-related atrophy. RPE and photoreceptor atrophy tends to spread around the central fovea in a horseshoe-like fashion. Drusen-related atrophy appears as separate patches that enlarge and coalesce, resulting in absolute and relative scotomas depending on the extent of damage. The distribution of geographic atrophy parallels known anatomic, topographic distributions of rods and lipofuscin and drusen formation in the posterior pole, and geographically and physiologically reflects the high turnover rate of rod discs compared with cone discs.

The size of the affected area of the macula is not indicative of visual function, thus patients may not seek care until the disease is quite advanced. A patient may lose 80% of photoreceptor–RPE complexes before the first line in Snellen acuity is lost. In many cases, by the time central fixation is compromised, atrophy has involved most of the fovea, and the patient may prefer a fixation point at the edge of atrophy, a point corresponding to the edge of an absolute scotoma, or to some distance away where the RPE and photoreceptors are still functional, i.e., at a relative scotoma. For these reasons, threshold Amsler grid testing, dark-adapted foveal red threshold sensitivity, contrast sensitivity, or short wavelength automated perimetry are more sensitive and specific than traditional Snellen acuity testing. Of these, threshold Amsler grid testing and contrast sensitivity are easily integrated into the array of clinical procedures for both office testing and home self-assessment.

In all likelihood, current instrumentation will not be sufficiently sensitive to measure subtle changes in visual function required for future nutrition or supplementation studies. Recently, it has been shown that foveal flicker sensitivity at low and midtemporal frequencies was highly sensitive to pre-exudative functional changes, showing significant changes up to 4 years in advance of neovascularization. The device uses a red light source with a stimulus wavelength of 660 nm, which largely bypasses confounding attenuation by the crystalline lens. Additionally, dark adaptation and pupil dilation are not required, and the test is relatively simple to administer. Foveal cone electroretinograms and digital imaging characterization of progressive RPE changes are other promising nascent research technologies that may someday be used clinically to determine subtle functional and pathologic changes in early AMD.

The presumed salutary health benefits of multivitamins and minerals combined with the minimal risk involved in their use has prompted some geriatric experts to establish the need for nutritional supplements in elderly patients. For example, a group of healthy, elderly adults who took a daily vitamin supplement for a year averaged only 23 days of infection-related illness compared with 48 days among a placebo group. The long-held belief that a good diet is all that is needed to maintain cardiovascular health is being questioned for vitamin E, as 100 IU per day of vitamin E has been shown to reduce the risk of heart attack by 45%. One would have to consume 4 cups of olive oil or a pound of almonds just to obtain 100 IU of vitamin E, an amount recommended by cardiologists.

Supplement Formulas*

In making recommendations to patients and interpreting double-blind study results, the clinician needs to discern the difference between recommended daily allowance (RDA) levels of nutrients to prevent historical deficiency diseases and therapeutic levels to stabilize or reverse progression of chronic disease.

The clinician's recommendation to the patient regarding a nutritional supplement as a prophylactic measure among high-risk individuals or to retard progression of AMD will most likely include a formulation that exceeds the current recommendations of the U.S. RDA. The formula should contain, for example, vitamins A, C, and E at levels a few times higher than the RDA. Such moderately higher levels are independently recommended by institutions such as the U.S. Department of Agriculture Center for Nutrition at Tufts University and the University of California at Berkeley School of Public Health newsletter to retard chronic disease such as cataracts. I-Caps Plus (LaHaye Labs), Ocuvite Plus (Storz Ophthalmics), and Maxilife (Twin Laboratories, Inc., Ronkonkoma, NY) are three examples of such formulations. Capsules should be taken in divided doses with meals and should not achieve total levels of zinc above 45 mg/day.

The appendix presents 23 current formulations organized by manufacturer, ingredient, and dose. It appears that in many instances clinicians are recommending nutrient formulas for eye disorders that do not differ significantly from that of daily over-the-counter vitamin formulas. A careful comparison will help the clinician make an informed recommendation for high-risk individuals. The clinician should realize that other products will likely appear on the market because a nutritional regimen or supplement formula has yet to be developed that incorporates all associated putative nutrient intake deficits matching the latest available scientific data. For example, none of the formulas listed contain the protective xanthophyll pigments or magnesium.

Nutritional supplements for the eyes are largely without serious side effects; however, clinicians should be aware of these minor side effects:

- Temporary diarrhea may occur if the patient is not used to taking vitamin C.
- Nausea may occur when taking nutrients on an empty stomach.

*This discussion is limited to the dry, insidious form of AMD, which results in atrophy of photoreceptor–RPE complexes and which represents 90% of all macular degeneration.

- Beta carotene in excess is stored in the skin appearing as a "beta carotene tan" in patients with liver disease.
- Dark yellow urine occurs with formulas containing riboflavin.

Patient-centered, computerized dietary food frequency questionnaires and office automated computational software are available to clinicians at low cost to simplify acquisition of dietary data. Such food frequency questionnaires are used in the treatment of other chronic diseases. However, an attempt to measure "serum levels" of antioxidant vitamins at one point in time does not provide a historical record of serum levels over the period when damage accumulated, nor does it reflect homeostatic compensatory mechanisms. In other words, serum values only reflect short-term nutrient intake.

In conclusion, basic science, epidemiologic, and non-double-blinded clinical trials to date suggest that AMD is a nutrition-responsive disease. There is evidence that vitamin and mineral supplementation combined with a low-fat diet, exercise, smoking cessation, and UVB solar filtration may prevent or postpone the morbidity of AMD. A balanced, sensible approach to dealing with this issue is recommended. Patient education and advice by way of brochures, pamphlets, and U.S. Department of Agriculture and RDA information will keep the patient abreast of attitudes and developments in this important area of nutrition.

SUGGESTED READING

Alexander LJ. Ocular vitamin therapy. Optom Clin 1992;2:1–34.

Dyrka B, Sabine I, Buchi ER. Arteriosclerotic changes in orbital arteries supplying the human eye. Neuro-ophthalmology 1994;14:121–126.

Eye Disease Case Control Study. Antioxidant status and neovascular age-related macular degeneration. Arch Ophthalmol 1992;111:104–109.

Hampton GR, Nelsen PT. Medical Treatment of ARM in Age-Related Macular Degeneration. In D Newsome (ed), Ophthalmology: Principles and Practice. New York: Raven, 1992;183–189.

Richer SP. Is there a prevention and treatment strategy for macular degeneration? J Am Optom Assoc 1993;64:838–850.

Sarks JP, Sarks SH, Killingsworth MC, et al. Evolution of geographic atrophy of the retinal pigment epithelium. Eye 1988;2:552–577.

Seddon JM, Ajani VA, Sperduto RD, et al. Dietary carotenoids, vitamins A, C, and E, and advanced age-related macular degeneration. JAMA 1994;272:1413–1420.

Vannas S, Orma H. On the treatment of arteriosclerotic chorioretinopathy. Acta Ophthalmol 1958;36:601–611.

Appendix

CURRENTLY AVAILABLE OCULAR ANTIOXIDANT/MINERAL FORMULAS

Product (manufacturer)	*Vitamin A/ beta carotene (IU)*	*Vitamin C (mg)*	*Vitamin E*	*L-Glutathione*	*L-Cysteine/ N-Acetylcysteine (mg)*
Bright Eyes (Futurebiotics)	500/Palmitate 10,000 Beta-C	333	67 IU	—	100
Eyebright Formula (Nutri-West)	9,996 Beta-C	100	25 IU	100 μg	—
Eye Formula (KAL Inc.)	2,500/Palmitate 6,250 Beta-C	200	100 IU	2 mg	50
Eye Power (Nature's Herbs)	10,000 Beta-C	400	160 mg	2 mg	40
Eye Support (Naturade)	5,000 Beta-C	75	15 IU	—	—
I-Caps Time Release (LaHaye Labs)	7,000 Beta-C	200	100 IU	—	—
I-Tone (Enzymatic Therapy)	1,250/Palmitate 1,250 Beta-C	67	10 IU	—	—
Lipotriad (Numark Labs)	5,000 Beta-C	60	30 IU	—	—
Macu Caps (Vita Source)	5,000 Beta-C	250	50 IU	—	—
Nutrivision (Bronson Pharmaceuticals)	5,000 Beta-C	300	100 IU	—	—
Ocucaps (Akorn Inc.)	5,000 Beta-C	400	200 mg	5 mg	—
Ocucare (Nature's Plus)	2,500/Palmitate	250	100 IU	—	25
OcuDyne (Allergy Research)	1,875/Palmitate	60	42 IU	—	31.3
Ocuguard (Twinlab)	10,000 Beta-C	375	100 IU	2.5 mg	50
Ocuvite (Storz/Lederle)	5,000 Beta-C	60	30 IU	—	—
Oxy-Vision (Nature Made/PharmaVite)	5,000 Beta-C	120	60 IU	—	—
See (Quantum)	12,500/Palmitate 2,500 Beta-C	500	100 IU	—	—
Vital Eyes (Allergan)	10,000 Beta-C	200	100 IU	—	—
VitalEyez (Metabolic Maintenance Products)	8,333 Beta-C	333	133 IU	33 mg	—
Vizion (Solaray)	833/Palmitate 3,333 Beta-C	333	67 IU	—	33
ZincACE (Royal Nutrition)	5,000 Beta-C	60	30 IU	500 μg	20

Vitamin B_2 (riboflavin) (mg)	Vitamin B_2 (niacin or niacinamide) (mg)	Vitamin B_6 (pyrodoxine) (mg)	Vitamin B_{12} (μg)	Folic acid (μg)	Zinc (mg)
13	3.3	1.6	—	—	5
10	—	—	—	125	5.4
10	2.5	2	5	100	5
10	—	—	—	—	6
5	—	3	—	200	7.5
20	—	—	—	—	40
1.5	15	—	—	—	2.5
1.7	20	2	6	—	30
10	—	—	—	—	20
—	—	—	—	—	30
—	—	—	—	—	40
—	—	—	—	—	10
3.0	7.1	3.6	6.2	100	10
12.5	—	—	—	—	6.25
—	—	—	—	—	40
—	—	—	—	200	40
20	—	—	—	—	12.5
—	—	—	—	—	40
5	—	5	—	—	10
—	—	—	—	—	1.6
25	—	—	—	—	40

Product *(manufacturer)*	*Chromium glucose tolerance factor (μg)*	*Manganese (mg)*	*Copper (mg)*	*Selenium (μg)*	*Taurine (mg)*
Bright Eyes (Futurebiotics)	67	—	—	33	—
Eyebright Formula (Nutri-West)	10	—	—	5	—
Eye Formula (KAL Inc.)	50	—	—	25	37.5
Eye Power (Nature's Herbs)	40	—	—	40	40
Eye Support (Naturade)	100	—	—	25	—
I-Caps Time Release (LaHaye Labs)	—	—	2	—	—
I-Tone (Enzymatic Therapy)	—	—	—	25	—
Lipotriad (Numark Labs)	—	—	2	40	—
Macu Caps (Vita Source)	—	5	1	20	—
Nutrivision (Bronson Pharmaceuticals)	25	—	1.5	50	—
Ocucaps (Akorn Inc.)	—	—	2	40	—
Ocucare (Nature's Plus)	—	—	—	—	—
OcuDyne (Allergy Research)	—	—	3.75	25	62.5
Ocuguard (Twinlab)	50	—	—	25	50
Ocuvite (Storz/Lederle)	—	—	2	40	—
Oxy-Vision (Nature Made/PharmaVite)	—	—	2	50	—
See (Quantum)	100	—	—	56	—
Vital Eyes (Allergan)	—	5	2	40	—
VitalEyez (Metabolic Maintenance Products)	67	1.6	2	33	—
Vizion (Solaray)	17	—	—	17	33
ZincACE (Royal Nutrition)	10	—	2	40	—

Glycine/ glutamic acid (mg)	*Pantothenic acid B_5 (mg)*	*L-Glutamine (mg)*	*L-Lysine (mg)*	*Quercetin (mg)*	*Bilberry (mg)*
—	13	25	—	33	3.3
—	—	—	—	—	—
—	—	—	—	—	25
—	—	—	—	50	16
—	—	—	—	—	25
—	—	—	—	—	—
—	—	—	—	—	—
—	—	—	—	—	—
—	—	—	—	—	—
—	—	—	—	—	—
—	—	—	—	—	—
—	50	—	25	See "Other flavonoids"	See "Other flavonoids"
6.25	25	—	—	37.5	5
—	—	—	—	25	2.5
—	—	—	—	—	—
—	—	—	—	—	—
—	20	—	—	See "Other flavonoids"	See "Other flavonoids"
—	—	—	—	—	—
—	—	—	—	—	—
—	—	33	—	—	—
—	—	—	—	—	—

***Product** (manufacturer)*	*Rutin (mg)*	*Citrus bioflavonoid (mg)*	*Ginkgo biloba (mg)*	*Other flavonoids (mg)*
Bright Eyes (Futurebiotics)	33	33	—	67
Eyebright Formula (Nutri-West)	18	—	—	5
Eye Formula (KAL Inc.)	25	—	—	75
Eye Power (Nature's Herbs)	—	—	4	—
Eye Support (Naturade)	—	—	—	12.5
I-Caps Time Release (LaHaye Labs)	—	—	—	—
I-Tone (Enzymatic Therapy)	12.5	15	—	—
Lipotriad (Numark Labs)	—	—	—	—
Macu Caps (Vita Source)	—	—	—	—
Nutrivision (Bronson Pharmaceuticals)	—	—	—	—
Ocucaps (Akorn Inc.)	—	—	—	—
Ocucare (Nature's Plus)	See "Other flavonoids"	See "Other flavonoids"	See "Other flavonoids"	190
OcuDyne (Allergy Research)	—	—	7.5	—
Ocuguard (Twinlab)	25	62.5	—	—
Ocuvite (Storz/Lederle)	—	—	—	—
Oxy-Vision (Nature Made/PharmaVite)	—	—	—	—
See (Quantum)	See "Other flavonoids"	See "Other flavonoids"	See "Other flavonoids"	180
Vital Eyes (Allergan)	—	—	—	—
VitalEyez (Metabolic Maintenance Products)	67	—	—	167
Vizion (Solaray)	—	23	—	23
ZincACE (Royal Nutrition)	—	—	—	—

Coenzyme Q10 (mg)	*Eyebright herb (mg)*	*Raw eye tissue (mg)*	*Other (see labels)*
—	167	—	Chamomile, pantothenic acid
—	300	—	Many others
—	—	—	—
—	See other ingredients	—	Eyebright base
—	25	—	Pantothenic acid, Eyebright, others
—	—	—	—
—	100	80	Potassium, inositol, others
—	—	—	Thiamine B_1
—	—	—	—
—	—	—	—
—	—	—	Pyruvate
—	—	—	Pantothenic acid
—	—	—	Thiamine B_1, calcium/magnesium, others
—	—	—	—
—	—	—	—
—	—	—	Vitamin D
—	—	—	OMEGA-3, 250 mg, pantothenic acid
—	—	—	—
10	—	—	—
—	—	—	Glycine
—	—	—	Calcium, thiamine

MANUFACTURER INFORMATION

Bright Eyes Tablets, Futurebiotics, 48 Elliott Street, Brattleboro, VT 05301, (802) 257-5691

Eyebright Complex Tablets, Nutri-West, P.O. Box 950, Douglas, WY 82633, (800) 443-3333

Eye Formula Capsules, KAL, Inc., P.O. Box 4023, Woodland Hills, CA 91365, (818) 340-3035

Eye Power Capsules, Nature's Herbs, P.O. Box 336, Orem, UT 84059, (800) HER-BALS

Eye Support Tablets, Naturade Products Inc., 7110 Jackson Street, Paramount, CA 90723, (310) 531-8120

I-Caps Plus and **Time Release** Tablets, LaHaye Laboratories, Inc., 2205 152nd Avenue, N.E., Redmond, WA 98052, (206) 644-2020

I-Tone Tablets, Enzymatic Therapy, P.O. Box 22310, Green Bay, WI 54305, (800) 783-2286

Lipotriad Tablets, Numark Laboratories, Inc., P.O. Box 6321, Edison, NJ 08818, (800) 331-0221

Macu Caps Caplets, Vita Source, 1377 East Citrus, Suite 339, Redlands, CA 92374, (800) 332-8180

Nutrivision Tablets, Bronson Pharmaceuticals, 1945 Craig Road, St. Louis, MO 63146, (800) 732-3323

OcuCaps Capsules, Akorn, Inc., 100 Akorn Drive, Abita Springs, LA 70420, (504) 893-1257

OcuCare Tablets, Nature's Plus, 548 Broad Hollow Road, Melville, NY 11747, (516) 293-0030

OcuDyne Capsules, Allergy Research Group/Nutricology, 400 Preda Street, San Leandro, CA 94577, (800) 545-9960, (800) 782-4274

Ocuguard Capsules, Twinlab, 2120 Smithtown, Ronkonkoma, NY 11799, (516) 467-3140

Ocuvite Tablets, Storz Ophthalmics/Lederle, 3365 Tree Court, St. Louis, MO 63122, (314) 225-5051

Oxy-Vision Tablets, Nature Made, 15451 San Fernando Mission Boulevard, Mission Hills, CA 91346, (818) 837-3633

See Capsules, Quantum, 754 Washington Street, Eugene, OR 97402, (503) 345-5556, (800) 448-1448

Vital Eyes Capsules, Allergan, Irvine, CA 92715, (800) 366-6554

VitalEyez Capsules, Metabolic Maintenance Products, P.O. Box 3600, Sisters, OR 97759, (800) 772-PURE

Vizion Capsules, Solaray, 2815 Industrial Drive, Ogden, UT 84401, (800) 669-8877

ZincACE Tablets, Royal Nutrition International, 4071 E. La Palma Avenue, Suite F, Anaheim, CA 92807, (800) 524-3727

Source: Reprinted with permission from Health Spectrum Publishers, 8851 Central Avenue G-620, Montclair, CA 91763. (800) 809-2219. Publishers of *Nutrition and the Eyes*.

CHAPTER

31 Ophthalmic Lasers

John L. Henahan

There has been a revolution in eye care since the first optical ruby laser was developed in 1960. Laser technology has advanced from the early days of ruby panretinal photocoagulation (PRP) to treat severe cases of proliferative diabetic retinopathy to include a flood of new technologies that has resulted in laser applications in nearly all areas of eye care, including retinal disease, glaucoma, and refractive surgery.

The pace of development continues to accelerate with new and ever more advanced lasers entering clinical trials. The result of this has been twofold: first, laser intervention is being considered earlier in eye disease; second, practicing optometrists are becoming more involved in deciding when laser intervention should be considered as they take more control of patients who require medical treatment.

Nowhere has the impact of laser technologies been more dramatic than in the treatment of retinal diseases. This is especially true of retinal vascular diseases including diabetic retinopathy and venous occlusive disease. Before the advent of lasers as a viable mode of treatment, the majority of these patients went untreated. Now, thousands have had their vision saved from severe loss and even total blindness. As our understanding of how lasers affect tissue deepens, we can expect significant advances to be made in treating various retinal diseases.

LIGHT AND LASER

To understand how lasers produce their effect, we first need to review some basic principles of light.

Visible light makes up only a small portion of the electromagnetic spectrum (Figure 31.1), which also includes ultraviolet (UV), infrared, and microwaves. Electromagnetic radiation is characterized by both *wave* and *particle* properties. Particle properties are responsible for molecular effects (i.e., photon absorption or emission), whereas waves produce larger scale phenomenon (i.e., reflection and refraction). Some lasers use visible light, whereas others use shorter (UV) or longer infrared wavelengths.

What are the characteristics of lasers that they should have such a powerful impact on ocular tissues, since they are simply a type of electromagnetic radiation that we are already exposed to constantly?

To answer that question, we need to review a bit of college physics with respect to the characteristics of "normal" light in addition to the unique properties that characterize laser light (Table 31.1).

Wavelength

Normal light is made up of many wavelengths. White light usually has wavelengths that cover most of the visible spectrum from red to violet. Lasers, on the other hand, consist (for all practical purposes) of a single wavelength. Wavelength is a crucial element in determining the nature of laser–tissue interactions.

Collimation

Laser light is highly collimated, which means there is virtually no divergence of the light over distance. Normal light (except for light from sources as far away as the sun) diverges rapidly as it moves away from its source. This causes the light's energy to spread out over a large area, therefore, the energy at any given point is minimal. By contrast, a laser delivers all of its energy to a very small spot, which depends on the spot size selected. Consequently, the energy is very intense at that location (Figure 31.2).

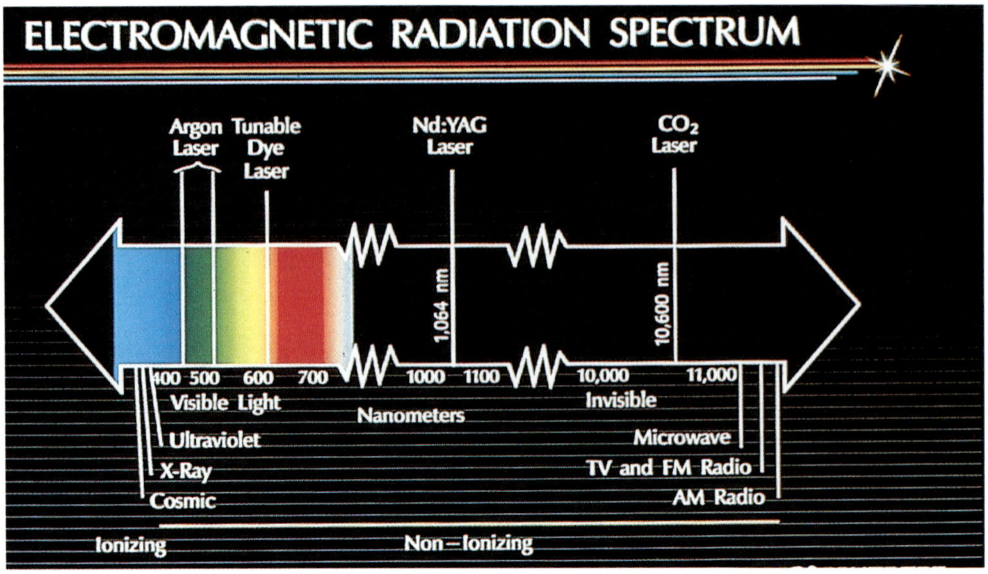

FIGURE 31.1. A schematic illustration of the electromagnetic spectrum. Notice that visible light makes up only a small portion of the total spectrum.

TABLE 31.1. Characteristics of Normal Versus Laser Light

Normal light	*Laser light*
Many wavelengths	Monochromatic
Divergent	Collimated
Incoherent waves	Coherent waves

Coherence

Even if collimated light from a nonlaser source (such as a star) could be harnessed, the effect would be less than a laser, because the incoherence of the waves reduces its power. Keep in mind that two equal waves that are out of phase cancel each other. Therefore, in order to be coherent, all the waves must be uniform and in phase (which magnifies the effect) (Figure 31.3). Therefore, a laser needs to be able to develop coherent, collimated, and monochromatic light to be effective. But how does a laser produce light with these properties?

To answer that question we need to look at some of the molecular *particle* properties of light. Laser stands for:

Light
Amplification by
Stimulated
Emission of
Radiation

Atoms have electrons surrounding them, which can orbit at various distinct distances from the nucleus. The farther from the nucleus an electron is, the farther it can fall back toward the nucleus. When it falls one orbit, it releases energy in the form of a *photon* (Figure 31.4). On the other hand, a photon must be absorbed by an atom in order to push it one orbit further from the nucleus. The question is, how can a laser have so much power if for every photon absorbed, one photon is emitted? The answer lies in the number of photons being absorbed.

When only a single photon of energy is absorbed, an electron is briefly elevated by one orbit. It then quickly falls back to a lower orbit (releasing a photon). But, if *another* photon hits the atom before the electron can fall back, two photons of equal energy and frequency are released (Figure 31.4). Moreover, these two photons travel in the same direction and are perfectly in phase (coherent). This interaction is the basis of the laser effect. Once this effect begins, there is a cascade effect that results in a large number of photons traveling through the laser cavity.

The question remains, however, how does one supply the energy to produce such an effect, and what determines the wavelength produced?

Atoms are excited by either an electrical current passing through the laser media or a flashlamp. The wavelength of the emitted photons is determined by the nature of the media (atoms) within the laser cavity. This may be either solid, liquid, or gas (Table 31.2).

LASER TYPES AND TISSUE RESPONSES

The nature of the laser–tissue interaction is determined by (1) wavelength and (2) the amount of energy delivered. How much energy is delivered depends on three things: the power used, exposure time, and spot size.

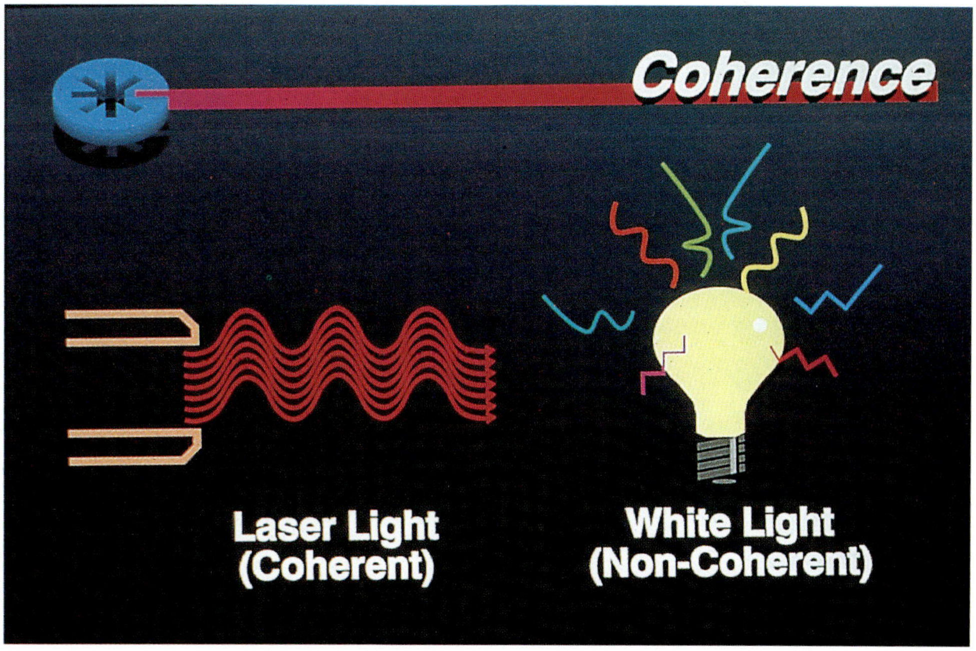

FIGURE 31.2. Noncoherent light is highly divergent from a source such as a light bulb, whereas laser light shows almost no divergence from its source.

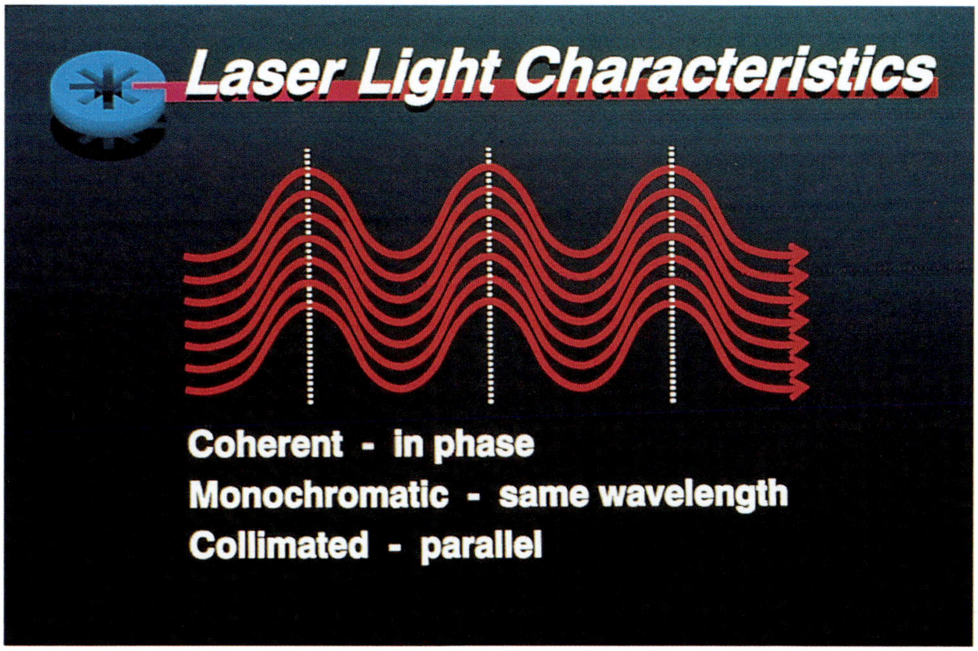

FIGURE 31.3. Normal light has many wavelengths, and waves of the same length are not all in phase. All the waves produced by a laser are the same length and in phase (they peak at the same spot).

There are three general types of laser–tissue responses to laser light exposure. These include thermal effects, photochemical effects, and ionizing effects.

Laser Effects

Photocoagulation is the most important clinical result of thermal effects. Generally, lasers in the visible wavelengths are used to produce this effect. The primary types used in ophthalmic procedures include argon blue-green, argon green, krypton yellow, krypton red, and tunable dye (Table 31.3).

As the name suggests, thermal effects are the result of increased temperature in the tissue targeted. A temperature increase of 10–20°C results in denaturation of biomolecules. Blood vessel and capillary closure probably results from heating of the red blood cells in the vessel with subsequent thrombus formation and collagen

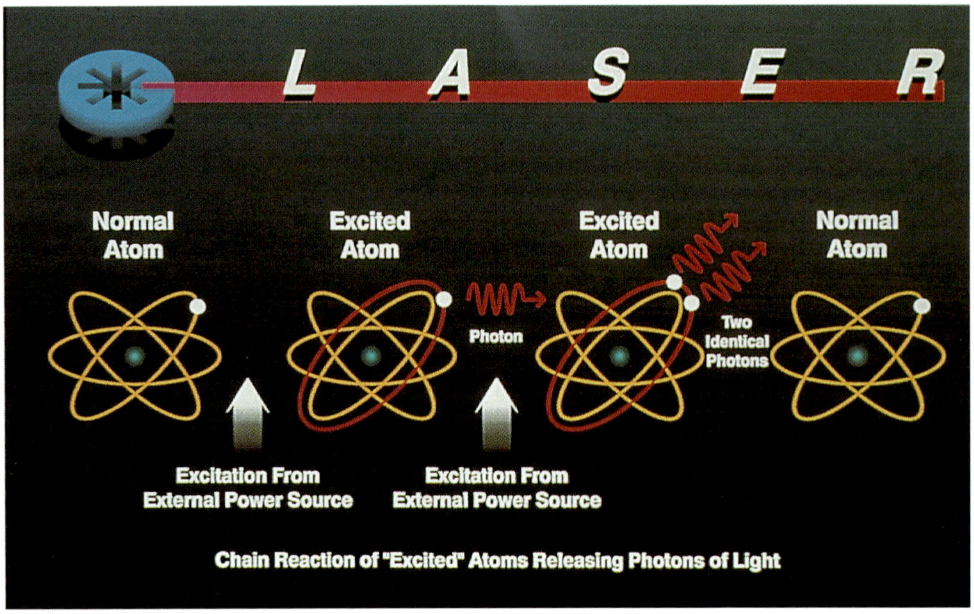

FIGURE 31.4. The fundamental laser effect is demonstrated. When an atom absorbs a photon of energy, its electron moves to a higher orbit. When it releases that energy, it falls back to its original orbit or ground state. However, if an energized atom absorbs another photon before falling back to the ground state, it will release two in-phase photons simultaneously that are traveling in the same direction.

TABLE 31.2. Laser Types

Media	*Examples*
Solid	Ruby, Nd:YAG
Liquid	Carbon dioxide
Gas	Argon, krypton, excimer

Nd:YAG = neodymium-yttrium-aluminum-garnet.

TABLE 31.3. Lasers Used in Ophthalmic Procedures

Laser types	*Wavelength (nm)*
Argon blue	488
Argon green	514.5
Krypton yellow	468.2
Krypton red	647.1
Tunable dye	570–630

shrinkage in the vessel wall itself. These two effects combine to "seal" the vessel.

Photocoagulating lasers have enjoyed the most widespread application of any type of ophthalmic laser system. Their applications include glaucoma management (open and closed angle), retinal vascular disease, age-related macular degeneration (AMD), and other retinal conditions.

The amount of energy delivered and the wavelength used determine which layer(s) of tissue are affected. As the wavelength increases, the penetration depth of the laser also tends to increase.

Photocoagulating lasers depend on absorption by melanin, macular xanthophyll, and hemoglobin pigments. In the absence of pigment, no significant effect can be achieved. Different wavelengths are absorbed to a greater or lesser degree by each of these pigments (Figure 31.5).

In certain disease states, specific layers of tissue are selected for laser treatment, whereas in other conditions, a more generalized, full-thickness burn is desired. When determining which wavelength and intensity to use for a specific condition, the tissue layers to be treated are of prime concern. However, the selectivity of various wavelengths for certain layers decreases as the intensity of the burn is increased. Therefore, powerful burns can affect all layers of the tissue, regardless of the wavelength chosen. Additionally, increased energy, especially from longer exposure times, causes increased thermal spreading to the surrounding tissue (increasing the amount of tissue affected).

Blue wavelengths are rapidly absorbed by macular xanthophyll and therefore have most of their effect on the inner retinal layers (closest to the vitreous). This is generally not desirable in macular procedures as it excessively damages the sensory layers of the retina. However, these lasers are effective in a blue-green mixture when a full-thickness burn is desired, such as in PRP.

Green wavelengths are less absorbed by xanthophyll than blue. Green is a good wavelength for many retinal procedures where an intraretinal effect is desired, such as focal treatment for diabetic maculopathy. Nevertheless, the absorption of green energy by xanthophyll may be undesirable when extremely precise burns are needed close to the fovea.

Krypton yellow and red are not significantly absorbed by macular xanthophyll pigment. This makes

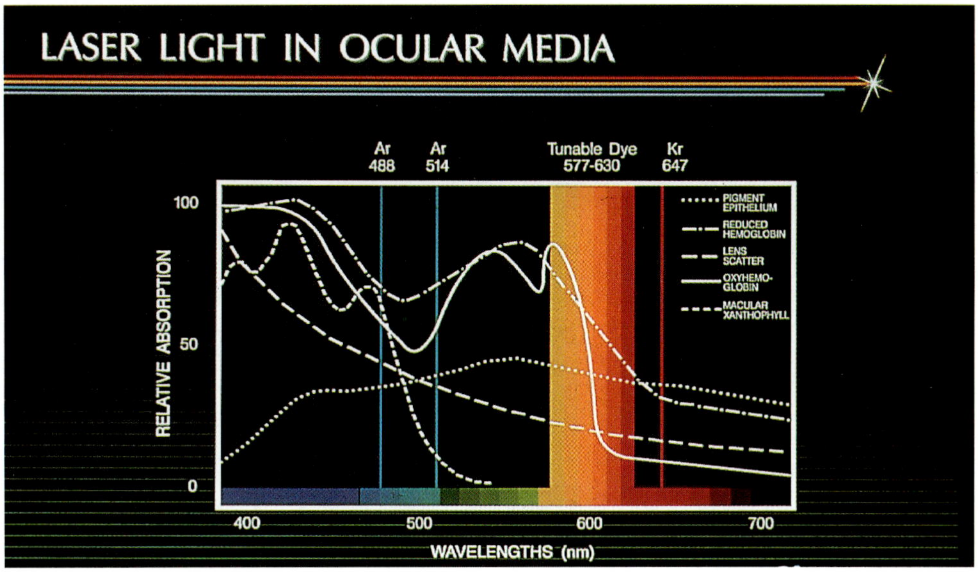

FIGURE 31.5. Melanin, oxygenated hemoglobin, and macular xanthophyll each have wavelength absorption profiles that differ from one another. This means you may selectively target different structures (and depths) or target all of them depending on the wavelength you choose.

them desirable for certain treatments in the macula. The choice of yellow versus red depends on the layer one wants to most affect. Yellow is used to treat intraretinal problems (such as backround diabetic retinopathy [BDR]), while red is used for subretinal and choroidal anomalies (subretinal or choroidal neovascularization). In addition, the red beam can penetrate media opacities and retinal hemorrhages to treat problems underneath the blood. A drawback of krypton red arises from its poor absorption in lightly pigmented eyes. When this problem occurs, many practitioners use a tunable dye laser.

Tunable dye lasers use organic dyes that allow a choice of wavelengths between 570 and 630 nm. Thus, when krypton red is not available, or minimal pigmentation of the fundus is of concern, a wavelength that balances absorption and deep penetration may be selected.

Photochemical effects include *photoradiation* and *photoablation*. Photoradiation is primarily used in the treatment of ocular tumors, especially large choroidal melanomas. A compound called hematoporphyrin derivative (HpD) is placed into the bloodstream by intravenous administration. HpD is selectively absorbed by active tumor tissue; consequently, it becomes heavily concentrated in the tumor's cells. Light between 625 and 635 nm is readily absorbed by HpD. When irradiated by light in this range, HpD and oxygen interact to create cytotoxic oxygen singlets that destroy hemorous cells. Therefore, it is possible to destroy HpD-laden tumor cells selectively by exposing them to a 630-nm rhodamine B dye laser.

Photoablation results from exposure to short (<300 nm) wavelength laser light in the UV portion of the electromagnetic spectrum. Lasers using these wavelengths, especially the 193 nm excimer laser, have their effect on tissues by causing breakdown of larger molecules into smaller ones. These small molecules, such as CO_2, are ejected from the surface in what literally appears to be a puff of smoke.

The clinical utility of short-pulsed excimer lasers results from their ability to remove tissue with submicron precision *without any thermal damage* to surrounding tissue. These "clean" removals are thought to incite less of an inflammatory and healing reaction, which is desirable in refractive and glaucoma surgery (Figures 31.5 and 31.6).

CLINICAL APPLICATION OF OPHTHALMIC LASERS

Photocoagulators in Retinal Disease

The retina is free from pigmentation (except for macular xanthophyll pigment) to the depth of the retinal pigment epithelium (RPE). However, blood corpuscles passing through the intraretinal capillary beds can absorb laser energy. When studying Figure 31.5, one can see that the absorption for most of the pigmented structures drops off quickly, with the exception of melanin. This fact, along with an understanding of retinal-choroidal anatomy, helps explain why longer wavelengths penetrate more deeply to the RPE and choroid.

The clinical appearance of the condition being treated determines which techniques of retinal laser photocoagulation are used. The following list summarizes the most commonly performed retinal laser treatments.

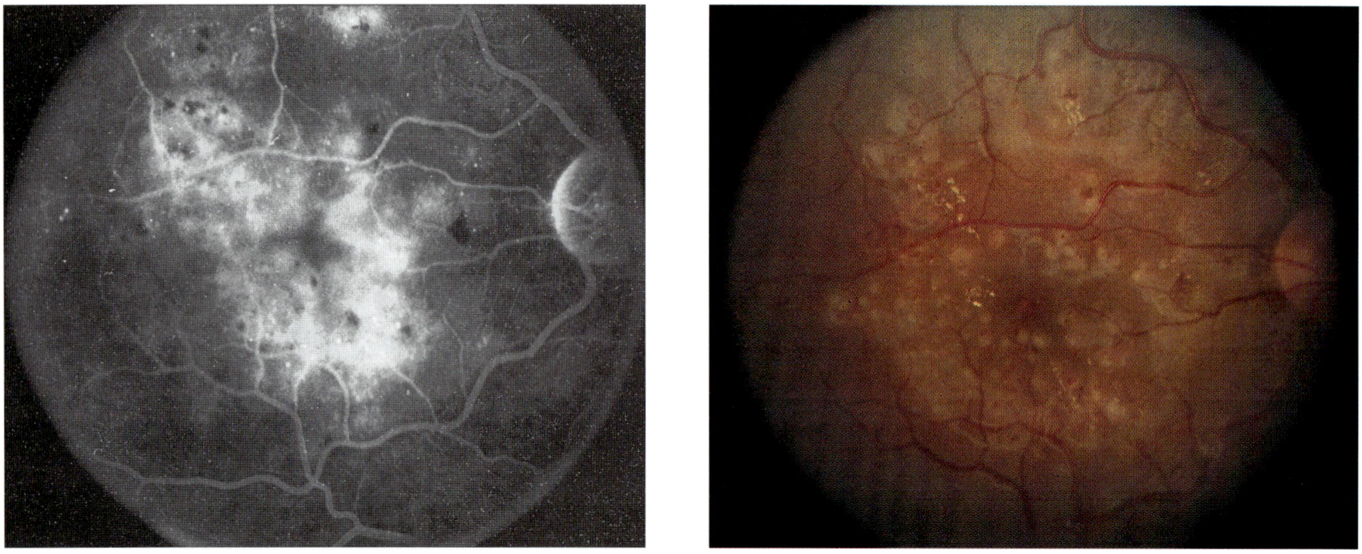

A B

FIGURE 31.6. This 20-year-old juvenile diabetic is suffering from diabetic maculopathy in the right eye. A. The fluorescein angiogram demonstrates diffuse leakage in the late phases. B. By treating those vessels that are leaking, the process can be arrested. Over the next few months the fluid will resorb, potentially improving vision. However, the main goal of treatment is to prevent further visual loss, not to improve vision.

Retinal Photocoagulation Techniques

- Macular treatment for BDR
- Panretinal/sectorial treatment
- Grid macular treatment
- Subretinal neovascular membrane treatment
- AMD membrane treatment
- Sealing retinal holes

Focal treatment for diabetic retinopathy is the most common form of retinal laser treatment in diabetics. This technique involves placing selected burns, usually of small size (50 μ), directly to leaking blood vessels. The wavelength used varies from practitioner to practitioner but argon green is most commonly used (514.5 nm). However, a growing number of practitioners prefer krypton yellow (568.2 nm) due to its reduced macular xanthophyll absorption and the fact that it causes less damage to the RPE. This is especially advantageous when working close to the foveal avascular zone, where preservation of the RPE is crucial. In nonproliferative diabetic retinopathy (NPDR), most practitioners reserve treatment until the macular area is directly threatened (Figure 31.6). Treatment for severe NPDR may also involve some degree of PRP. In cases of macular edema, some type of focal or macular grid laser pattern is used depending on the specific case.

PRP is a technique where large (250–500 μ) burns are placed throughout the posterior pole and equator. The macular area is spared. The goal of treatment is to selectively destroy less vital areas of the retina. This is believed to reduce production of a "vasoproliferative factor" that arises from ischemic retinal tissue and prompts the formation of neovascular nets. Complications due to neovascularization are the main cause of profound visual loss in diabetic retinopathy. While most practitioners agree that performing full PRP (usually 1,200–2,000 burns) at one session increases the risk of visual loss, there is less consensus regarding how to stage the treatment (Figure 31.7). Nevertheless, a general rule is that a blue-green laser with just enough power to blanch the treated spot and a spacing that leaves one spot size between burns is acceptable. Sectorial PRP is also used in some types of venous occlusive diseases.

Sectorial treatment is similar to PRP, except that the treatment area is limited. This is most commonly used in patients suffering from a branch retinal vein occlusion or regional ischemia from another cause.

Grid macular treatment is just as the name implies; a series of light burns are placed throughout the parafoveal region in a grid pattern in hopes of reducing diffuse macular edema. Typically, a green-only or yellow beam is used to perform this procedure. Again, the yellow wavelength is minimally absorbed by xanthophyll pigment distributed in the macula; therefore, use of a yellow beam is less harmful to the sensory retinal layers.

Subretinal neovascularization, by definition, arises from the deeper layers of the retina–choroid complex. Consequently, treatment is aimed at the source of the problem in the deeper layers of the retina. Most commonly a krypton red or tunable dye laser in the red range

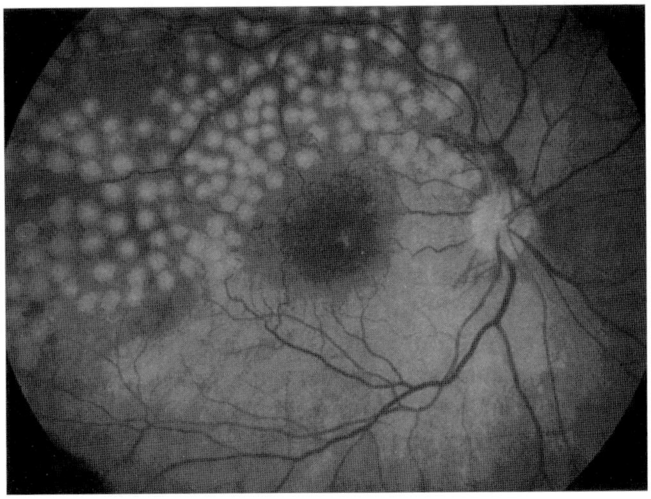

FIGURE 31.7. The pattern of burns in full superior temporal panretinal photocoagulation. Notice how the major vessels and macular area are spared.

is used to treat these conditions. By directing a moderate intensity burn to the abnormal area, it is possible to coagulate the diseased vessels, without excessive damage to the overlying retina and nerve fiber layer.

Treatment strategies for wet macular degeneration continue to rapidly evolve, and considerable controversy about when, what, and how to treat persists. The goal is to halt the development of abnormal blood vessels under the macula. These vessels leak fluid profusely and often hemorrhage, resulting in profound central vision loss and macular scarring. Of the three main categories of neovascularization in AMD, extrafoveal membranes are the most successfully treated. Unfortunately, even these patients have a 60% recurrence rate of neovascularization. Treatment of subfoveal and recurrent neovascularization does not enjoy a very favorable prognosis; however, treatment can be effective in minimizing the size of the central blind spot. This may be crucial when providing low vision rehabilitation.

A variety of other macular conditions are amenable to treatment with lasers. These include macroaneurysms, neovascularization in angioid streaks, presumed ocular histoplasmosis, choroidal rupture, and other conditions.

SIDE EFFECTS

In addition to the problems of misdirected burns to the center of the patient's fovea, a number of potentially serious side effects arise as a result of the thermal nature of photocoagulation. These include damage to the sensory retina, resulting in vision loss, and tissue shrinkage, which can result in retinal detachment, epiretinal membrane formation, and retinal edema secondary to an inflammatory reaction incited by the laser. Hemorrhaging may also occur.

SUMMARY

Lasers play an essential role in the treatement of macular disease. Patients suffering from retinal disease have been some of the main beneficiaries of ophthalmic laser applications. This trend may be expected to continue as the technology continues to evolve. Strides in the treatment of AMD, the nation's leading cause of blindness among those over 65 years of age, may be expected. Lasers will be used more in "surgical procedures" to treat glaucoma. Even those with corneal blindness may have new, less invasive options to cure their conditions.

It is essential that eye care providers keep abreast of these rapidly evolving modalities and seek access to this technology and its applicable techniques to ensure the best possible care for their patients.

SUGGESTED READING

Alexander L. Primary Care of the Posterior Segment. East Norwalk, CT: Appleton & Lange, 1989.

L'Esperance F. Opthalmic Lasers (3rd ed). St. Louis: Mosby, 1988.

Pflibson KP, Weiter J. Retinal Laser Surgery: Principles and Techniques. In SJ Ryan (ed), Retina. St. Louis: Mosby, 1989:129–138.

CHAPTER

32

Visual and Rehabilitative Considerations

John L. Henahan and Gerald R. Friedman

In the past century, the size of our elderly population has quadrupled. This trend is continuing at an ever increasing pace. In fact, the number of persons with severe vision impairment is currently estimated at approximately 2.9 million. That number is projected to double in the next 35 years.

Clearly, we are on the cusp of an exploding problem of severely visually impaired persons in our society, many of whom are suffering from macular disease. The problem of vision impairment is highly personal and traumatic for the individual suffering from it. This is especially true of patients without a family member or friend to assist them with activities of daily living. These patients are more likely to require institutionalization or other costly remedies. However, even patients with a strong family support system may suffer from depression or other psychological conditions when they lose vision.

As providers of eye health care, optometrists and ophthalmologists are in the unique position of delivering the news of vision loss to their patients. The manner in which this is handled, or too often not handled, may have a profound effect on how the patient copes with his or her vision loss.

The purpose of this chapter is to provide the practitioner dealing with macular diseases with an awareness of the importance of addressing the patient's fears and concerns in a sensitive manner. In addition, an overview of services (low vision and other services) that patients with vision loss may use is presented. This chapter is not, however, meant to be a course on low vision or the physiology and psychology of vision loss.

COUNSELING THE PATIENT WITH VISION IMPAIRMENT

One of the greatest fears people have is of "going blind." The emotional power that phrase carries cannot be understated. Most people also have no concept or understanding of *legal blindness*. When a patient hears the word *blind* in any context, an image of eternal night, helplessness, and despair may overcome him or her. As the messengers of this news, we can avoid triggering this response in our patients by explaining their condition sensitively and presenting low vision alternatives when appropriate. By providing these patients with an opportunity to continue reading and performing other tasks through the use of their remaining vision, we do them the greatest possible service. Low vision treatment or rehabilitation can be the vehicle by which this is achieved.

When counseling patients with macular disease regarding their vision loss, it is essential to reassure the patient (when appropriate) that they will never go blind. Many patients even with 20/200 or 20/400 are greatly reassured with this news; a sense of hopelessness is averted and a strata on which to initiate a rehabilitative effort is provided.

When explaining the role of low vision treatment to patients, one should emphasize that the low vision specialist cannot cure the underlying problem. The particular treatment could, however, help restore functional vision to some degree.

A discussion of legal blindness could follow. It may be emphasized that legal blindness only means that the patient is entitled to certain tax benefits and other services. An unfortunate scenario, all too common, is the patient realizing his or her predicament only when confronted by a stranger from the government representing an agency or commission for the blind. Once again, the problem of definition is complicated by poor communication.

LOW VISION EVALUATION

As with any complicated medical condition, the history is vital, and, as in life, history often repeats itself. In today's ever changing health care delivery system, a comprehensive history can serve to reduce or eliminate duplication of testing and treatment, making it an important part of total treatment. Whether the low vision evaluation is provided in the office or referred out, a more comprehensive history may be necessary in order to approach the treatment of the patient appropriately.

Medical Information and Significant Tests

- Diagnosis
- Previous retinal laser therapy
- Review of visual fields
- Previous ocular surgery
- General medical history
- Overall mental status
- Review of electroretinograms/visual evoked potential
- Review of fundus photographs and fluorescein angiograms
- Review of scanning laser ophthalmoscopy
- Review of neuroimaging studies

In addition, the presence of certain systemic diseases (see following list) may have an impact on the evaluation and management options available. In the low vision evaluation, the importance of understanding the patient's overall mental and physical health cannot be overstated.

Select List of Systemic Diseases That Influence the Low Vision Consultation

- Trauma
- Peripheral vascular disease
- Alzheimer's disease
- Cancer
- Parkinson's disease
- Other neuromuscular disease
- Diabetes mellitus
- Inherited diseases
- Stroke
- Congenital defects
- Inflammatory disease
- Acquired immunodeficiency syndrome

When determining the patient's visual needs, the systemic review and other factors, such as age, education level, employment status, and presence or absence of family supports, are crucial in determining the patient's requirements. In the subsequent evaluation, the examination may be geared toward meeting the patient's expectations. For patients suffering from macular disease, the problems of reading and writing are usually foremost, although they may assume a secondary role to driving and other aspects of daily living. The ability to keep driving a car is indisputably foremost in the minds of those who wish to maintain independence.

OPTICAL AIDS

Low vision aids (LVA) may be divided into optical (Figure 32.1) and nonoptical devices. Categories of optical aids are listed below.

- Near LVA
  - Spectacle microscopes
  - Hand magnifiers
  - Stand magnifiers
  - Illuminated magnifiers
  - Loupes
  - Telemicroscopes
  - Closed circuit television (CCTV)
- Distance LVA
  - Galilean telescopes
  - Keplerian telescopes
- Other LVA
  - Absorptive filters
  - Lamps with magnifiers

The nature of the patient's presenting problem, visual demands, medical history, and level of visual function all influence treatment with LVA. As a general guideline, a simple, basic approach is favored in patients first confronted with a simple need. By minimizing the number of devices, the patient is most likely to be able to adapt to the device prescribed. Moreover, additional, more complex devices may be added later when the patient has become proficient in using less complex aids. However, although a seeming paradox, one must keep in mind that a key failure in vision rehabilitation is use of simple LVA to solve complicated problems.

NONOPTICAL AIDS

Everything from talking watches to CCTV to large-print books and special computer software is available to persons with vision impairment. It is often left to the patient and his or her family or adaptation to daily living counselor to select those items that are most appropriate. The main exceptions to the rule are light sources, computer software, and CCTV. Here, the low vision practitioner is better equipped to make a determination.

Lighting is one of the most underrated of all elements in successfully managing visual impairment. By providing a patient with an appropriate light source, the practitioner may greatly ease most near tasks. Many patients have success using adjustable gooseneck lamps with a 60 W incandescent bulb (Figure 32.1A). This design provides a warm, well-directed light source with much less of the blue wavelengths

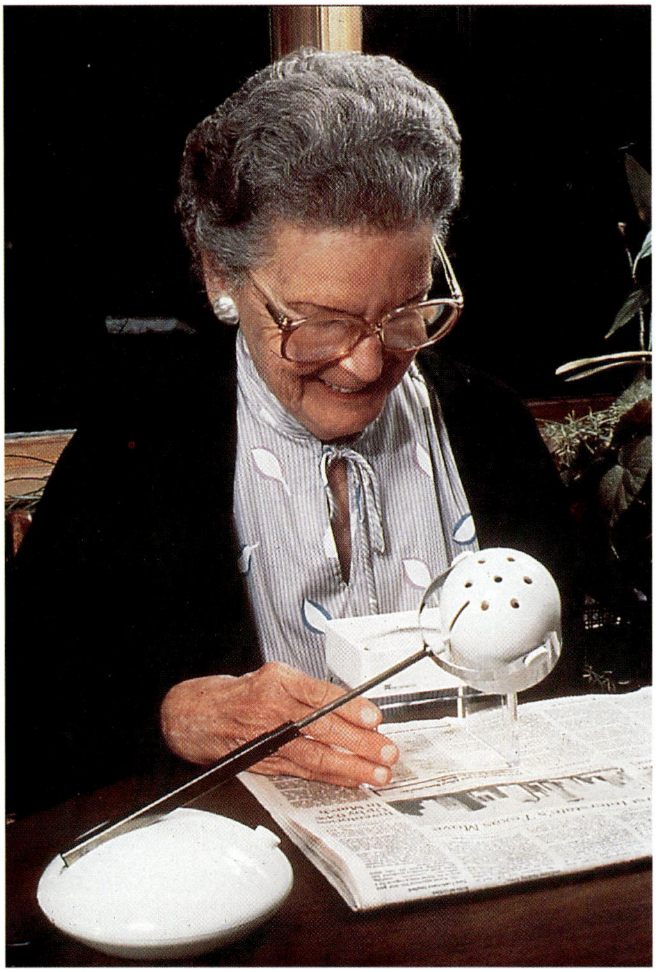

A

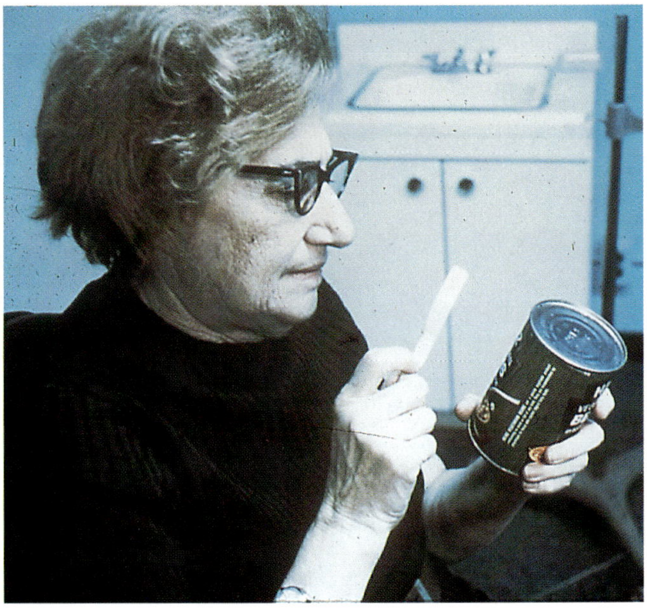

B

FIGURE 32.1. Optical aids. A. Gooseneck lamp with stand magnifier. B. Hand-held magnifier. C. Illuminated bar magnifier.

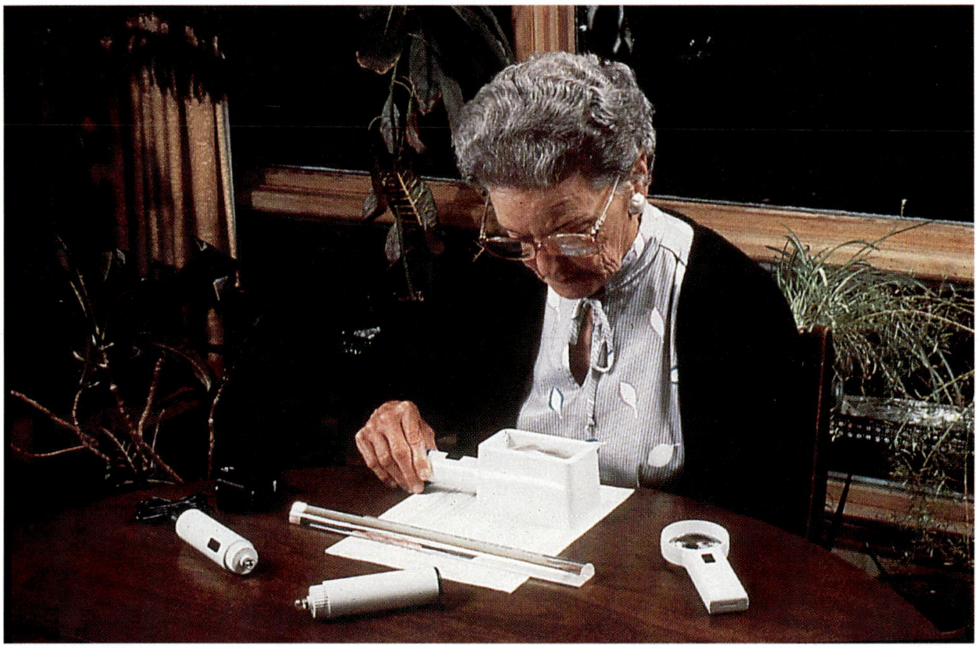

C

found in fluorescent lights. Blue wavelengths are highly scattered by optical media, and media opacities can result in significant glare.

CCTVs allow magnification of written materials without optical aberration. In fact, they can provide magnification up to 80×, although the practicality of the upper range is suspect from a functional standpoint. Other aspects of CCTVs to bear in mind are summarized below.

Important Aspects of CCTV Design

- Increased contrast/glare reduction with figure-ground reversal
- Ability to network with computers
- Advantageous in writing (normal working distance)
- Field-limiting margins
- Movement of material through a limited field (object acceleration)

Unfortunately, CCTVs are also very costly, not readily portable, and somewhat difficult to master. Nevertheless, for a certain group of patients they are worth the expense.

OTHER RESOURCES FOR THE VISUALLY IMPAIRED

While the need for low vision services for patients suffering from macular disease is clear, there are a variety of other services that may be of benefit to patients with vision impairment. These services can help patients deal with the complex social, vocational, and psychological issues facing them.

Mental Health

Among the services that must be considered is a referral to a mental health specialist. One must keep in mind the devastating emotional impact vision loss can have on a person. This may be especially true for persons without adequate support from family or friends, or both. The prospect of lost independence and helplessness can result in severe depression, anger, or other psychological problems. The psychological crisis may be severe enough to compromise the entire rehabilitation effort.

Adaptation to Daily Living

Adaptation to daily living counselors are specially trained "teachers" who provide assistance to persons suffering from visual loss in the area of personal management. For example, they help the person develop organizational schemes for their dishes, food, closets, etc. This allows the impaired person to work with confidence in his or her home. They may also suggest nonoptical visual aids, such as color-coded items, voice-activated equipment, and so forth.

While traditionally geared toward children and younger adults, the services provided by rehabilitation teachers are now expanding to include older adults in "independent living programs" aimed at helping people maintain their independence and avoid the need for institutional settings.

Orientation and Mobility Instruction

While primarily of benefit for patients suffering from diseases that affect more than just the macula, orientation and mobility instruction may be of benefit to some patients with macular disease. Orientation and mobility instructors teach patients how to navigate successfully with the use of LVA or without the benefit of visual cues.

Techniques include use of a cane or guide dog, along with techniques for counting intersections, etc., which allow the visually impaired person to maintain awareness of their position. For patients with macular disease, less complex techniques may often be used if they are unable to use their peripheral vision to remain oriented.

Vision Teacher

Federal law requires that children with vision impairment between 3 and 21 years of age receive special educational services. Often these services are provided at schools for the blind, although in some instances they are delivered within the public school system. This instruction is individually geared toward the patient's needs and problems and may include some elements of all the aforementioned services. Additionally, braille instruction and other educational techniques may be employed.

Support Groups

Support groups provide assistance to people suffering from vision loss. In certain cases, the value of commiserating with others suffering from similar problems cannot be overstated. In addition to the psychological support that may be derived, the hints and strategies for working with vision loss provided by patients with similar problems may be of great help.

SUMMARY

The low vision consultation should provide answers to heretofore unanswered questions in the eye examination. The application of these answers to the physical loss of vision should dictate the final treatment modality and carry the treatment into the functional environment.

Maximizing the residual vision is obviously not only good but also the key to the formulation of treatment and the ultimate rehabilitation effort. Obviously, the management strategy is disease specific; it must also be environmentally task specific.

The use of magnification, minification, and image relocation must be applied in the context of manipulating environmental factors, such as lighting, contrast, and other specific influences. Physical, psychological, emotional, and motivational complications must be carefully factored in. Only then may the concept of a realizable goal or goals be formulated and a rehabilitative effort mounted to achieve it. The patient usually must be followed in order to modify any significant changes in condition.

Today, unfortunately, there are few treatment modalities available for many visually devastating disorders, and the patient's best hope must lie with the use of residual vision by an intense, well-managed rehabilitative effort. Fortunately, with maculopathy, low vision treatment and rehabilitation have proven successful and efficient means of managing a complex problem.

SUGGESTED READING

Barney JL. The prerogative of choice in long-term care. Gerontology 1977;17:309–314.

Crews JE. The demographic, social and conceptual contexts of aging and vision loss. J Am Optom Assoc 1994;65:63–68.

Nelson KA. Projected increases in the prevalence of severe vision impairment among elderly Americans. Personal communication, 1991.

Weisse F. Providing Services for People with Vision Loss, A Multidisciplinary Perspective. Lexington, MA: Resources for Rehabilitation, 1989.

Index

Note: Page numbers in italics indicate figures; page numbers followed by t indicate tables.